EVERY VICTORY COUNTS®

Essential Information and Inspiration for a Lifetime of Wellness with Parkinson's Disease

By Monique Giroux, MD
& Sierra Farris, PA-C, MPAS

And by 40 leading Parkinson's specialist contributors

*With encouragement and inspiration
from people who are living with Parkinson's*

FIFTH EDITION, EIGHTH PRINTING

This publication is supported in part by grants and donations from:

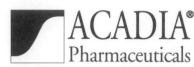
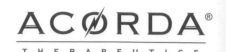

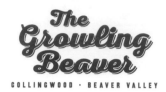
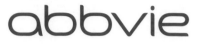
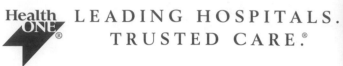

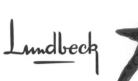
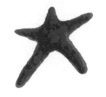
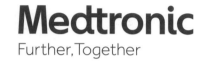

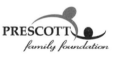
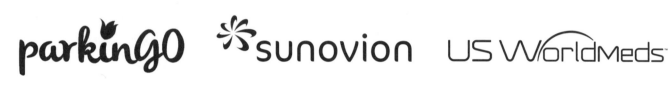

Larry Christensen
Family

Disclaimer:

TABLE OF CONTENTS

INTRODUCTION

A MESSAGE FROM DAVIS PHINNEY 9

    What is Self-Care? 10

    This Manual is Your Roadmap for Living Well Today 11

MEET YOUR PARKINSON'S GUIDES 12

LEAD AUTHORS 20

CONTRIBUTING AUTHORS 21

WHAT YOU NEED TO KNOW ABOUT PARKINSON'S

PARKINSON'S: AN OVERVIEW 43

    What is Parkinson's? 43

        Shame and Parkinson's 44

    How is Parkinson's Diagnosed? 45

    What Causes Parkinson's? 47

    Who Gets Parkinson's? 50

    When Does Parkinson's Start? 50

    What Premotor Symptoms May Occur? 51

    What Motor Symptoms May Occur? 51

        Early Symptoms of Parkinson's 52

    What Non-Motor Symptoms May Occur? 53

    How Does Parkinson's Change Over Time? 54

AFTER DIAGNOSIS 57

    Assembling Your Wellness Team 57

        Virtual House Calls: The Promise of Telemedicine for High-Quality Parkinson's Care .. 57

        Your Parkinson's Wellness Team 60

        Palliative or Supportive Care and Parkinson's 62

    Take Control 66

        The Importance of Self-Efficacy 67

    How Can I Get Involved in Research? 70

        The Process of Research in Parkinson's: A Long and Winding Road 70

        My Perspective: Participating in Clinical Trials 74

    Managing Emotions 77

    Initial Treatment 78

    Family, Relationships and Work 82

Workplace Issues..86
   Disability Options for People with Parkinson's................................87
   Legal Issues with Respect to Employment: What to Consider When You've Been
   Diagnosed with Parkinson's..92

CORE PARKINSON'S SYMPTOMS 96

Motor Symptoms..96
   Balance: So Automatic, So Vulnerable, So Re-Trainable......................98
   Fall Prevention in Parkinson's Disease....................................100

Non-Motor Symptoms..102
   Parkinson's Psychosis: The Elephant in the Room...........................104
   Depression and Anxiety in Parkinson's.....................................108
   Neurogenic Orthostatic Hypotension (nOH) in Parkinson's...................118
   Talking to Your Doctor About Sex..122

YOUNG ONSET PARKINSON'S 125

Employment..127
Family..128

LIVING WELL NOW

LIVING WELL WITH PARKINSON'S 131

There <u>Are</u> Things You Can Do to Live Well <u>Today</u>.........................131
   Living Well: Then and Now...131
Parkinson's Self-Care...132
General Health..135
Preventative Screening..136
Acute Change in Parkinson's Motor or Cognitive Symptoms.......................137
Bone Health...137
Heart Health..137
   Dental Health...138
   Vision Health...140
Fatigue...142
Sleep...142
Mood Changes and Cognitive Problems...143
   Cognitive Changes Related to Parkinson's..................................145
Gastrointestinal, Bowel and Bladder Changes...................................144
Constipation..144
Overactive Bladder and Incontinence...147
Excessive Sweating..147
Weight Management...148
Smoking Cessation...148
Alcohol Use...148

EXERCISE 149

  A Stronger Body Leads to Better Movement 149

    Exercise Is Medicine for the Brain 150

    Research Summary: The Positive Effects of Physical Activity on Parkinson's Disease .. 151

    Move It! Exercise and Physical Activity are Key to Living Well with Parkinson's 153

  Common Questions Before Starting an Exercise Routine 154

    Three Ways to Get Maximum Benefit from Your Exercise Routine 156

    Staying on Track with Your Exercise Routine 160

DIET AND NUTRITION 165

  General Nutrition 165

  Dietary Recommendations for Specific Parkinson's Symptoms 171

  Protein Interference with Medication 173

  Nutrition for a Healthy Brain 174

    Sample Menus for Living Well with Parkinson's 177

EMOTIONAL HEALTH 182

  Mind-Body Connection 182

    Mindfulness 182

  Depression 185

    Depression in Parkinson's 184

    Practical Strategies for Managing Depression and Anxiety 186

  Anxiety 190

    Promoting Emotional Health and Wellness in Parkinson's 191

  Counseling 193

  Connecting with Your Community 195

    Community and Social Capital 194

    Help Others, Help Yourself: The Importance of Getting Involved in Your Community .. 196

  Creativity 198

    Art Therapy for People Living with Parkinson's 199

  Spirituality and Personal Beliefs 202

    Spiritual Care as a Path to Living Well with Parkinson's 201

  Hope 203

    Choosing to Make a Difference 203

MEDICATION 205

  Medication Overview 205

  Medication for Motor Control 205

  Medication for Non-Motor Control 214

SURGICAL THERAPIES 221

  Enteral Suspension Medication Delivery: The Levodopa Stomach Pump 221

    Duopa: Help for Motor Fluctuations in Advanced Parkinson's 221

  Deep Brain Stimulation: The Brain Pacemaker 222

    When to Consider DBS as a Treatment Option 224

    Deep Brain Stimulation for Parkinson's: A Surgeon's Perspective 226

COMPLEMENTARY THERAPIES 234

    Complementary Therapies for Parkinson's 234

  Physical Therapy 237

    Balancing Life, Exercise and Function for Optimal Health 238

  Occupational Therapy 241

    Driving 241

    Warning Signs of a High Risk Driver 242

    Occupational Therapy for People Living with Parkinson's 243

  Speech-Language and Swallowing Therapy 245

    The Benefits of Speech-Language Therapy in Parkinson's 246

    Addressing Speech Challenges in Parkinson's 249

  Creative Therapists 251

WHAT TO KNOW ABOUT HOSPITAL STAYS AND EMERGENCY ROOM VISITS 252

  Questions to Ask Before Discharge 253

  Medications to Avoid 253

  Hospital Tips for Individuals with Duopa or Deep Brain Stimulation 254

  Medical Alert Bracelet 254

PARKINSON'S AND THE FAMILY

    How Parkinson's Affects the Family 256

PARKINSON'S AND CARE PARTNERS 259

  Care Partner Health: A Medical Perspective 259

  Stress and Strain of Caring for Someone Living with Chronic Illness 259

  Coping Strategies are Not Created Equal 260

  Parkinson's in My House 261

  Caregiver Strain: A Medical Syndrome 263

    Caregiver Strain 264

  Risks to the Relationship with Your Loved One with Parkinson's 265

  Tools to Prevent Caregiver Burnout 266

  Coping Strategies for Parkinson's Care Partners 267

  Notes from the Trenches: An Experienced Care Partner's Perspective 271

  Care Partner Support: Learning to Find What You Need 277

6

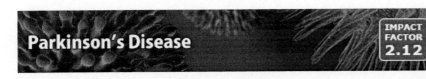

Parkinsons Dis. 2010; 2010: 480260.
Published online 2011 Feb 7. doi: 10.4061/2010/480260

PMCID: PMC3038575
PMID: 21331376

Treatment of Advanced Parkinson's Disease

Sara Varanese, [1,*] Zoe Birnbaum, [1] Roger Rossi, [2] and Alessandro Di Rocco [1]

[1] New York University School of Medicine, Department of Neurology, Division of Movement Disorders, New York, NY 10016, USA
[2] Robert Wood Johnson Medical School, Johnson Rehabilitation Institute, Edison, NJ 08818, USA
*Sara Varanese: sara.varanese@nyumc.org
Academic Editor: Ray Chaudhuri

Received 2010 Aug 13; Accepted 2010 Dec 20.

Abstract

Patients at late stage Parkinson's disease (PD) develop several motor and nonmotor complications, which dramatically impair their quality of life. These complications include motor fluctuations, dyskinesia, unpredictable or absent response to medications, falls, dysautonomia, dementia, hallucinations, sleep disorders, depression, and psychosis. The therapeutic management should be driven by the attempt to create a balance between benefit and side effects of the pharmacological treatments available. Supportive care, including physical and rehabilitative interventions, speech therapy, occupational therapy, and nursing care, has a key role in the late stage of disease. In this review we discuss the several complications experienced by advance PD patients and their management. The importance of an integrative approach, including both pharmacological and supportive interventions, is emphasized.

1. Introduction

Advanced Parkinson's disease (PD), stage 4 or 5 of the Hoehn and Yahr Scale [1], is characterized by very limited mobility without assistance, severe motor deficits, risk of falls, and cognitive and psychotic problems. The mean time from disease onset to wheelchair-dependence is estimated at 14 years [2], although about a third of patients seem to have a relatively milder disease and remain stable for many years [3]. With the advent of the L-Dopa and other dopaminergic treatments, the progression of PD has become markedly slower. However, over the years treatment loses its efficacy, while a number of complications, such as motor fluctuations and dyskinesia, develop, probably due to the progressive loss of dopaminergic neurons and their striatal and cortical connections [4]. These complications are observed in 50% of patients after 5 years of disease and in 80% of patients after 10 years of treatment [5, 6]. However, the response to L-Dopa therapy predictability decreases over the years.

While worsening of motor function and the drug-induced motor complications represents a major challenge in patients with mid to advanced disease, in the advanced stage of PD the most troublesome and distressful complications are usually in the area of non-motor symptoms, including psychiatric and cognitive disorders, autonomic disturbances, and sleep disorders that significantly increase the need for supportive. These symptoms are frequently neglected in clinical practice due to limited consultation time, perception of the patient and caregivers that their symptoms are unrelated to the disease, or insufficient awareness of the clinicians who generally focus the consultation towards motor symptoms [7].

Psychosis and dementia are frequent and share a common pathophysiology in a significant proportion of patients [8, 9], where the impact on patients and family is variable. Dementia is associated with reduction in quality of life [10] and patient lifespan [11], psychosis is a risk factor for nursing home placement [12], and both are important sources of caregiver distress [13].

Management of motor and non-motor complications should be tailored to the individual patient. This implies a careful assessment of whether the symptom is a side effect of the medications or is related to the progression of the disease. In advanced disease, patients may also experience an enhanced sensitivity to small changes in L-Dopa or become more prone to adverse reactions to antiparkinsonian drugs.

Proper supporting care becomes increasingly important in advanced PD. Rehabilitative and support services for patients and family also become key interventions as the disease reaches its more debilitating stages and pharmacological or surgical treatment becomes less relevant.

In this article we discuss the spectrum of the motor and non-motor complications seen in advanced stage PD and present an evidence-based review of current therapeutic options in the management of these complications.

2. Motor Disability

PD is defined as advanced when the patient is severely disabled. As per Hoehn and Yahr classification, patients in stage 4 are still able to walk and stand unassisted, but they are markedly incapacitated in their ability to perform activities of daily living (ADL). Patients in stage 5 are confined to bed or wheelchair unless aided.

Many patients in advanced stage range from stage 4 to 5 during the day because of the inconsistent and limited response to their medications.

Even when patients are still able to ambulate without assistance, limited motor ability due to marked bradykinesia and inability to perform fine and alternate movements lead them to dependency in ADLs, being unable to provide for basic personal care like dressing, bathing, and often feeding.

Advanced patients are frail individuals exposed to high risk of several unfavorable circumstances during daily activities, like falls.

The incidence of falls in advanced PD is high (40–70%) [14], even when patients are optimally medicated. Falls in advanced PD occur because of very unstable gait, loss of center of gravity, poor balance, orthostatic hypotension, side effects of medications like antidepressants and benzodiazepines, and disturbances of posture like camptocormia or retropulsion. Falls lead to injuries and fracture that further reduce patient independence and increase the risk of nursing home admission. Patients with previous falls often develop fear of falling which further limits their mobility, contributing to increased weakness and deterioration.

Because of the devastating consequences, an assessment of falls risk should be taken in all advanced PD patients. A combination of both disease-specific and balance- and mobility-related measures is necessary to accurately predict falls in patients with PD [15].

Treatment of falls implies a complex approach aimed at reducing all the potential risk factors, muscle strengthening, range of motion exercise and balance, and postural control training.

Although there is still insufficient evidence for effective prevention of falls, exercise interventions have shown to be effective at improving physical functioning, leg strength, balance, and walking [16]. Thus, physical interventions should be emphasized in advanced stages of disease, particularly as falls are currently not well addressed either by pharmacotherapy nor by subthalamic nucleus deep-brain stimulation (DBS) surgery.

The neuroanatomical substrates of posture and gait are poorly understood but a number of important observations suggest a major role for the pedunculopontine nucleus and adjacent areas in the brainstem. A recent double-blinded study reported a significant reduction in falls in the on and off medication states both at 3 and 12 months after pedunculopontine nucleus DBS as captured in the Unified Parkinson's Disease Rating Scale part II scores in six advanced Parkinson's disease patients with significant gait and postural abnormalities [17].

It has to be noted, however, that advanced patients are at high risk of short- and long-term complications from the DBS procedure, and surgical treatment is generally contraindicated in these patients. Furthermore, literature on pedunculopontine nucleus DBS is still limited, and long-term follow-up studies investigating safety and efficacy are unavailable.

3. Motor Complications

Long-term motor complications of PD are due to duration of disease and treatment, and to cumulative intake of L-Dopa, with several central and peripheral mechanisms involved. The progressive degeneration of the nigrostriatal dopaminergic transmission results in fewer and fewer terminals capable of taking up exogenously administered L-Dopa and converting it to dopamine for subsequent storage and release [6]. Unlike early and mid-stage PD patients advanced- and end-stage patients experience an enhanced sensitivity to small changes in plasma L-dopa levels [18, 19], that narrow the therapeutic window and negatively impact motor function.

3.1. Wearing-Off, On-Off Fluctuations, and Management Strategies

"Wearing-off" refers to the recurrence of motor and non-motor symptoms preceding the scheduled dose of L-Dopa, while the on-off fluctuations are sudden unpredictable shifts between "well-" or "over-" treated status (on) and an undertreated state with severe Parkinsonism symptoms (off).

"Wearing-off" and on-off fluctuations overlap in advanced patients.

"Wearing-off" is a direct consequence of the nonphysiological, pulsatile dopaminergic stimulation, and its occurrence is generally predictable following the L-Dopa administration with progressive therapeutic window progressively narrowing over the years.

A plethora of sensory, psychiatric, and autonomic symptoms may be associated with the motor fluctuation. Patients, indeed, may present with paresthesia, pain, anxiety, shortness of breath, sweating, and other symptoms that may not be recognized as part of the L-Dopa response pattern [20].

Management strategy for "wearing-off" phenomena is focused on prolonging the effect of individual L-Dopa doses without increasing the pulsatile dopaminergic stimulation.

Strategies include fragmentation of dosing, with more frequent administration of lower doses, and use of COMT inhibitor (entacapone and tolcapone), MAO inhibitor (selegiline and rasagiline), and use of dopamine agonists.

Adjunctive therapy with a COMT inhibitor extends the duration of the L-Dopa effect, hence ameliorating wearing off, by blocking the COMT enzyme in the peripheral catabolism of L-Dopa. Potential adverse event, however, may arise from the COMT inhibitors. Increasing synaptic dopamine levels may also be associated with dyskinesia and increased L-Dopa toxicity leading to worsening of dementia and psychosis.

Fragmentation of oral therapy, with L-Dopa administered up to 6-7 times a day at about 3-hour intervals, is a commonly used and effective strategy [21]. However, lowering individual doses of L-Dopa may increase the risk of occasional drug failure or delayed response.

Substitution of regular with controlled-release L-dopa preparations may be particularly reasonable in end-stage patients [22], but the available extended release formulations are not always affective and reliable.

The use of dopamine-agonists (DAs), although theoretically useful in regulating fluctuations by direct stimulation of the postsynaptic receptors, is generally contraindicated in late-stage disease in order to avoid hallucinations and psychosis, and worsening of autonomic dysfunction.

The main challenge in controlling the on-off response is to improve the "on" time without increasing the dyskinesia.

In very late-stage PD this can be achieved using liquid formulations of L-Dopa [23], which can be prepared by dissolving ten 25/100 mg standard-release carbidopa/levodopa tablets and 2 g of ascorbic acid in 1 L of tap water [24].

Gastrointestinal dysfunction, with erratic gastric emptying worsening over the years, is a common cause of poor absorption of L-Dopa in PD. There is no gastric absorption of L-Dopa, indeed; so gastric emptying and transit via the pyloric sphincter are critical factors for regular intestinal absorption [25].

The liquid effervescent levodopa formulation of melevodopa (methyl-ester levodopa) plus carbidopa is a prodrug with a high solubility (about 250 times more than L-Dopa) in small volume of water, and it is able to reach quickly the small intestine where it is absorbed in a more regular and rapid way compared to solid formulations [26]. One clinical advantage of this formulation is that it avoids erratic absorption and the related unpredictability in the plasma L-Dopa concentration curve [27]. The drug is approved in certain European countries and currently under phase II investigation in the US.

Continuous infusion of levodopa/carbidopa gel through portable duodenal systems (Duodopa) using percutaneous endoscopic gastrostomy (PEG) can be a practical alternative [28, 29]. The infusion provides constant plasma levodopa concentration and continuous dopamine availability and receptor stimulation. This solution may be particularly reasonable in very advance patients with severe dysphagia, as the PEG may also be used for nutrition. Intrajejunal L-dopa/carbidopa gel infusion is effective in reducing off time, severity and duration of dyskinesia in advanced PD [30, 31]. Most importantly, a recent multicenter study demonstrated that intrajejunal L-dopa/carbidopa infusion provides a beneficial effect on several nonmotor complications, including cardiovascular, gastrointestinal, and urinary symptoms, sleep/fatigue, attention/memory, and pain [32]. Adverse event can occur, however, from the procedure or from the dislocation or occlusion of the intestinal tube. Advanced patients may also experience local complications at the site of entry, particularly inflammation and infections.

Apomorphine subcutaneous infusion is also an effective option for patients with severe fluctuations poorly controlled by oral treatment [33]. Apomorphine infusion is often limited by the development of skin reaction at the site of injections after few years of treatment.

3.2. Dyskinesias

Dyskinesias are involuntary choreiform, twisting and turning movements invariably occurring in patients undergoing long-term L-Dopa treatment. Dyskinesias usually occur in "on" state, as chorea, myoclonus or dystonic movement. In end-stage patients dyskinesia may appear in off state as dystonic posture, especially in the lower limbs. Off dystonia is generally most troublesome upon morning awakening but in advanced disease may also develop complex twisting dystonic movements during the day. Because of the narrow therapeutic window at this stage it is also not uncommon for patients to experience diphasic dyskinesia. These are usually repetitive alternating movements occurring at the beginning as well as at the end of the interval between two L-Dopa doses [34].

Management of dyskinesias implies detailed understanding of the L-Dopa cycle.

The most common approach is to lower the single L-Dopa dose. Controlled-release levodopa may worsen dyskinesias, especially later in the day due to cumulative effect. Amantadine in doses between 100 mg and 400 mg can be effective, but side effects are frequent in more advanced patients and should be carefully monitored. These include edema, livedo reticularis, and confusional state or hallucinations and psychosis.

Clozapine, an atypical dopamine receptor antagonist, has been found to be effective in reducing dyskinesia in advanced patients [35, 36], and it may be particularly useful when hallucinations are also present. Advanced patients, however, are particularly prone to develop agranulocitosis, with high risks of infections, and thus the white cell count should be regularly monitored.

Recent evidence suggests that memantine is also effective in reducing dyskinesia when other options are contraindicated [37, 38].

Despite limited evidence-based data high-frequency subtalamic DBS (DBS-HFS) has been shown by several reports to be surgically safe and able to produce improvements in dopaminergic drug-sensitive symptoms and reductions in subsequent drug dose and dyskinesias are well documented. However, the procedure is associated with adverse effects, mainly neurocognitive, with side-effects created by spread of stimulation to surrounding structures, depending on the precise location of electrodes. The occurrence of cognitive complications limits the motor improvements induced by STN-HFS to a short period of time, because patients' quality of life is greatly impaired by the progressing cognitive disorder. In late stage of disease the rate of patients eligible for surgical treatment of PD is extremely low, due to age and general debilitation that significantly increase the risks of short- and long-term complications.

3.3. Drug Failure Response

As the disease progresses, the efficacy of L-Dopa progressively decreases and patients may not respond at all to administered doses. This phenomenon is more pronounced later during the day and may be related to poor gastric emptying and insufficient intestinal absorption. Domperidone is an effective option, where available. The neutral aromatic amino acids contained in dietary proteins may compete with L-Dopa for intestinal absorption and transport across the blood-brain barrier, thus limiting its efficacy and being responsible for the occurrence of motor fluctuations. Low-protein dietary regimens with protein redistribution by shifting protein intake to the evening are an effective strategy to ameliorate the response to L-Dopa. Low-protein products designed for chronic renal failure patients are also a safe, well-tolerated, and useful option for end-stage patients [39].

4. Nonmotor Complications

The neuroanatomical and neurochemical substrates of the majority of non-motor symptoms are still unclear, although the concept of Parkinson's disease as a six-stage pathological process introduced by Braak and collegues [40] provided critical information to understand the physiopathology of several nonmotor symptoms, such as sleep disorder, autonomic dysfunction, and visual hallucinations.

Several studies have shown that non-motor symptoms impact significantly on quality of life and institutionalization is greater than for the motor symptoms [41, 42]; so in recent year attention was focused on the development of measures specifically designed to recognize and quantify these symptoms in advanced patients, and they are now also widely used in the clinical trials.

The development of clinical measures useful in recognizing and quantifying these symptoms deeply improved the clinical care as well as the clinical trials.

The Non-Motor Symptoms Scale, for instance, is a 30-item scale for assessment of nine dimensions (cardiovascular, sleep/fatigue, mood/cognition, perceptual problems, attention/memory, gastrointestinal, urinary, sexual function, and miscellany), that has proven to be a valid, reproducible, and accurate tool in rating severity and frequency of non-motor symptoms in PD [43, 44].

4.1. Dementia

Community-based studies of dementia in patients with PD have reported a prevalence between 28% and 44%, with longitudinal studies estimating that dementia occurs in up to 75% of patients [45]. The pattern of deficits is similar to dementia with Lewy bodies and differs from that in Alzheimer's disease for the predominant involvement of executive, visuospatial, and attention dysfunction and for the presence of cognitive fluctuations [46–49].

The cognitive symptoms are a consequence of dopaminergic depletion [50] in the corticostriatal loop and of dysfunction of the cholinergic system [51]. Serotoninergic and noradrenergic mechanisms may also be involved, though their role is not well defined.

Dopaminergic replacement does not lead to cognitive improvement or may even worsen it, but cholinergic enhancement can instead be helpful. Cholinesterase inhibitors, in fact, may be effective in ameliorating cognition, but their tolerability seems variable due to peripheral cholinergic adverse effects and in some case can worsen motor functions. Rivastigmine seems the most useful agent [52], while more controversial is the benefit produced by donepezil [53, 54].

Avoiding the medications that can possibly worsen dementia, like anticholinergics and DA-agonists, as well as maintaining L-Dopa at the lowest effective doses, is certainly a key strategy to contain confusion, hallucinations, and psychosis in advanced patients [55].

4.2. Hallucinations and Psychosis

Behavioral disorders, and especially hallucinations, illusions, and other psychotic symptoms, are also frequent in advanced PD with frequency rates ranging from 25 to 30%. Resembling very closely those seen in dementia with Lewy bodies, psychotic symptoms in PD are represented by delusions (false and fixed beliefs maintained despite evidence to the contrary) and, particular, hallucinations (abnormal perceptions that can involve any sensory modality in the absence of a physical stimulus). Visual hallucinations, simple or complex in form, are the most common psychotic symptom in advanced PD patients, typically occurring in dim surrounding, but often occurring through the entire day in late-stage patients [56].

A range of factors contributes to the development of hallucinations and psychosis in PD, including

intrinsic pathology and dopaminergic replacement therapy.

In the treatment of these complications the first step should always be to evaluate the role of drugs that can potentially induce or worsen psychosis, such as amantadine, anticholinergics, COMT-inhibitors, and DA-agonists. These drugs should be tapered off, balancing the effect on psychosis with worsening of motor function.

All precipitating events, like urinary and pulmonary infections, cerebrovascular events, and metabolic dysfunctions, should be also carefully investigated and treated if possible, as even mild metabolic imbalance or infection can profoundly affect the development of psychotic symptoms.

Decreasing the dose of L-Dopa should also be considered when severe psychosis persists, even though this action could worsen parkinsonim.

All traditional antipsychotic drugs, such as haloperidol, aripriprazole, and chlorpromazine, should be avoided because of the high sensitivity of PD patients to the motor adverse effects induced through potent antagonisms of D_2 receptors.

Clozapine and quetiapine are the only two newest antipsychotic that should be considered atypical, thus safe in PD, due to their predominant affinity for D_1 and D_4 receptor and low affinity for D_2 receptors.

There is a wealth of evidence demonstrating the efficacy and tolerability of clozapine in PD, but its use is limited by the need of weekly blood testing for the initial 6 months of treatment [57]. A more practical alternative is represented by quetiapine. Unlike clozapine, quetiapine does not require monitoring of blood cell counts and it is effective in suppressing hallucinations and psychosis in the majority of patients at relatively low doses, ranging from 12.5 mg to 100 mg.

Main side effects of quetiapine and clozapine are sedation and postural hypotension.

4.3. Depression and Anxiety

Depression affects 40–60% of patients with PD and appears to be a major determinant of health-related quality of life in PD [58].

In some cases depression occurs during off periods; thus controlling the on-off fluctuation can improve depression.

Sedating antidepressants, like tricyclic (TCA), and more activating antidepressants, like selective serotonin reuptake inhibitors (SSRIs) and serotonin-norepinephrine reuptake inhibitors (SNRIs), are useful but significantly limited in advanced patients by the ancticholinergic and orthostatic negative effects. SSRIs are also contraindicated in patients receiving slelegiline, because of the potential drug-drug interation leading to "serotonin syndrome".

S-Adenosyl-methionine (SAMe), a natural molecule present in all eucaryotic cells that participates as methyl group donor to a number of metabolic events, is reported to have an effective antidepressant effects [59], without worsening of Parkinsonism [60].

Anxiety often occurs during "off" periods and improves with better control of motor symptoms but can be a major source of distress for patients even during "on" state. Low doses of benzodiazepines are effective when anxiety is persistent and debilitating but may cause amnesia and confusion in advanced patients and are a risk factor for falls.

4.4. Sleep Disorders

Sleep disorders occur in almost all patients with advanced PD, and they consist of sleep fragmentation,

REM sleep behavior disorders (RBDs), excessive daytime sleepiness, and altered sleep-wake cycle.

Sleep fragmentation can be caused by difficulty turning in bed or nocturnal dystonia and can be ameliorated with controlled-release levodopa. Increased nocturnal urinary frequency can also affect sleep and can be controlled by reducing the amount of liquids in the evening, when anticholinergic drugs are contraindicated.

RBD is a disruption of the normal REM sleep cycle, in which the paralysis that normally occurs during REM sleep is incomplete or absent, making the patient "act out" their dreams, that usually are vivid, intense, and violent. Dream-enacting behaviors can be complex, including talking, yelling, punching, kicking, jumping from bed, and grabbing, with great distress for the patient and bed partner. RBD also prevents physiological nocturnal restoration of dopamine reseverve in cells, with worsening of parkinsonian symptoms. RBD improves when dopaminergic medications are reduced at bedtime. When RBD persists, low doses of clonazepam are effective and should be considered.

Modafinil, a wake promoting agent approved for narcolepsy, is effective in ameliorating daytime sleepiness induced by dopamine-agonists without significant side effects [61] and can be helpful in ameliorating alertness in advanced PD.

4.5. Autonomic Dysfunction

4.5.1. Orthostatic Hypothension (OH) OH is defined as a fall in systolic blood pressure below 20 mmHg and I diastolic pressure below 10 mmHg within 3 minutes of standing. Orthostatic intolerance related to OH results from a reduction of cerebral perfusion when upright and presents in severe cases with lightheadedness or syncope, exposing the patient to high risk of fall.

Careful education of patients and caregivers on factors that can trigger the OH symptoms, like avoiding rapid changes of position or straining during micturition or defecation, is essential in the management of OH.

Fluid intake, particularly in the morning, should be maintained at around 2 L of water daily and at least 8 g of sodium chloride is recommended to ensure adequate hydration [62].

Antihypertensive therapy, when present, should be reconsidered and eventually discontinued. Thromboembolic elastic stocking and abdominal binders can be helpful and should be encouraged.

When OH becomes more severe, it is necessary to start pharamchological agents such as plasma volume expander, like fludrocortison, and vasoactive agents, like midodrine.

4.5.2. Dysphagia, Nutrition, and Hydration Severe dysphagia occurs frequently at late stage of disease causing weight loss, malnutrition, dehydration, and significantly increasing the risk of inducing aspiration pneumonia and death.

In order to make the swallow safer and more effective swallowing maneuvers, like the supraglottic swallow maneuver, the super supraglottic swallow maneuver, the Mendelsohn maneuver, and the effortful swallow maneuver, should be taught to patients.

Dysphagia for fluid can be controlled adding thickening agents, or thickeners, to liquids, increasing their viscosity without substantially modifying their other properties, such as taste. They provide body, increase stability, and improve suspension of added ingredients. Some thickening agents are gelling agents, forming a gel that can be swallowed by patients significantly reducing the risk of chocking.

When dysphagia becomes more severe, PEG should be considered. In this phase PEG could be a useful solution to guarantee to patients' adequate food and fluid intake as well as dopaminergic therapy through infusion.

4.5.3. Genitourinary and Elimination Constipation is a common and early manifestation of PD but in late stage can become particularly severe due to the combination of anti-PD medications, slowed intestinal motility, immobility, and dehydration. Constipation should be well managed in order to avoid bowel occlusion and in order to ensure proper absorption of L-dopa and other medications. Dietary supplementation of fibers that stimulate intestinal motility should be encouraged as well as increased fluid intake. A conservative therapeutic option is administration of macrogol (polyethylene glycol), which can lead to marked improvement [63].

Many late-stage PD patients face urinary problems such as urgency or frequency or stress incontinence, which can cause anxiety and feelings of social isolation. Overactive bladder is the result of loss of normal inhibition by the basal ganglia and the frontal cortex to the sacral spinal cord [64]. Anticholinergics are commonly used to inhibit the overactive bladder, although their use should be discouraged in late-stage patients due to cognitive and other central anticholinergic adverse effects [65]. Newer generation of peripheral anticholinergics, like trospium, is better tolerated and can be used sometimes even in advanced patients. Recently, botulinum toxin injections in the detrusor muscle have demonstrated marked efficacy in reducing the urinary frequency with no side effects [66].

Reduced mobility and difficulty toileting often lead to the use of urinary pads or catheters at end stage of disease, exposing the patients to high risk of urinary dangerous infections when hygienic measures are not appropriate.

5. Supportive Care

Supportive care in advanced PD patients should include physical and rehabilitative therapy, occupational therapy, speech therapy, social work, and nursing care. These care services could greatly benefit late-stage patients by prolonging independency in the ADL and reducing complications like pain, decubiti, and falls.

5.1. Mobility

Full mobility should be encouraged and maintained as long as possible. Occupational and physical therapy should be encouraged whenever possible. Individual rehabilitative therapy sessions should be encouraged two to three times weekly for 30- to 40-minute durations even at late-stage when the patient is able to safely ambulate. Falls are perhaps the greatest concern for late stage PD patients who are still mobile, and patients should be discouraged to stand or walk without assistance at very late stage of disease. If patients are bedridden, residual mobility should be maintained through active and passive movement exercises, frequent position changes, and breathing exercises to prevent complications associated with being bedridden, such as decubitus, contracture, pain, and pneumonia [67].

5.2. Nutrition, Hydration, and Genitourinary Care

Malnutrition is a common problem in advanced PD patients. It is caused by difficulty feeding, altered satiety mechanism, diminished gastric and intestinal motility, inactivity, lack of appetite, dysphagia, and metabolic syndrome. In patients still able to eat independently, meal and portion sizes should be monitored in order to provide sufficient nutrition. Any effort, including compensatory strategies, should be considered to delay the PEG placement. Adequate hydration is another concern for late-stage PD patients, since even mild temperature change can lead to relative dehydration and exacerbate confusion and OH and cause syncope. Many patients become embarrassed when eating or drinking, and nursing assistance, can assure adequate nutrition and hydration through a nonjudgmental caregiver that assist patients with the administration of meals.

5.3. Communication

Difficulty with speech with severe dysarthria, hypophonia, tachylalia, and freezing of speech is another problem associated with late-stage PD and leads to significant source of frustration for patients and families. Speech therapy should be encouraged whenever possible. The Lee Silverman Voice treatment has been shown, clinically and scientifically, to be a powerful method of improving speech and related functions such as swallowing and facial expression in PD, with documented Improvement in vocal loudness, voice quality, prosody, and speech articulation, sustained at 1-year and 2-year follow-ups [68]. Simplified and codified communications (like asking yes/no questions, or by using alphabet boards or speaking dictionaries) can become the only way of effective communication [69] and should be considered.

6. End of Life Care

When patients with advanced PD encounter a medical illness requiring an extended rehabilitation stay, they are often transferred to subacute rehabilitation facilities with no expertise in treating Parkinson's disease. These transfers often lead to an inevitable decline due to worsening of dementia, psychosis, and social withdrawal. Nursing home placement should be delayed as long as possible, because of the well-known risk of reduced survival. As death approaches for late-stage PD patients, it is important to provide them with the best care possible in a passionate environment. Many patients choose to do this through hospice care. Support to families, through social work and psychological counseling, should be offered at this time.

7. Conclusion

The management of end-stage PD challenges clinicians, patients, and families in many ways.

The main goal should be to maintain acceptable levels of functioning through careful balance not limited to drug management, but including strong and supportive services.

Many patients with advanced PD, in fact, benefit from a more intensive intervention to address the complexity of the disease. Medication management can become arduous with on/off fluctuations and dyskinesias, frequent falls, constipation, blood pressure instability, cardiac problems, and other medical complications of PD developing and becoming more severe as the disease progresses. The process is further complicated when speech is affected, and swallowing becomes difficult with malnutrition and risk of developing aspiration pneumonia. Psychological problems often accompany these later stages of the disease, including anxiety, depression, and insomnia. Cognitive problems and hallucinations also are prominent.

There comes a time when it becomes too difficult to manage all these complexities at home. Patients and caregivers become overwhelmed, often with unnecessary catastrophic consequences. Institutionalization typically follows the dramatic period of declining health and diminished ability to cope. For most persons with advanced PD the quality and dignity of a life at home are much superior to what they can ever expect in a nursing home. A well-designed interdisciplinary intervention can, in most cases, resolve many problems and render the care of patients much more manageable at home. Unfortunately, medical facilities are unprepared to accommodate the needs of the neurologically frail and complex PD patients.

References

1. Hoehn MM, Yahr MD. Parkinsonism: onset, progression and mortality. *Neurology.* 1967;17(5):427–442. [PubMed] [Google Scholar]

2. Hoehn MM. Parkinsonism treated with levodopa: progression and mortality. *Journal of Neural Transmission*. 1983;19, supplement:253–264. [PubMed] [Google Scholar]

3. Poewe WH, Wenning GK. The natural history of Parkinson' disease. *Annals of Neurology*. 1998;44(3):S1–S9. [PubMed] [Google Scholar]

4. Poewe WH, Lees AJ, Stern GM. Low-dose L-dopa therapy in Parkinson's disease: a 6-year follow-up study. *Neurology*. 1986;36(11):1528–1530. [PubMed] [Google Scholar]

5. Schrag A, Quinn N. Dyskinesias and motor fluctuations in Parkinson's disease: a community-based study. *Brain*. 2000;123(11):2297–2305. [PubMed] [Google Scholar]

6. Chase TN, Mouradian MM, Engber TM. Motor response complications and the function of striatal efferent systems. *Neurology*. 1993;43(12):S23–S27. [PubMed] [Google Scholar]

7. Chaudhuri KR, Healy DG, Schapira AHV. Non-motor symptoms of Parkinson's disease: diagnosis and management. *Lancet Neurology*. 2006;5(3):235–245. [PubMed] [Google Scholar]

8. Williams-Gray CH, Foltynie T, Lewis SJG, Barker RA. Cognitive deficits and psychosis in Parkinson's disease: a review of pathophysiology and therapeutic options. *CNS Drugs*. 2006;20(6):477–505. [PubMed] [Google Scholar]

9. Aarsland D, Marsh L, Schrag A. Neuropsychiatric symptoms in Parkinson's disease. *Movement Disorders*. 2009;24(15):2175–2186. [PMC free article] [PubMed] [Google Scholar]

10. Schrag A, Jahanshahi M, Quinn N. What contributes to quality of life in patients with Parkinson's disease? *Journal of Neurology Neurosurgery and Psychiatry*. 2000;69(3):308–312. [PMC free article] [PubMed] [Google Scholar]

11. Nussbaum M, Treves TA, Inzelberg R, Rabey JM, Korczyn AD. Survival in Parkinson's disease: the effect of dementia. *Parkinsonism and Related Disorders*. 1998;4(4):179–181. [PubMed] [Google Scholar]

12. Goetz CG, Stebbins GT. Risk factors for nursing home placement in advanced Parkinson's disease. *Neurology*. 1993;43(11):2227–2229. [PubMed] [Google Scholar]

13. Aarsland D, Larsen JP, Karlsen K, Lim NG, Tandberg E. Mental symptoms in Parkinson's disease are important contributors to caregiver distress. *International Journal of Geriatric Psychiatry*. 1999;14(10):866–874. [PubMed] [Google Scholar]

14. Pickering RM, Grimbergen YAM, Rigney U, et al. A meta-analysis of six prospective studies of falling in Parkinson's disease. *Movement Disorders*. 2007;22(13):1892–1900. [PubMed] [Google Scholar]

15. Kerr GK, Worringham CJ, Cole MH, Lacherez PF, Wood JM, Silburn PA. Predictors of future falls in Parkinson disease. *Neurology*. 2010;75(2):116–124. [PubMed] [Google Scholar]

16. Goodwin VA, Richards SH, Taylor RS, Taylor AH, Campbell JL. The effectiveness of exercise interventions for people with Parkinson's disease: a systematic review and meta-analysis. *Movement Disorders*. 2008;23(5):631–640. [PubMed] [Google Scholar]

17. Moro E, Hamani C, Poon YY, et al. Unilateral pedunculopontine stimulation improves falls in Parkinson's disease. *Brain*. 2010;133(1):215–224. [PubMed] [Google Scholar]

18. Lang AE, Lozano AM. Medical progress: Parkinson's disease—I. *The New England Journal of Medicine*. 1998;339:1044–1055. [PubMed] [Google Scholar]

19. Lang AE, Lozano AM. Medical progress: Parkinson's disease—II. *The New England Journal of Medicine*. 1998;339:1130–1143. [PubMed] [Google Scholar]

20. Riley DE, Lang AE. The spectrum of levodopa-related fluctuations in Parkinson's disease. *Neurology*. 1993;43(8):1459–1464. [PubMed] [Google Scholar]

21. Waters CH. Managing the late complications of Parkinson's disease. *Neurology*. 1997;49(1):S49–S57. [PubMed] [Google Scholar]

22. Koller WC, Pahwa R. Treating motor fluctuations with controlled-release levodopa preparations. *Neurology*. 1994;44(7):S23–28. [PubMed] [Google Scholar]

23. Metman LV, Hoff J, Mouradian MM, Chase TN. Fluctuations in plasma levodopa and motor responses with liquid and tablet levodopa/carbidopa. *Movement Disorders*. 1994;9(4):463–465. [PubMed] [Google Scholar]

24. Kurth MC, Tetrud JW, Irwin I, Lyness WH, Langston JW. Oral levodopa/carbidopa solution versus tablets in Parkinson's patients with severe fluctuations: a pilot study. *Neurology*. 1993;43(5):1036–1039. [PubMed] [Google Scholar]

25. Pierantozzi M, Pietroiusti A, Brusa L, et al. Helicobacter pylori eradication and L-dopa absorption in patients with PD and motor fluctuations. *Neurology*. 2006;66(12):1824–1829. [PubMed] [Google Scholar]

26. Stocchi F, Fabbri L, Vecsei L, Krygowska-Wajs A, Monici Preti PA, Ruggieri SA. Clinical efficacy of a single afternoon dose of effervescent levodopa-carbidopa preparation (CHF 1512) in fluctuating Parkinson disease. *Clinical Neuropharmacology*. 2007;30(1):18–24. [PubMed] [Google Scholar]

27. Hardoff R, Sula M, Tamir A, et al. Gastric emptying time and gastric motility in patients with Parkinson's disease. *Movement Disorders*. 2001;16(6):1041–1047. [PubMed] [Google Scholar]

28. Kurlan R, Nutt JG, Woodward WR, et al. Duodenal and gastric delivery of levodopa in parkinsonism. *Annals of Neurology*. 1988;23(6):589–595. [PubMed] [Google Scholar]

29. Samanta J, Hauser RA. Duodenal levodopa infusion for the treatment of Parkinson's disease. *Expert Opinion on Pharmacotherapy*. 2007;8(5):657–664. [PubMed] [Google Scholar]

30. Antonini A, Isaias IU, Canesi M, et al. Duodenal levodopa infusion for advanced Parkinson's disease: 12-month treatment outcome. *Movement Disorders*. 2007;22(8):1145–1149. [PubMed] [Google Scholar]

31. Devos D, Agid Y, Al Khedr A, et al. Patient profile, indications, efficacy and safety of duodenal levodopa infusion in advanced Parkinson's disease. *Movement Disorders*. 2009;24(7):993–1000. [PubMed] [Google Scholar]

32. Honig H, Antonini A, Martinez-Martin P, et al. Intrajejunal levodopa infusion in Parkinson's disease: a pilot multicenter study of effects on nonmotor symptoms and quality of life. *Movement Disorders*. 2009;24(10):1468–1474. [PubMed] [Google Scholar]

33. Tyne HL, Parsons J, Sinnott A, Fox SH, Fletcher NA, Steiger MJ. A 10 year retrospective audit of long-term apomorphine use in Parkinson's disease. *Journal of Neurology*. 2004;251(11):1370–1374. [PubMed] [Google Scholar]

34. Luquin MR, Scipioni O, Vaamonde J, Gershanik O, Obeso JA. Levodopa-induced dyskinesias in Parkinson's disease: clinical and pharmacological classification. *Movement Disorders*. 1992;7(2):117–124. [PubMed] [Google Scholar]

35. Bennett JP, Landow ER, Schuh LA. Suppression of dyskinesias in advanced Parkinson's disease. II. Increasing daily clozapine doses suppress dyskinesias and improve parkinsonism symptoms. *Neurology*. 1996;46:1059–1062. [PubMed] [Google Scholar]

36. Gomez Arevalo GJ, Gershanik OS. Modulatory effect of clozapine on levodopa response in Parkinson's disease: a preliminary study. *Movement Disorders*. 1993;43:1551–1555. [PubMed] [Google Scholar]

37. Hanagasi HA, Kaptanoglu G, Sahin HA, Emre M. The use of NMDA antagonist memantine in drug-resitant dyskinesia resulting from L-dopa. *Movement Disorders*. 2000;15:1016–1017. [PubMed] [Google Scholar]

38. Varanese S, Howard J, Di Rocco A. NMDA antagonist memantine improves levodopa-induced dyskinesias and "on-off" phenomena in Parkinson's disease. *Movement Disorders*. 2010;25(4):508–510. [PubMed] [Google Scholar]

39. Cereda E, Barichella M, Pezzoli G. Controlled-protein dietary regimens for Parkinson's disease. *Nutritional Neuroscience*. 2010;13(1):29–32. [PubMed] [Google Scholar]

40. Braak H, Del Tredici K, Rüb U, De Vos RAI, Jansen Steur ENH, Braak E. Staging of brain pathology related to sporadic Parkinson's disease. *Neurobiology of Aging*. 2003;24(2):197–211. [PubMed] [Google Scholar]

41. Aarsland D, Larsen JP, Tandberg E, Laake K. Predictors of nursing home placement in Parkinson's disease: a population-based, prospective study. *Journal of the American Geriatrics Society*. 2000;48(8):938–942. [PubMed] [Google Scholar]

42. Chaudhuri KR, Schapira AHV, Martinez-Martin P, et al. The holistic management of Parkinson's using a novel non-motor symptom scale and questionnaire. *Advances in Clinical Neuroscience and Rehabilitation*. 2004;4:20–24. [Google Scholar]

43. Chaudhuri KR, Martinez-Martin P, Brown RG, et al. The metric properties of a novel non-motor symptoms scale for Parkinson's disease: results from an international pilot study. *Movement Disorders*. 2007;22(13):1901–1911. [PubMed] [Google Scholar]

44. Martinez-Martin P, Rodriguez-Blazquez C, Abe K, et al. International study on the psychometric attributes of the non-motor symptoms scale in Parkinson disease. *Neurology*. 2009;73(19):1584–1591. [PubMed] [Google Scholar]

45. Williams-Gray CH, Foltynie T, Lewis SJG, Barker RA. Cognitive deficits and psychosis in Parkinson's disease: a review of pathophysiology and therapeutic options. *CNS Drugs*. 2006;20(6):477–505. [PubMed] [Google Scholar]

46. Emre M. Dementia associated with Parkinson's disease. *Lancet Neurology*. 2003;2(4):229–237. [PubMed] [Google Scholar]

47. Aarsland D, Litvan I, Salmon D, Galasko D, Wentzel-Larsen T, Larsen JP. Performance on the dementia rating scale in Parkinson's disease with dementia and dementia with Lewy bodies: comparison with progressive supranuclear palsy and Alzheimer's disease. *Journal of Neurology, Neurosurgery and Psychiatry*. 2003;74(9):1215–1220. [PMC free article] [PubMed] [Google Scholar]

48. Ballard CG, Aarsland D, McKeith I, et al. Fluctuations in attention: PD dementia vs DLB with parkinsonism. *Neurology*. 2002;59(11):1714–1720. [PubMed] [Google Scholar]

49. Varanese S, Perfetti B, Monaco D, et al. Fluctuating cognition and different cognitive and behavioural profiles in Parkinson's disease with dementia: comparison of dementia with Lewy bodies and Alzheimer's disease. *Journal of Neurology.* 2010;257(6):1004–1011. [PubMed] [Google Scholar]

50. Rinne JO, Portin R, Ruottinen H, et al. Cognitive impairment and the brain dopaminergic system in Parkinson disease. *Archives of Neurology.* 2000;57(4):470–475. [PubMed] [Google Scholar]

51. Dubois B, Ruberg M, Javoy Agid F. A subcortico-cortical cholinergic system is affected in Parkinson's disease. *Brain Research.* 1983;288(1-2):213–218. [PubMed] [Google Scholar]

52. Emre M, Aarsland D, Albanese A, et al. Rivastigmine for dementia associated with Parkinson's disease. *New England Journal of Medicine.* 2004;351(24):2509–2518. [PubMed] [Google Scholar]

53. Aarsland D, Laake K, Larsen JP, Janvin C. Donepezil for cognitive impairment in Parkinson's disease: a randomised controlled study. *Journal of Neurology Neurosurgery and Psychiatry.* 2002;72(6):708–712. [PMC free article] [PubMed] [Google Scholar]

54. Leroi I, Brandt J, Reich SG, et al. Randomized placebo-controlled trial of donepezil in cognitive impairment in Parkinson's disease. *International Journal of Geriatric Psychiatry.* 2004;19(1):1–8. [PubMed] [Google Scholar]

55. Factor SA, Molho ES, Podskalny GD, Brown D. Parkinson's disease: drug-induced psychiatric states. *Advances in Neurology.* 1995;65:115–138. [PubMed] [Google Scholar]

56. Ravina B, Marder K, Fernandez HH, et al. Diagnostic criteria for psychosis in Parkinson's disease: report of an NINDS, NIMH Work Group. *Movement Disorders.* 2007;22(8):1061–1068. [PubMed] [Google Scholar]

57. The Parkinson Study Group. Low dose clozapine for the treatment of drug-induced psychosis in parkinson's disease. *The New England Journal of Medicine.* 1999;340:757–763. [PubMed] [Google Scholar]

58. Schrag A, Barone P, Brown RG, et al. Depression rating scales in Parkinson's disease: critique and recommendations. *Movement Disorders.* 2007;22(8):1077–1092. [PMC free article] [PubMed] [Google Scholar]

59. Kagan BL, Sultzer DL, Rosenlicht N, Gerner RH. Oral S-adenosylmethionine in depression: a randomized, double-blind, placebo-controlled trial. *American Journal of Psychiatry.* 1990;147(5):591–595. [PubMed] [Google Scholar]

60. Rocco AD, Rogers JD, Brown R, Werner P, Bottiglieri T. S-adenosyl-methionine improves depression in patients with Parkinson's disease in an open-label clinical trial. *Movement Disorders.* 2000;15(6):1225–1229. [PubMed] [Google Scholar]

61. Hauser RA, Wahba MN, Zesiewicz TA, Anderson W. Modafinil treatment of pramipexole-associated somnolence. *Movement Disorders.* 2000;15(6):1269–1271. [PubMed] [Google Scholar]

62. Lahrmann H, Cortelli P, Hilz M, Mathias CJ, Struhal W, Tassinari M. EFNS guidelines on the diagnosis and management of orthostatic hypotension. *European Journal of Neurology.* 2006;13(9):930–936. [PubMed] [Google Scholar]

63. Jost WH. Gastrointestinal dysfunction in Parkinson's Disease. *Journal of the Neurological Sciences.* 2010;289(1-2):69–73. [PubMed] [Google Scholar]

64. Blackett H, Walker R, Wood B. Urinary dysfunction in Parkinson's disease: a review. *Parkinsonism and Related Disorders.* 2009;15(2):81–87. [PubMed] [Google Scholar]

65. Andersson KE, Chapple CR, Cardozo L, et al. Pharmacological treatment of overactive bladder: report from the International Consultation on Incontinence. *Current Opinion in Urology.* 2009;19(4):380–394. [PubMed] [Google Scholar]

66. Jankovic J. Disease-oriented approach to botulinum toxin use. *Toxicon.* 2009;54(5):614–623. [PubMed] [Google Scholar]

67. Calne SM, Kumar A. Nursing care of patients with late-stage Parkinson's disease. *The Journal of Neuroscience Nursing.* 2003;35(5):242–251. [PubMed] [Google Scholar]

68. Sapir S, Spielman JL, Ramig LO, Story BH, Fox C. Effects of intensive voice treatment (the Lee Silverman Voice Treatment [LSVT]) on vowel articulation in dysarthric individuals with idiopathic Parkinson disease: acoustic and perceptual findings. *Journal of Speech, Language, and Hearing Research.* 2007;50(4):899–912. [PubMed] [Google Scholar]

69. Calne DB, Calne S. Treatment of Parkinson's disease. In: Ancil RJ, Holliday SG, Mithani AH, editors. *Therapeutics in Geriatric Neuropsychiatry.* Chichester, England: John Wiley & Sons; 1997. pp. 1–12. [Google Scholar]

PARKINSON'S AND CHILDREN 284

Kids at Home 285

Adult Children 286

Grandkids 286

My Perspective: Kids as Care Partners 287

PARKINSON'S WHEN YOU LIVE ALONE 288

PRACTICAL PLANNING FOR THE FUTURE 289

Planning for the Financial Impact of Parkinson's 290

Long-Term Care Planning for People with Parkinson's 293

WORKSHEETS AND RESOURCES

♥ **WELLNESS AND LIFESTYLE SELF-ASSESSMENTS** 299

Parkinson's Care Questionnaire 299

Goal Summary for Doctor Visits 302

Daily Medication Log 305

Overall Medication Log 306

Wellness Self-Assessment 307

Pre-Exercise Self-Assessment 309

Exercise Journal 313

Nutrition Self-Assessment 314

Parkinson's Psychosis Self-Assessment 317

Deep Brain Stimulation (DBS) Self-Assessment 318

Our Relationship Self-Assessment 320

☑ **SYMPTOM CHECKLISTS** 321

My Symptoms Worksheet 321

Bladder Worksheet 324

Cognitive Wellness Worksheet 325

Constipation Worksheet 326

Dental Worksheet 328

Dyskinesia and "Off" Time Log 330

Emotional Wellness: Anxiety 331

Emotional Wellness: Depression 333

Fatigue Worksheet 335

Gait, Balance and Freezing Worksheet 337

Insomnia and Sleep Worksheet 340

Low Blood Pressure and Dizziness Worksheet 342

Speech and Communication Worksheet 344

Swallowing Worksheet 346

Sexual Dysfunction Worksheet 348

📷 **MEDICAL INFORMATION SNAPSHOTS** 350

    Clinical Appointments Summary 350

    Current Symptoms Summary 355

    Wellness Team Contact Information 357

    Medical Providers 358

    DBS Medical History 359

    Prepare for Your Hospital Stay 363

    Medical Summary for Your Doctor Appointment 366

    Medical Summary for Dentists 367

GLOSSARY

KEY PARKINSON'S TERMS 369

8

A MESSAGE FROM DAVIS PHINNEY

My background is one of sport; cycling, specifically. The Olympics and the Tour de France are my former domains. I learned much about myself through years of competing successfully in tough, demanding events. I came to understand the importance of focus, and purpose; that paying attention to and being engaged in the process are just as important as the achievement of goals. I came to understand that victory – that elusive, electric moment of triumph – was not exclusive to those who crossed the finish line first.

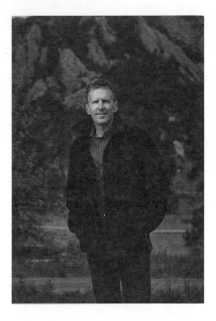

These are lessons that are rooted in me, and they help me now in the much more challenging race against Parkinson's. This race, a no-holds-barred winner-take-all type of event, demands everything from me. Let down my guard, and it'll knock me flat – but by refusing to give in, by exercising daily, by eating well and most especially, by maintaining a positive attitude – I find ways to win.

I've had Parkinson's since 2000 (plus another 10 or so years pre-diagnosis), and what I also know is this: We can improve our quality of life. It takes work and commitment. It takes patience and support. It takes education and understanding. It takes a road map, which is exactly what this manual is meant to be for living well with Parkinson's.

If there's an upside to Parkinson's, it's that I'm constantly meeting members of the Parkinson's tribe who are exploring new ways to live better with this disease. People who are climbing mountains, running marathons and even riding their bikes across the country – and others who find victory in spending time with their loved ones or walking around the block. I've met singers and songwriters, painters and poets. The commonality is their motivation to keep living an inspired life.

Ultimately, it's not the size of victory that counts, but the acknowledgment of the victory and the incentive it provides us to keep seeking ways to win. It's about what we can do today to improve our lives. And that is a victory in itself.

— DAVIS PHINNEY

9

When the Davis Phinney Foundation was established in 2004, Davis was clear that he wanted its mission to be different from that of other existing Parkinson's organizations. While a cure is what we all want for Parkinson's disease, it was also clear that in the meantime, people desperately needed better information about how to live with Parkinson's right now.

So, the Foundation's mission — then and now — is to help people with Parkinson's live well today. The *Every Victory Counts* manual is an important part of fulfilling that mission. First published in 2010, it broke new ground as the only resource of its kind, devoted solely to the principle of proactive self-care and a holistic approach to managing Parkinson's. In subsequent editions, it has gained international notoriety as a superb and comprehensive resource for changing the way people live with Parkinson's.

The manual embraces the Davis Phinney Foundation's philosophy of taking action to improve your quality of life with Parkinson's. Within these pages, we hope you'll feel like you've found your people, your tribe. Here, we'll acknowledge loss, but we won't dwell on might-have-been. Rather, we'll turn our attention to what is yet to be and how we will make the most of today and every day. Most people with Parkinson's will live for many years, and there are things that you can do to live well and, indeed, to thrive.

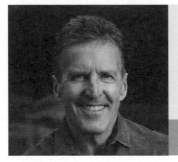

❝ *I can't control that I have Parkinson's, but I can control how I live with Parkinson's.*❞

— DAVIS

WHAT IS SELF-CARE?

Self-care refers to a person taking a central role in the management of their own health and well-being. Self-care requires you to be educated about your health so that you and anyone closely involved in your care can make informed decisions related to your treatment. Self-care helps you to make good choices that will improve the way you feel and help you better manage the symptoms you experience.

Self-care is proactive: you, the person living with Parkinson's, are in the driver's seat. If your medication isn't working as you think it should, contact your doctor and ask for a consultation. Instead of waiting for a cure to come, find out what you can do now to maintain mobility, strength and balance. By embracing the self-care approach, you'll take steps to improve your diet, to begin or continue exercising and generally focus on your physical, cognitive and emotional well-being.

Self-care is an effective strategy no matter how old you are or how long you have been living with Parkinson's. There is always something that you can do, even if it's simply choosing to focus on the positive. Set one or two goals for yourself at a time, and then go after them, using the tools in this manual to guide you.

THIS MANUAL IS YOUR ROADMAP FOR LIVING WELL TODAY. THE ROUTE YOU CHOOSE IS UP TO YOU.

Parkinson's changes over time, and your experiences, needs and treatments will change direction from time to time, too. The *Every Victory Counts* manual is designed to provide the information you need to make choices about how you manage your Parkinson's today and in the future. As your needs evolve, so will your approach. Armed with essential knowledge and inspired by the successful experiences recounted in these pages by clinicians and people with Parkinson's alike, you can create your own self-care plan and build in the flexibility to adjust course over time. Though your symptoms will inevitably change, your commitment to living well is a constant. Remember, whatever your current situation, it *is* possible to live well with Parkinson's *today*.

Think of this manual and the additional material located on the *Every Victory Counts* companion website (⌂ **dpf.org/evc-connect**) as a living resource to help you take steps to preserve or improve your quality of life after a Parkinson's diagnosis. Share a favorite essay, video, podcast, worksheet or this entire manual with family and friends to start a conversation about your experience or to help them learn more about Parkinson's.

This is material you can turn to again and again — when you need a little extra motivation or hope, or when you want to dig deeper into a specific topic that's especially important to you right now. Keep the manual out where you'll see it and where it will serve as a daily reminder of your commitment to living well with Parkinson's. Use the worksheets to log your activities and keep notes about which changes you've made have a positive effect on your symptoms. Complete the self-assessments to help you become more aware of your physical, cognitive and emotional state and to prepare for and get the most benefit from your next appointment with your doctor or member of your wellness team.

The key to living well today with Parkinson's is actively choosing to do the things that will result in your best possible quality of life. Be informed, be engaged, be connected, be courageous and be active. Each day will bring new challenges and opportunities for positive change. Remember, your daily triumphs, large or small, are worth celebrating: *Every Victory Counts*!

11

MEET YOUR PARKINSON'S GUIDES

Throughout this manual and on the *Every Victory Counts* companion website ⮔ dpf.org/evc-connect, you'll get to know 17 individuals who are living with or caring for someone who has Parkinson's. These "Parkinson's Guides" are here to share their experiences and lend context to the topics covered by the manual's authors and contributors.

They are real people, just like you, speaking candidly about how they're living well today with Parkinson's. They are women and men, some with young children at home, some with grandchildren, some living with care partners and others living alone. They'll be the first to say that some days are better than others, but their long-term commitment to enhance their well-being doesn't waver.

The stories from our Parkinson's Guides reflect a snapshot in time. Chances are, you'll find one of our Guides who is treading a similar path to your own, right now. Take a moment to read about the Guides living with Parkinson's below, then look for their contributions throughout the manual, as well as on the companion website: ⮔ dpf.org/guides.

JOHN ALEXANDER

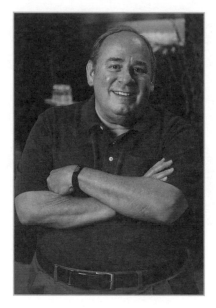

John was diagnosed with Parkinson's in 2010 at the age of 59. Following his diagnosis, John took up cycling and has since ridden more than 3,000 miles in the past several years, in addition to climbing a mountain in Scotland and completing two triathlons. John and his son Brian rode the last day of *Ride with Larry* in 2011, a transformative experience that introduced John to the team behind the documentary film of the same name as well as the Davis Phinney Foundation.

John sees Parkinson's as "both a blessing and a calling." He explains, "Parkinson's is a blessing because it has allowed me to meet the most inspirational and amazing people, which in turn has caused me to accept and deal with this condition in a positive, optimistic way." A natural connector, John enjoys building relationships while providing the Parkinson's community with resources to "lighten their burden and bring them joy," believing that the Davis Phinney Foundation's philosophy "gives people hope and skills to cope with this condition like no other group." John has written a book about his Parkinson's experience entitled, *The Journey Begins With 1,000 Miles – Thriving with Parkinson's Disease Through Hope, Optimism, and Perseverance*. In it, he shares how staying active, seeking inspiration from others and serving as an advocate have helped him to live with Parkinson's.

Meet John: ⮔ dpf.org/john

EDIE ANDERSON

Edie was diagnosed with Parkinson's in 2013 at the age of 60. She developed Parkinson's symptoms after undergoing several surgeries and chemotherapy in her earlier battle with breast cancer. After a year-long "pity party," Edie found the help she needed through a local support group where she met another person living with Parkinson's who shared his passion for exercising. "I became a workout junkie," she says. "I have benefited physically, mentally and emotionally from my active lifestyle."

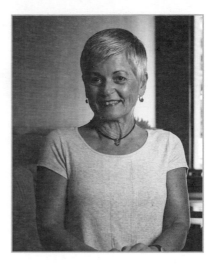

Now retired, Edie is passionate about helping others with Parkinson's discover the benefits of exercise to live well with the disease. She teaches at a variety of support groups and other Parkinson's educational events about developing a proactive approach to wellness. "I want to give hope to people living with Parkinson's and their caregivers by telling my story," she explains. "And showing that exercise works to improve our ability to function, which translates into a happier life for all of us!" Edie and her husband, Scott, split their time between the Blue Ridge mountains of Virginia and the sunny southern coast of Florida. Snowbirding is an integral part of Edie's wellness program because the Florida sunshine warms her heart, body and mind, helping her stay active year-round. Edie's husband, Scott, is also featured in the *Every Victory Counts* manual.

Meet Edie: dpf.org/edie
Meet Scott: dpf.org/scott

JILL ATER

Jill was diagnosed with Parkinson's in 2005 at the age of 42. She had young children at the time and was running a successful staffing company in the Denver metro area. She soon discovered she carries a mutated gene associated with Parkinson's, LRRK2, shared with her mother and sister who are also living with Parkinson's. "Like most, I would prefer to not have to deal with Parkinson's," Jill says, "but since that is not an option, the choice I do have is to live as fully as possible and make my 'lemonade' by helping others to keep going. It's all about information, empowerment and an end to the isolation that often comes for those living with Parkinson's disease."

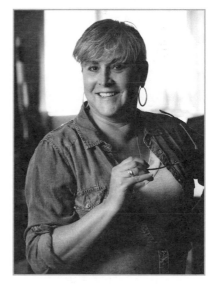

Jill and her husband have moved 19 times over the past 25 years through six states and two foreign countries. Now retired and living in Tacoma, Washington, Jill assists with Parkinson's support groups and events throughout the greater South Puget Sound area. "So many people living with Parkinson's focus on what they can no longer do," Jill explains. "I want to help people to focus on what they can do." Her plan is to move overseas once her youngest graduates from high school in 2019 and travel as long as possible, explaining, "Parkinson's gave me a gift: to live fully now, not wait for someday."

Meet Jill: dpf.org/jill

LIZ EASTERLY

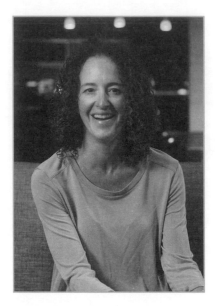

Liz was diagnosed with Parkinson's in 2010 at the age of 40. A mom to two young boys with a successful career as a writer and marketer, Liz has found a supportive group through Parkinson's boxing classes. She's continually amazed and reminded by those she meets at Parkinson's boxing classes that no matter your age or stage of Parkinson's, it's never too late to start moving and improving how you feel. "It's important for me to surround myself with others who are optimistic and taking an active role in their treatment," she says. "The goal of giving my kids a normal childhood has motivated me to take control of things I can manage, like exercise and healthy lifestyle choices."

"When I got the *Every Victory Counts* manual, it was like I had just been handed a life preserver," she explains. "It was the first time I heard that it was possible to live well with Parkinson's, and while I had no control over having Parkinson's disease, there were plenty of things I could control! It was full of hope and optimism, and changed my whole outlook on my disease." Surrounding herself with optimism and actively participating in her own treatment provides Liz with a strong sense of empowerment. Liz's husband, Dave, is also featured in the *Every Victory Counts* manual.

Meet Liz: dpf.org/liz
Meet Dave: dpf.org/dave

TIM HAGUE, SR.

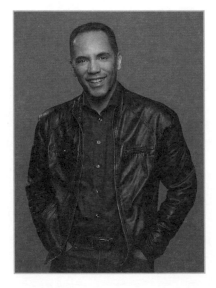

Tim was diagnosed with Parkinson's in 2011 at the age of 46. He is the Founder and Executive Director of U-Turn Parkinson's, a registered Canadian charity whose mission is to help people living with Parkinson's live their best through the practice of wellness. Tim's previous career as a registered nurse (retired) spanned over 20 years and encompassed both work at the bedside and in management. Tim's diagnosis of young onset Parkinson's led to Tim and his son, Tim Jr., being selected to participate in the inaugural season of *The Amazing Race Canada*. In spite of the difficulties of Parkinson's, "The Tims" went on to win season one of the race.

Tim maintains a busy speaking schedule traveling across North America encouraging Parkinson's groups as well as a corporate motivational keynote speaker. Tim has had the opportunity to speak for TEDx and has spoken at a number of The Victory Summit events. He is a keen supporter of the Davis Phinney Foundation's work to "live well today." Tim's wife, Sheryl, is also featured in the *Every Victory Counts* manual.

Meet Tim: dpf.org/tim

STEVE HOVEY

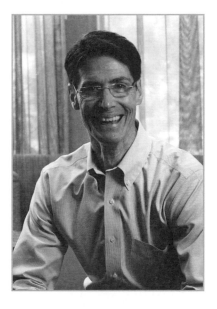

Steve was diagnosed with Parkinson's in 2007 at the age of 50. At the time of diagnosis, Steve did not know anyone with Parkinson's, so he and his wife, Nancy, took it upon themselves to learn as much as they could about Parkinson's symptoms and treatment. Their search soon led them to the Davis Phinney Foundation, where they learned about the importance of exercise and a healthy lifestyle, something Steve credits as significantly impacting the quality of life he continues to enjoy. Steve sold his business and retired in June of 2015, so he could spend more time focusing on his personal wellness, family and volunteer work. Steve and Nancy recently moved to Saratoga Springs, New York, to be closer to their two daughters, two sons-in-law and especially their two granddaughters, Rylan and Haddie.

Steve enjoys sharing the message that there are things people can do to manage Parkinson's. "When I was diagnosed, the focus of treatment was on medicine. The doctors never mentioned the benefits of dealing with the disease on a more holistic level – exercise, good nutrition and a healthy lifestyle," Steve says. "I am happy to say that through careful observation and research, the medical community now embraces the clear benefits of exercise for people with Parkinson's. Our job is to get out there and reinforce this message throughout the Parkinson's community." Nancy is also featured in the *Every Victory Counts* manual.

Meet Steve: dpf.org/steve
Meet Nancy: dpf.org/nancy

BRENDA HUTCHINSON

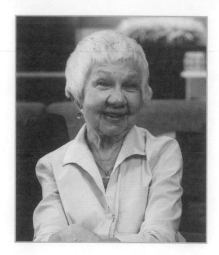

Brenda was diagnosed with Parkinson's in 2010 at the age of 72. A retired teacher living in Boulder, Colorado, Brenda was an avid traveler and athlete, skiing, cycling and hiking across the United States, Canada, Europe and Asia at the time of her diagnosis. As shocking as it was hearing the words, "You have Parkinson's," she remembers also feeling relief, as there was now a direction to follow. She realized immediately that coping with this degenerative disease would be a lifelong challenge, especially as someone living alone.

In a relatively short time, Brenda became active in the local Parkinson's community, taking advantage of the many exercise classes like boxing, dance, yoga and boot camp, as well as attending the local support group, informal coffee discussions and a women's support group. She was inspired by the determination and stamina of many of the participants to fight Parkinson's, as well as their refreshing sense of humor. Brenda's goal is to continue challenging herself in order to live independently, staying disciplined in exercising, informed on recent research and programs and involved by reaching out to others to give support as well as to receive it. She acknowledges the positive changes this unexpected disease has brought, explaining: "Parkinson's has forced me to slow down, become more mindful of my surroundings, more compassionate and less demanding of myself and others. I am more appreciative of what I can still do as well as all that I experienced in the past."

Meet Brenda: dpf.org/brenda

COREY KING

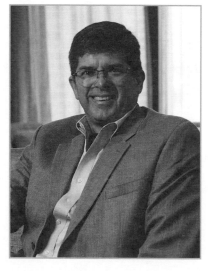

Corey was diagnosed with Parkinson's in 2009 at the age of 47. He is president and chairman of the board of directors for the San Antonio Area Parkinson's Disease and Movement Disorder Foundation (SA Moves), a nonprofit educational foundation chartered to improve quality of life and quality of care for people challenged with movement disorders. He also is a past member of the board of directors of the Lone Star Parkinson Society in Texas, and the past president and chairman of the board of the Alamo Area Parkinson's Support Group. Corey is a US Air Force veteran and served as a space operations and engineering officer. After his Air Force career, Corey was an engineer and business executive in the high-tech world. After being diagnosed with young onset Parkinson's in 2009, Corey retired from his professional career in 2011.

Corey currently volunteers as an advocate for the Parkinson's and movement disorders communities. Corey writes a blog about his experiences in life and with Parkinson's at ⬚ thecrookedpath.net and has published two books: *Walking the Crooked Path* in 2013 and *Stumbling Toward Victory: Living in Defiance of Early-Onset Parkinson's Disease* in 2016. He and his wife Amy live in San Antonio, Texas with their standard poodle Izzy and two recovering stray cats (Skitter and Honeybee), who actually run the whole operation. They have two grown children.

Meet Corey: ⬚ dpf.org/corey

BRIAN REEDY

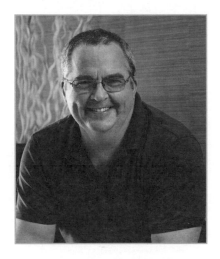

Brian was diagnosed with Parkinson's in 2010 at the age of 49. Brian is a former high school teacher. In his twenty years as a teacher, he taught English, theatre arts, computer literacy, video production and photography. His students won many state and national awards. While teaching, Brian also worked with Adobe for ten years as an Adobe Education Leader, where he received special training and went around the country teaching at conferences and seminars. The greatest blessing of his life was found in the high school library, as his wife Lily was a library assistant. She is the absolute love of his life! She told him after he was diagnosed with Parkinson's that she is not his caregiver, but his care *partner*. When Lily was diagnosed with breast cancer in 2016, Brian found out what it means to be a care partner and Lily found what a lot of Brian's health issues, like daily fatigue, were really like. This shared awareness has made them ready to give back to others.

Last year they became co-directors of their community's Parkinson's support group. They attended in the World Parkinson's Congress in 2013 and 2016, and have been to numerous other Parkinson's conferences. A few years ago, Brian and Lily appeared in the PBS documentary out of CPBN in Connecticut, "Living With Parkinson's." This year they also both appear in the new book, *Faces of Parkinson's: Global Reflections*. They are actively finding ways to make a positive difference in the Parkinson's world and love sharing what they learn so others can see the positives to be found when entering the world of Parkinson's. Brian and Lily do not let Parkinson's define them, rather they are actively defining it in their lives. Lily is also featured in the *Every Victory Counts* manual.

Meet Brian: ⬚ dpf.org/brian
Meet Lily: ⬚ dpf.org/lily

LINDA SWANSON

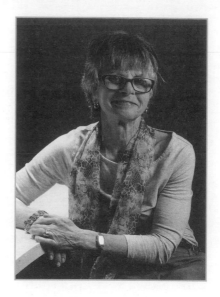

Linda was diagnosed with Parkinson's in 2009 at the age of 56. She and her husband, Mike, celebrated their 44th wedding anniversary in 2016 and have three grown children and four grandchildren. After Mike semi-retired 10 years ago, they relocated back to Texas to be closer to their family. They both continued to work after the move, but Linda retired from teaching after over twenty years in 2010. She completed her master's in education/reading specialist just before she celebrated her 50th birthday and she still occasionally tutors privately.

Linda was diagnosed with Parkinson's in 2009 after she hurt her back while training to do the Chicago Marathon, which would have been her third marathon. However, she has continued being active and has completed 10 half marathons since 2011. Her mission is to help change the "face" of Parkinson's by being an active advocate in the Parkinson's community. Linda has attended Dance for PD regularly since 2011, is an active member of Parkinson Voice Project's LOUD CROWD, as well as a Parkinson Voice advocate. She is also active in the local Dallas Area Parkinsonism Society and was an assistant state director for the Parkinson's Action Network. She also attends a weekly Bible study and has recently joined a book club. She spends her time at home working in her flower garden and enjoys doing jigsaw puzzles. Linda's husband, Mike, is also featured in the *Every Victory Counts* manual.

Meet Linda: dpf.org/linda
Meet Mike: dpf.org/mike

RYAN TRIPP

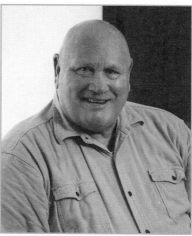

Ryan was diagnosed with Parkinson's in 1996 at the age of 47. He worked as a physical education teacher and administrator for 23 years. Two and a half years after being diagnosed with Parkinson's, he was forced to take a long-term disability health leave from his profession. This led to a major slip into depression, a fractured marriage and a stage of "Who am I and what is happening to me?!?" After joining a Parkinson's support group, improved medication and some valuable counseling, he found a renewed focus on life and living with Parkinson's.

His active involvement in events and speaking engagements outside of Parkinson Canada has brought him a wealth of information, contacts and experiences that are extensive and invaluable. Within Parkinson Canada, he has been a strong, consistent fundraiser, an active committee volunteer, an enthusiastic advocate in the community both on Parliament Hill and at Queen's Park in Canada, plus he started and led a local support group in Muskoka, Ontario. Finally, during the past decade, he has committed much of his time to the World Parkinson Coalition. He has attended all four of the past World Parkinson Congresses and been a global ambassador for the past two. This is the very best extended family any Parkinsonian could ever have. His personal code is to remain positive, be grateful and smile daily! "Carpe Diem!"

Meet Ryan: ☐ dpf.org/ryan

LEAD AUTHORS

MONIQUE GIROUX, MD

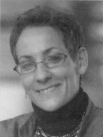

Dr. Monique Giroux is medical director and co-founder of the Movement & Neuroperformance Center of Colorado in Fort Collins, CO and executive director of The Healthy Living Institute, a nonprofit focused on healthy lifestyle programs for people with chronic illness (thehealthylivinginstitute.com). Dr. Giroux received her medical degree from Ohio State University, completed her neurology residency at Yale, her movement disorders fellowship at Emory University and completed a fellowship in holistic health and integrative medicine at the University of Arizona. She is board certified in neurology and specializes in lifestyle medicine, integrating non-medical approaches with traditional medical and surgical treatment, including deep brain stimulation and neurorehabilitation programs, which she developed.

She has received training in mindfulness-based stress reduction, which she has adapted to create wellness programs for neurological conditions. Dr. Giroux's latest book, *Optimizing Health with Parkinson's: A Guide to Integrating Lifestyle, Alternative and Conventional Medicine*, is the first comprehensive book to be published that reviews the scientific rationale and practical considerations for integrating complementary therapy for Parkinson's disease.

SIERRA FARRIS, MPAS, PA-C

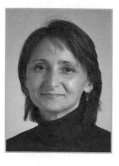

Ms. Farris is the director of Deep Brain Stimulation Services and Research at the Movement and Neuroperformance Center of Colorado and an assistant clinical professor and clinical instructor at the University of Colorado School of Medicine. She specializes in the interdisciplinary care of people living with Parkinson's disease, focusing on deep brain stimulation (DBS) management and research with extensive experience in troubleshooting unsatisfactory results after DBS surgery. Ms. Farris believes that one day a cure will be discovered, but until then, people should utilize all available strategies to live their best with Parkinson's every day.

Ms. Farris is a certified physician assistant and an American College of Sports Medicine-certified clinical exercise specialist and health fitness specialist. She holds master's degrees in philosophy, with concentration in bioethics and in physician assistant studies, with concentration in neurology. Ms. Farris has published medical articles regarding deep brain stimulation, Parkinson's disease and medical ethics.

Ms. Farris and Dr. Giroux were awarded the 2006 National Paragon Award from the American Academy of Physician Assistants for teamwork in patient care, and Ms. Farris was chosen as Alumna of the Year by the State University of New York at Stony Brook, Physician's Assistant program in 2006. Sierra has written patient empowerment books, including *A Patient Guide to DBS*, and manages an online DBS advocacy blog: dbsprogrammer.com.

CONTRIBUTING AUTHORS

JAY L. ALBERTS, PhD (p. 150)

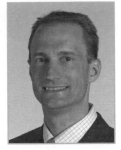

Dr. Jay Alberts is the vice chair of the Office of Clinical Transformation, the director of the Concussion Center, and the Edward F. and Barbara A. Bell Family Endowed Chair at the Cleveland Clinic. Dr. Alberts' research is focused on understanding the effects of exercise on the motor and non-motor symptoms associated with Parkinson's. He has led a research team that demonstrated the benefits associated with "forced-exercise" in people with Parkinson's. In addition, he studies how Parkinson's impacts cognitive and motor function under dual-task conditions in order to develop rehabilitation strategies that improve these declines.

Within clinical transformation, Dr. Alberts develops technology to objectively quantify Parkinson's symptoms using consumer electronic devices and to develop subsequent models of clinical care. He serves as the principal investigator on a number of studies, including ones supported by the National Institutes of Health, Department of Defense and the Davis Phinney Foundation. He was presented with an Alumni Achievement Award from Iowa State University in 2011 for his translational research related to Parkinson's and was awarded the prestigious Sones Award for Innovation in 2013 from the Cleveland Clinic.

RABBI RENA ARSHINOFF, BCC (p. 201)

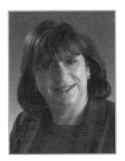

Rabbi Rena Arshinoff obtained her nursing training in Montreal. She completed a master of health science degree in epidemiology at University of Toronto and worked for 20 years in clinical research prior to entering rabbinical school in 2003. Following rabbinic ordination in 2008, she trained in hospital chaplaincy. She currently works with the Krembil neuroscience program as the spiritual care provider with that program at Toronto Western Hospital of the University Health Network, and at Baycrest as rabbi and chaplain with the palliative care and rehabilitation programs.

Her main areas of interest are spiritual needs in Parkinson's disease and movement disorders, professional grief and bereavement and healing in children and adults. She volunteers with Bereaved Families of Ontario with the children's program and the infant loss program as a group facilitator and professional advisor. She does rabbinic work in the community with Jewish Family and Child Services and Darchei Noam Congregation, as well as lifecycle events and teaching in the area of bereavement. She is currently pursuing a PhD in palliative care from Lancaster University in England focusing on Parkinson's. Her thesis topic is: "Experiences of Mutuality in the Spousal/Common Law Relationship in Advanced Parkinson's Disease from the Perspective of the Caregiving Partner." Rabbi Arshinoff lives in Toronto with her husband Stephen. They have three children and one grandchild.

JOHN BAUMANN, JD (p. 92)

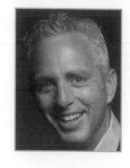

John Baumann has had many "successes" in his life, overcoming challenge after challenge. After years as a successful attorney, John was diagnosed in 2002 with Parkinson's disease at 41 years old. John has successfully reinvented himself, writing a critically-acclaimed book entitled, *DECIDE SUCCESS*, and becoming an internationally-recognized, inspirational success speaker. From Malaysia to France, from Vermont to Tucson, from Portland to Miami, and over 100 places in between, John has presented to audiences from 15 to 1,500. His informative, inspirational and surprisingly funny presentations address subjects as varied as how to successfully live a full life with a chronic illness to successfully building a workplace proactive prevention culture to success as a supervisor by simply being respectful and appreciative. John now makes himself available as a keynote speaker, a workshop facilitator and a success coach.

As to his Parkinson's, John has gotten himself in the best shape of his life via a combination of positive thinking, a healthy diet and vigorous exercise. His healthier lifestyle has allowed him to successfully minimize the progression and degenerative effects of this chronic illness. Learn more about John at JohnBaumann.com.

KARA BEASLEY, DO (p. 226)

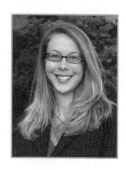

Dr. Kara Beasley is a neurosurgeon with Boulder Neurosurgical & Spine Associates (BNA). She completed a dual degree in medicine with a MA in biomedical ethics at Midwestern University in Glendale, AZ and is one of only a few dually credentialed neurosurgeon bioethicists in the world. She completed a general neurosurgery residency at Philadelphia College of Osteopathic Medicine in Philadelphia, PA. Before joining BNA, Dr. Beasley also completed fellowships in stereotactic radiosurgery at Cooper University Hospital in Camden, NJ, and functional and restorative neurosurgery at The Cleveland Clinic Foundation in Cleveland, OH.

Dr. Beasley decided to dedicate her career in part to the surgical treatment of Parkinson's disease after meeting Parkinson's patients and learning about deep brain stimulation during her training. Upon moving to Boulder, Dr. Beasley began working with the Davis Phinney Foundation to support community outreach and education and has spoken at The Victory Summit symposia. She is currently the chair of the Davis Phinney Foundation's board of directors.

NANCY BIVINS, LMSW (p. 256)

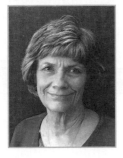

Nancy Bivins received her master of social work degree from Arizona State University. Her career choice has been to serve seniors and the disabled. Eight years ago, she joined the community outreach team at the Muhammad Ali Parkinson Center in Phoenix, Arizona. This position has allowed her the opportunity to interface with people living with Parkinson's and their families and to provide encouragement, support and information as they face the challenge of living well with Parkinson's.

BASTIAAN BLOEM, MD, PhD (p. 100)

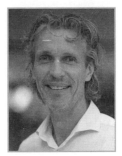

Professor Bas Bloem is a consultant neurologist at the department of neurology, Radboud University Nijmegen Medical Centre, the Netherlands. He received his MD degree (with honors) at Leiden University Medical Centre in 1993. In 1994, he obtained his PhD degree in Leiden, based on a thesis entitled: "Postural reflexes in Parkinson's disease." He was trained as a neurologist between 1994 and 2000, also at Leiden University Medical Centre. He received additional training as a movement disorders specialist during fellowships at The Parkinson's Institute, Sunnyvale, California (with Dr J.W. Langston), and at the Institute of Neurology, Queen Square, London (with Prof. N.P. Quinn and Prof. J.C. Rothwell).

In 2002, he founded and became medical director of the Parkinson Centre Nijmegen (ParC), which was recognized from 2005 onwards as a center of excellence for Parkinson's disease. Together with Dr. Marten Munneke, he also developed ParkinsonNet, an innovative healthcare concept that now consists of 66 professional networks for Parkinson patients covering all of the Netherlands (parkinsonnet.nl). Because of the evidence-based quality improvement and significant cost reduction, ParkinsonNet has received multiple awards, including the prize "Best Pearl for Healthcare Innovation" in 2011 and "Value Based Health Care" prize in 2015.

In September 2008, Professor Bloem was appointed as professor of neurology, with movement disorders as a special area of interest. He has published over 550 publications, including over 400 peer-reviewed international papers.

MELANIE M. BRANDABUR, MD (p. 184)

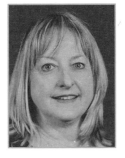

Dr. Melanie Brandabur received her BA degree from the University of Illinois in Urbana and her MD degree from Rush Medical College in Chicago. She completed her neurology residency at Rush-Presbyterian-St. Luke's Medical Center in Chicago. While there, she completed a fellowship in movement disorders and pharmacology under the direction of Doctors Harold Klawans and Christopher Goetz. This was followed by a post-doctoral basic sciences fellowship in neurodegenerative diseases with Dr. Elliott Mufson. She also studied at the Hospital de la Salpetriere in Paris, France under Dr. Yves Agid.

Dr. Brandabur is a member of the Movement Disorder Society and the American Academy of Neurology. She served as the medical director of three separate National Parkinson Foundation Centers of Excellence: the University of Illinois, Alexian Neurosciences Institute and the Parkinson's Institute. As a clinician, Dr. Brandabur offered a multidisciplinary approach, with an emphasis on exercise and nutrition, in addition to medication and served as an investigator on over 40 clinical trials. Following twenty years of experience as a clinician and clinical researcher, Dr. Brandabur is currently a senior medical director at Ultragenyx Pharmaceuticals, where she works as a clinical scientist on the development of therapeutic agents for rare diseases. In addition, she is an adjunct faculty member at UCSF, where she continues to see movement disorders patients in the Surgical Movement Disorders Clinic.

HELEN BRONTE-STEWART, MD, MSE (p. 98)

Dr. Helen Bronte-Stewart is the John E. Cahill Family Professor in the department of neurology and neurological sciences and in the department of neurosurgery (by courtesy) at the Stanford University School of Medicine, Stanford, California. She received her bachelor's degree in mathematics and physics at the University of York, England and a master of science in bioengineering (MSE) from University of Pennsylvania School of Engineering in Philadelphia, Pennsylvania. Dr. Bronte-Stewart received her MD degree from University of Pennsylvania School of Medicine.

Dr. Bronte-Stewart's research goal is to understand how the brain controls movement. She is also very interested in balance and gait disorders and maintains an active research program in this area. With a background in ballet and modern dance, she initiated the idea and helped to design a dance studio in the new Stanford Neurosciences Health Center. She has also authored and co-authored over 90 peer-review manuscripts, book chapters and other materials on Parkinson's-related issues. Throughout her career she has held many teaching positions, beginning during her undergraduate years with directorships of two dance companies. Her research has been supported by numerous foundations devoted to Parkinson's disease awareness. She currently serves as a member of the Davis Phinney Foundation's board of directors.

JANE BUSCH, DDS (p. 138)

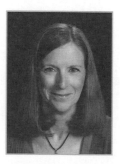

Dr. Jane Busch is a former practicing dentist in Cross Plains, WI, and a current fitness instructor with a focus on Parkinson's. She completed her undergraduate degree at the University of Wisconsin-Madison and went on to complete a bachelor of science in dentistry and doctorate of dental surgery at the University of Minnesota School of Dentistry-Minneapolis. After completing her education, Dr. Busch worked in a private dental practice for nearly 17 years, leaving in 1999 to become director of education for the Academy for Excellence in Dental Technology, an academic training program for dental technicians through D&S Dental Laboratory, Inc. For several years, she also was a post-graduate dental instructor at Madison Area Technical College.

Dr. Busch is a member of several professional societies including Omicron Kappa Upsilon National Dental Society, the American Dental Association, the Wisconsin Dental Association and the Dane County Dental Society. She is the founder, CEO and chair of the LIFE Foundation (Lifestyles Initiative for Fitness Empowerment), a community-based health initiative fostering healthy lifestyles with evidence-based strategies.

SOPHIE CANADÉ, ATR, LPC (p. 199)

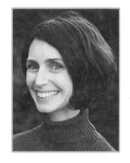

Sophie Canadé is a registered art therapist and licensed professional counselor working for the Institute for Therapy through the Arts, Gilda's Club Cancer Support Community and Creatively Empowered Women (CEW). A graduate of the master of arts in art therapy program from the School of the Art Institute in Chicago, she works in Chicago and surrounding areas of Cook County, IL.

Ms. Canadé's clinical experience has specialized in work with older adults who are challenged by age-related cognitive, emotional and physical issues, including symptoms from stroke, Parkinson's and Alzheimer's disease. For Northwestern Memorial Hospital, she facilitates the weekly Parkinson's art therapy support group, the Pi Delts, so named to communicate the supportive fellowship of the group in the spirit of fraternity and sorority.

CONNIE CARPENTER PHINNEY, MS (p. 261)

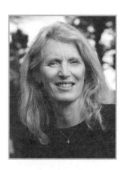

Connie is an entrepreneur, author, artist and lifelong athlete, and is extremely passionate about her work as a founding board member of the Davis Phinney Foundation. Connie particularly enjoys sharing her experiences via the written word, and she is an eloquent and humorous public speaker. She has two adult children, Taylor and Kelsey, with her husband Davis Phinney.

TIM COLLIER, PhD (p. 70)

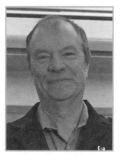

Dr. Tim Collier is a professor in the department of translational science & molecular medicine, Edwin A. Brophy Endowed Chair in Central Nervous System Disorders and past director of the Udall Center of Excellence in Parkinson's Disease Research at Michigan State University. He trained at the University of Minnesota, Northwestern University and the University of Rochester, and has been a faculty member at Rush University Medical School in Chicago and the University of Cincinnati. He is a past president of the American Society for Neural Therapy and Repair, past chairperson of the NIH CNNT study section, associate editor of the European Journal of Neuroscience and has published over 100 peer-reviewed scientific reports.

More than fifteen years ago, Dr. Collier became a member of a four principal investigator collaborative team that has been studying issues of dopamine neuron biology as they apply to aging, Parkinson's disease and experimental therapeutics. In 2010, the team was recruited to the Michigan State University College of Human Medicine, where they continue to study issues related to Parkinson's disease in cell culture, rodent and nonhuman primate models, with interests in cell transplantation, growth factors, stem/progenitor cell biology, gene transfer and dietary/exercise interventions, among others.

AL CONDELUCI, PhD (p. 194)

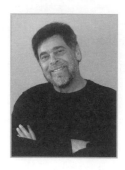

Dr. Al Condeluci has been an advocate, a catalyst for building community capacities and leader in understanding social culture since 1970. Al Condeluci serves as CEO of Community Living and Support Services (CLASS), a full service nonprofit organization supporting people with disabilities, where he has worked for the past 44 years. He has also held faculty appointments with the University of Pittsburgh's School of Health and Rehabilitation Sciences and School of Social Work.

Dr. Condeluci received his masters and doctorate degrees at the University of Pittsburgh and is a lifelong resident of Pittsburgh, Pennsylvania. Dr. Condeluci's books, *Interdependence* (1991, 1995), *Beyond Difference* (1996), *Cultural Shifting* (2002), *Advocacy for Change* (2004), *Together is Better* (2008) and *Social Capital* (2014) have been used around the world.

DIANE G. COOK (p. 67)

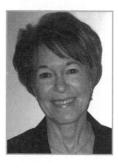

Diane was diagnosed with Parkinson's disease in 2008 and has founded and facilitated four groups for newly diagnosed people with Parkinson's. She has participated in 15 clinical trials, serves as patient consultant to a number of studies and is an active advocate for greater patient participation in the clinical research process. Nationally, Diane serves as a patient representative to the FDA, a Parkinson's Disease Foundation (PDF) research advocate and has just completed terms as a member of PDF's People with Parkinson's Advisory Council and the Steering Committee of the Clinical Trials Transformation Initiative (CTTI).

Diane pioneered the application of the science of self-efficacy to newly diagnosed Parkinson's patients and has presented in that regard at the Montreal World Parkinson's Congress, at both the Sydney and the Berlin International Movement Disorders Congresses and at the New York Academy of Sciences. The Colorado Neurological Institute (CNI) Foundation funded her initial research on the impact of self-efficacy on disease outcomes in newly diagnosed Parkinson's people with Parkinson's and she has since trained people with Parkinson's/healthcare professional teams to deliver the PD SELF (Self-Efficacy Learning Forum) program she developed in 10 metropolitan areas across the US. PDF designated PD SELF one of their national pilot programs.

TAMARA RORK DeANGELIS, PT, DPT, GCS (p. 160)

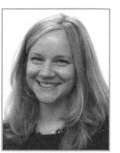

Dr. Tami DeAngelis is a senior physical therapist at the Center for Neurorehabilitation at Boston University, where she has been providing physical therapy services, contributing to research and implementing educational programs to persons with Parkinson disease over the last decade. Dr. DeAngelis is also the coordinator for the American Parkinson Disease Association (APDA) National Rehabilitation Resource Center at Boston University, providing information and resources on exercise and rehabilitation to persons with Parkinson's, families and healthcare providers nationwide. She co-authored the BE ACTIVE & BEYOND booklet, an exercise program for people with Parkinson disease, distributed by the APDA, Inc.

She lectures in the Doctor of Physical Therapy program at Boston University, Parkinson's support groups, professional conferences and symposia about the benefits of rehabilitation for persons with Parkinson disease. Dr. DeAngelis received a Bachelor of Arts degree in Biology from Lafayette College, a Master of Science degree in Physical Therapy from Boston University College of Health and Rehabilitation Sciences: Sargent and her Doctorate in Physical Therapy from Temple University. She is also a board certified specialist in Geriatric Physical Therapy and a member of the American Physical Therapy Association.

LEE DIBBLE, PT, PhD, ATC (p. 151)

Dr. Lee Dibble is a Professor at the University of Utah in the department of physical therapy and athletic training. For the past 15 years, he has been the co-director of the University of Utah Rehabilitation and Wellness Clinic, which provides community-based risk reduction programs for people with Parkinson disease.

He completed a bachelor's degree in animal physiology from UC Davis, a master's degree in physical therapy from Duke University and his PhD in exercise and sports science from the University of Utah. Dr. Dibble's research agenda focuses on the effects of rehabilitation interventions on hypokinesia, fall risk and quality of life in people with Parkinson disease and other disorders that affect balance and mobility.

ROSEANNE D. DOBKIN, PhD (p. 108, 186)

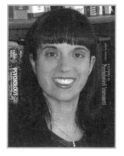

Dr. Roseanne Dobkin is an associate professor of psychiatry at Rutgers-Robert Wood Johnson Medical School, in Piscataway, NJ. She is also a practicing psychologist in New Jersey and Delaware. Dr. Dobkin received her PhD in clinical psychology from the Medical College of Pennsylvania-Hahnemann University in Philadelphia, PA in August 2002. She completed a postdoctoral fellowship in clinical psychopharmacology in the department of psychiatry at Robert Wood Johnson Medical School in September 2003.

The majority of her research and clinical work over the past 15 years has focused on the behavioral treatment of the psychiatric complications (i.e., depression, anxiety, insomnia, cognition) in Parkinson's disease. She has also begun to systematically examine barriers to mental health care utilization in Parkinson's, as well as the use of telemedicine to leverage patient access to specialized mental healthcare. Dr. Dobkin's research has been funded by the National Institutes of Health, the Patterson Trust Awards Program in Clinical Research, the Michael J. Fox Foundation for Parkinson's Research, the Parkinson's Unity Walk, the Parkinson's Disease Foundation and the Health Services and Research Development Division (HSR&D) of the Veteran Affairs Administration.

RAY DORSEY, MD, MBA (p. 57)

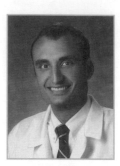

Dr. Ray Dorsey is David M. Levy professor of neurology and director of the CHET at the University of Rochester Medical Center. Dr. Dorsey is helping investigate new treatments for movement disorders and improve the way care is delivered for individuals with Parkinson disease and other neurological disorders. Using simple, web-based video conferencing, he and his colleagues are seeking to provide care to individuals with Parkinson and neurological diseases anywhere that they live.

Dr. Dorsey previously directed the movement disorders division and neurology telemedicine at Johns Hopkins and worked as a consultant for McKinsey & Company. He completed his undergraduate studies at Stanford University, medical school at the University of Pennsylvania and business school at the Wharton School. Dr. Dorsey's research has been published in the leading medical, neurology and economic journals and has been featured on National Public Radio, *The New York Times* and *The Wall Street Journal*.

GAMMON M. EARHART, PT, PhD (p. 153)

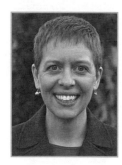

Gammon M. Earhart, PT, PhD, is a physical therapist and movement scientist. She is currently professor of physical therapy, neuroscience and neurology, as well as director of the program in physical therapy at Washington University in St. Louis.

Dr. Earhart is presently president of the American Physical Therapy Association Section on Research and has over 100 peer-reviewed publications. Since 2004, she has been working with people with Parkinson's disease to better understand and help address their movement challenges.

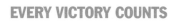

TERRY ELLIS, PhD, PT, NCS (p. 160)

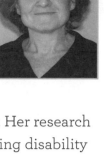

Dr. Terry Ellis is an assistant professor at Boston University College of Health and Rehabilitation Sciences: Sargent College in the department of physical therapy and athletic training and the director of the Center for Neurorehabilitation at Boston University. She has a PhD in behavioral neuroscience from Boston University School of Medicine and earned her degree in physical therapy from Springfield College.

In addition, Dr. Ellis is a board certified specialist in neurologic physical therapy. Her research focuses on investigating the effectiveness of exercise and rehabilitation in reducing disability and optimizing function and quality of life in people with Parkinson disease.

STEVE EMERSON, MA (p. 44)

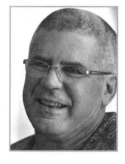

Steve was diagnosed with Parkinson's in 2007 at the age of 49. A former mental health therapist and current professional Christian life coach, Steve routinely meets with individuals and families living with Parkinson's and serves as a guest speaker for various organizations and events on the topic of living well with Parkinson's. For Steve, living well begins with attitude, and the building blocks of maintaining a strong, positive attitude include "exercise, good nutrition, prayer and getting into the stream of life, even when I don't feel like doing so."

"I have come to learn that the more I give, the more I get," Steve says. "I hope to become increasingly able to educate and support those living with Parkinson's, their care partners and the community at large that it is entirely possible to live a full, enriching and wonderful life not only with Parkinson's, but with any of life's obstacles that may arise."

Photograph ©Sharon Gekoski-Kimmel / The Parkinson's Project

MATTHEW P. FORD, PT, PhD (p. 156)

Dr. Matthew Ford is an associate professor and chair of the department of physical therapy in the College of Health Sciences at Samford University in Birmingham, Alabama. He holds a bachelor of science in physical therapy from Quinnipiac University, a master of arts in motor learning from Teachers College, Columbia University and a PhD in motor behavior from Pennsylvania State University. He previously held faculty positions in the departments of physical therapy at the University of Alabama at Birmingham (UAB) and Saint Francis University.

He has spent the past 10 years working with people with Parkinson's in both a research and service capacity in collaboration with the department of neurology – UAB, Center for Exercise Medicine – UAB, Lakeshore Foundation, Neuromuscular Rehab and Balance Center at Southeast Alabama Medical Center, the Parkinson's Association of Alabama and the Davis

Phinney Foundation. Matt is a regular speaker at The Victory Summit symposia on the subject of "exercising for the rest of your life" and is featured on the Foundation's "Parkinson's Exercise Essentials" DVD. He resides in Alabama with his wife and two sons. He currently serves as a member of the Davis Phinney Foundation's board of directors.

CYNTHIA FOX, PhD, CCC-SLP (p. 249)

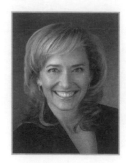

Dr. Cynthia Fox received her doctorate degree in speech and hearing sciences from the University of Arizona, Tucson. She is an expert on rehabilitation and neuroplasticity and the role of exercise in the improvement of function consequent to neural injury and disease. Dr. Fox is a leader in administration of LSVT LOUD® speech treatment for people with Parkinson disease and has been part of the LSVT research team for over 20 years. She was the first to apply this treatment to disorders other than Parkinson disease and pioneered the application to pediatric populations, including children with cerebral palsy and Down syndrome.

Dr. Fox worked closely on the development of a physical therapy program, LSVT BIG that was modeled after the speech treatment protocol. Dr. Fox has numerous publications in these areas of research and has presented extensively nationally and internationally. She is a co-founder and vice president of operations of LSVT Global, Inc., and a research associate at the National Center for Voice and Speech in Denver, Colorado.

DANIEL GOLD, DO (p. 140)

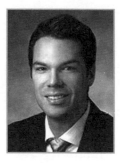

Daniel Gold, DO, is assistant professor of neurology, ophthalmology, otolaryngology – head & neck surgery and neurosurgery at The Johns Hopkins School of Medicine in Baltimore, Maryland. He is a neurologist with fellowship training in neuro-ophthalmology, which is the study of visual disorders or vision loss that are not primarily ocular in origin (i.e., disorders of the anterior or posterior pathways from the optic nerves to the occipital lobes); eye movement disorders including nystagmus; disorders of the pupils and eyelids; and double vision, among other conditions. Dr. Gold has additional training in vestibular neurology and also sees patients with dizziness and imbalance. He is the director of Urgent Neurology, and has a particular interest in the rapid diagnosis and treatment of acute neuro-ophthalmologic and vestibular disorders.

Dr. Gold completed his DO at the University of Medicine and Dentistry of New Jersey-School of Osteopathic Medicine. He went on to complete his residency in neurology at the University of Maryland and his fellowship in neuro-ophthalmology at the Hospital of the University of Pennsylvania.

DONALD L. HAISMAN, CFP® (p. 290)

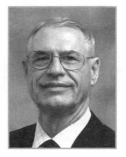

Donald Haisman is the managing director of Carnegie Investment Counsel in Fort Myers, Florida and is the president of Haisman Wealth Management, Inc. He shows successful families and organizations, many with charitable intent, how to simplify their financial lives and make smart money decisions, so they can achieve their goals and fulfill their values. He does this by helping them get their entire "financial house" in order to keep it that way forever. Mr. Haisman has previously served as the president of multiple organizations including the Financial Planning Association, the Institute of Certified Financial Planners, the International Association for Financial Planning and the Estate Planning Council of Lee County. He has also served on the Planned Giving Board of the Lee County American Cancer Society and the National Committee on Planned Giving.

Donald Haisman holds an MBA in finance and an undergraduate degree in mechanical engineering. He is a CFP-certified financial planner practitioner. He has produced and hosted hundreds of radio shows on various financial and investment topics, been a guest lecturer on cruise ships and is an occasional "on-air" guest at Waterman Broadcasting local NBC-V2 discussing current financial matters. Mr. Haisman has also authored multiple articles and presented on topics like money management, investing and charitable giving.

JOANNE HAMILTON, PhD, ABPP-CN (p. 191)

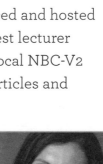

Dr. Joanne Hamilton is the director of adult neuropsychology at Advanced Neurobehavioral Health of Southern California and resident neuropsychologist at the Parkinson's Disease and Movement Disorders Center at Scripps Clinic. Dr. Hamilton received her bachelor's degree from Stanford University and her doctorate in clinical psychology with specialization in neuropsychology from the San Diego State University/ University of California, San Diego joint doctoral program in clinical psychology. She completed her postdoctoral fellowship at the University of California, Shiley-Marcos Alzheimer's Disease Research Center and was licensed to practice neuropsychology in 2003.

Dr. Hamilton became a diplomat in clinical neuropsychology from the American Board of Professional Psychology in 2010. She was a research neuroscientist at the Shiley-Marcos Alzheimer's Disease Research Center studying cognitive changes associated with Lewy body spectrum disorders, including Parkinson's disease and Dementia with Lewy bodies, until 2012.

KATHRYNNE HOLDEN, MS, RD (p. 177)

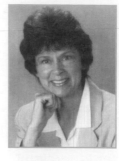

Kathrynne Holden (retired) has specialized in the nutritional concerns of Parkinson's disease for over 20 years. She has authored *Eat Well, Stay Well with Parkinson's Disease*, *Cook Well, Stay Well with Parkinson's Disease* and the National Parkinson Foundation booklet *Nutrition Matters*. See her website at ⮕ nutritionucanlivewith.com for more Parkinson-related nutrition information.

KAREN JAFFE, MD (p. 196)

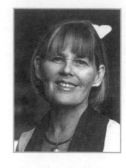

Dr. Karen Jaffe is a retired OB/GYN and Parkinson's advocate. She was diagnosed with Parkinson's at the age of 48. She is a member of the Michael J. Fox Foundation's Patient Advisory Council as well of the Brain Health Initiative at the CWRU-SOM in Cleveland, Ohio. She and her husband, Marc, founded Shaking With Laughter, a nonprofit foundation that has raised one million dollars for Parkinson's research.

Today she spends much of her time at InMotion (⮕ beinmotion.org). InMotion, for which she is a co-founder, is a center for Parkinson's disease and other movement disorders that strengthens lives through a holistic approach of education, exercise and healing arts. She was the recipient of the Red Cross Heroes award, the Irene Zehman award for Volunteerism, the World Parkinson's Program International Parkinson's Community Service award and the University Hospital Neurological Institute Champions for Parkinson's award.

Photograph ©Billy Delfs

CHERIAN KARUNAPUZHA, MD (p. 104)

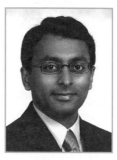

Dr. Cherian Karunapuzha completed his internship in internal medicine, residency in adult neurology and a fellowship in movement disorders at the University of Texas Southwestern Medical Center, Dallas. He is a member of the AAN and holds board certification from the American Board of Psychiatry and Neurology. Dr. Karunapuzha is an assistant professor of neurology at the University of Oklahoma Health Sciences center, Oklahoma City and is the director of the OU Parkinson's Disease & Movement Disorders Center.

Dr. Karunapuzha is a keen clinical educator who has received several teaching awards and is a frequently invited speaker for CME programs. Focused on community medicine, he has developed clinics for the uninsured in tandem with the patient support groups so as to improve statewide access to movement disorder specialists as well as access to research studies.

HORACIO KAUFMANN, MD (p. 118)

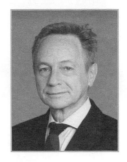

Dr. Horacio Kaufmann is professor of neurology and medicine and the director of the Dysautonomia Center at New York University. He is one of the world's leading experts in the diagnosis and management of patients with autonomic synucleinopathies (Parkinson disease and multiple system atrophy), a subject that has been the focus of his research and academic career over the last 25 years.

He has extensive experience as the principal investigator of national and international studies on autonomic dysfunction, including clinical trials for orthostatic hypotension, and identification and development of biomarker for early diagnosis and progression of Parkinson disease and related disorders.

PETER A. LEWITT, MD, MMedSc (p. 52)

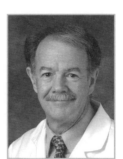

Dr. Peter A. LeWitt directs the Parkinson's Disease and Movement Disorders program at Henry Ford Hospital in West Bloomfield, Michigan. In 1989, he was appointed professor of neurology at Wayne State University School of Medicine. In addition to extensive experience in conducting clinical trials for Parkinson's disease and other neurological disorders, his research interests have included animal models and biomarkers of neurological disease, pharmacokinetic analysis of neurological drugs, and gene therapy. He is the author of more than 300 publications in basic and clinical neuroscience.

Dr. LeWitt attended Brown University and its medical school and completed his post-graduate medical training at the University of Pennsylvania and Stanford University School of Medicine. He is board certified in neurology. At the National Institute of Neurological Disorders and Stroke (National Institutes of Health), he served as a research fellow in the Experimental Therapeutics Branch and had an appointment as lieutenant commander in the US Public Health Service. Dr. LeWitt was a founding member of the Parkinson Study Group and in 1998 was elected to serve as secretary of the Movement Disorder Society (now the International Parkinson and Movement Disorder Society), for which he serves as a member of that organization's Task Force for the Development of Rating Scales for Parkinson's Disease. Dr. LeWitt has received research grants from the National Institutes of Health, the Michael J. Fox Foundation for Parkinson's Research, The Harris Foundation Neuroscience Program, the National Parkinson Foundation and other organizations. Since 2003, he has been editor-in-chief of *Clinical Neuropharmacology* and he has served on the editorial boards of *Movement Disorders*, *Journal of Neural Transmission*, *Journal of Parkinson's Disease* and *Translational Neurodegeneration*.

MARK MAPSTONE, PhD (p. 145)

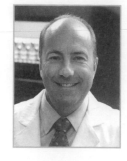

Dr. Mark Mapstone is professor of neurology at the University of California, Irvine School of Medicine where he is also a member of the Institute for Memory Impairments and Neurological Disorders (IMIND). He holds an adjunct appointment at the University of Rochester. His research focuses on early detection of neurological disease, especially Alzheimer's disease and Parkinson's disease using cognitive tests and biomarkers obtained from blood. He has a special interest in developing strategies to maintain successful cognitive aging. In the clinic, he specializes in cognitive assessment of older adults with suspected brain disease.

Dr. Mapstone earned a PhD in clinical psychology at Northwestern University and completed fellowship training in neuropsychology and experimental therapeutics at the University of Rochester. He has authored over 100 manuscripts and abstracts and is the recipient of a Career Development Award from the National Institute on Aging. His research has been funded by the National Institutes of Health, the Michael J. Fox Foundation and the Department of Defense.

MARTIN J. McKEOWN, BEng, MD, FRCP(C) (p. 221)

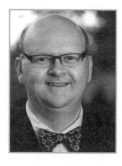

Dr. Martin McKeown is the PPRI/UBC chair in Parkinson's research, director at the Pacific Parkinson's Research Centre, professor in the department of medicine and adjunct professor in the department of electrical and computer engineering at the University of British Columbia, Canada. He did his engineering physics, medicine and neurology training at McMaster, University of Toronto, and University of Western Ontario, respectively. He did a three-year research fellowship at the computational neurobiology laboratory at the Salk Institute for Biological Studies in San Diego before being hired as an assistant professor of medicine and biomedical engineering at Duke University. He was recruited to the University of British Columbia in 2003.

Dr. McKeown has been responsible for a variety of peer-reviewed research projects funded through the National Institutes of Health, the National Parkinson Foundation, the Canadian Foundation for Innovation, the Natural Sciences and Engineering Research Council of Canada, the Canadian Institutes of Health Research, the International Association of Translational Neuroscience and the (US) Whitaker Foundation. He was a member of the Neuroscience A Canadian CIHR Scientific peer-review committee as well as a member of the Scientific Advisory Board of the Parkinson Canada. He has authored over 150 peer-reviewed papers and book chapters. In addition to seeing patients (>1700 patient visits per year) Dr. McKeown supervises graduate students in neuroscience and engineering and trains the next generation of doctors.

JANIS M. MIYASAKI, MD, MEd, FRCPC, FAAN (p. 62)

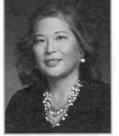

Dr. Janis Miyasaki is a graduate of the University of Toronto, completing medical school, residency and a movement disorders fellowship under Dr. Anthony Lang. She joined the University of Alberta faculty of medicine and dentistry in 2014 following 22 years at the University of Toronto. In 2015, Dr. Miyasaki became the director of the movement disorders program comprising seven neurologists and a dedicated interdisciplinary team.

She has held leadership positions at the University of Toronto, the University of Alberta, the International Parkinson Disease and Movement Disorder Society and the American Academy of Neurology. Dr. Miyasaki founded the first dedicated palliative care program for Parkinson's disease and related disorders at the University of Toronto in 2007. Since then, she has published original research on this topic and is viewed as the founder of palliative care for Parkinson's disease. In 2015, Dr. Miyasaki established the Complex Neurologic Symptoms Clinic at the Kaye Edmonton Clinic, University of Alberta with Dr. Wendy Johnston, an expert in ALS. This program provides care to all neurologic patients with palliative care needs.

JOSE-ALBERTO PALMA, MD, PhD (p. 118)

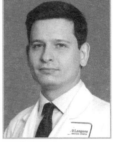

Dr. Jose-Alberto Palma is assistant professor of neurology and assistant director of the Dysautonomia Center at New York University. His work over the past years has been focused on the diagnosis, management and understanding on autonomic disorders in patients with autonomic synucleinopathies, such as Parkinson disease and multiple system atrophy, as well as in the search for biomarkers for early diagnosis of these disorders.

Dr. Palma has been involved in several studies and clinical trials to develop new treatments for autonomic dysfunction and to describe the premotor phase of Parkinson's disease.

DAVIS PHINNEY (p. 131, 182)

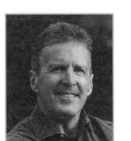

As an Olympic Bronze medalist and Tour de France stage winner, Davis Phinney has celebrated the most victories of any cyclist in American history. After nearly 20 years in professional cycling, he launched a successful second career as a television network sportscaster. In 2000, after years of feeling not quite right and a seemingly endless battery of tests, he was diagnosed with young onset Parkinson's disease at the age of 40.

Today, as founder of the Davis Phinney Foundation, he is a passionate and outspoken role model for living well with Parkinson's. He speaks to thousands of people with Parkinson's each year through his work with the Foundation and as a motivational speaker. Davis' personal journey, learning to redefine victory post-Parkinson's, serves as a powerful example for others living with the disease. Though the day-to-day challenges of Parkinson's are always present, he practices what he preaches and encourages others to join him in getting up, getting out and being active each day, savoring the Moments of Victory® as they come. Davis lives in Colorado with his wife, Connie Carpenter Phinney, and is the proud father of two grown children, Taylor and Kelsey.

DEANNA POWER (p. 87)

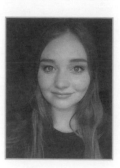

Deanna Power is the director of outreach for Disability Benefits Help, an independent organization dedicated to helping people of all ages receive the Social Security benefits they need. She initially began working with people with disabilities by volunteering with Best Buddies throughout college. She now specializes in helping Social Security claimants determine if they medically qualify for disability benefits.

Ms. Power's work has been published by hundreds of organizations, including the National Down Syndrome Society, the National Breast Cancer Foundation and the American Parkinson Disease Association. If you have any questions on qualifying, visit disability-benefits-help.org.

CYNTHIA RACZKO, OTR/L (p. 243)

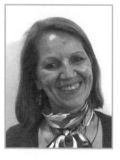

Ms. Cynthia Raczko attended Eastern Michigan University and received a bachelor of science in organizational communication. Following that, she pursued a second major in occupational therapy. Prior to her career in occupational therapy, she was a massage therapist for ten years and studied complementary and alternative medicines. She chose occupational therapy because it allows her to use all of her skills and training to help people who face health challenges to live a full and rewarding life. Occupational therapy supports people in being independent within their level of ability and it allows her to combine traditional, evidence-based practice with complementary and alternative approaches to healing.

Ms. Raczko's time is divided between the acute care hospital and the outpatient clinic. She works with a wide variety of neurological and orthopedic conditions. She also coordinates the occupational therapy intern program, including student learning, sharing knowledge, teaching techniques and maintaining a positive focus on student strengths to develop students' ability to recognize their areas of growth and help them grow.

LORRAINE RAMIG, PhD, CCC-SLP (p. 249)

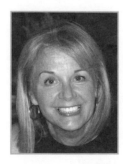

Dr. Lori Ramig obtained a doctorate in speech science from Purdue University following her clinical training in speech-language pathology at the University of Wisconsin-Madison. She currently holds the positions of research professor in the department of speech, language and hearing science at the University of Colorado-Boulder, senior scientist at the National Center for Voice and Speech, Denver and adjunct professor at Columbia University, New York City and co-founder of LSVT Global, Inc.

Dr. Ramig's research on voice treatment for Parkinson's disease has been funded by the National Institutes of Health for more than 20 years. She served on the National Institutes of Health Advisory Council for the Institute of Deafness and Communication Disorders and received Honors of the Association from the American Speech Language Hearing Association, the highest award granted from her professional association. Through LSVT Global, Inc., Dr. Ramig and her colleagues are implementing this research in clinical practice and today there are over 25,000 speech, physical and occupational therapists trained in LSVT LOUD and LSVT BIG Programs in 70 countries, improving quality of life in patients with Parkinson's globally. Learn more at: lsvtglobal.com.

ANGELA ROBB (p. 277)

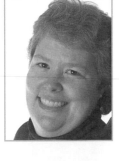

Angela Robb is a care partner for her husband, Karl, who has young onset Parkinson's disease. In 2015, she was honored as a White House Champion of Change in Parkinson's Disease. She is an advocate and frequent speaker on care partner issues at conferences and support groups. She is a certified Reiki master and with Karl, teaches Reiki to people with Parkinson's and their care partners and caregivers.

ISRAEL ROBLEDO (p. 74)

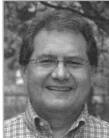

Israel works as a special education teacher. His family includes his wife, Chris, three daughters and two grandchildren. He was diagnosed with Parkinson's disease in 2007 at age 42. He soon became involved with the Parkinson's community as an advocate for increased clinical trial participation and health-related quality of life issues related to Parkinson's.

Israel is a member of the Patient Council for the Michael J. Fox Foundation for Parkinson's Research. He serves on the Executive Council for Parkinson's Movement – an initiative of the Cure Parkinson's Trust in England, the Integration Panel for the Congressionally Directed Medical Research Programs (Parkinson's Research Program), the Editorial Board of the Journal of Parkinson's Disease and as a patient reviewer for the British Medical Journal. Israel has also served in an advisory and support capacity for the Parkinson's Disease Foundation, the World Parkinson Congress and the Patient-Centered Outcomes Research Institute.

JEFFREY SHAW, PsyD, ABPP-CN (p. 122)

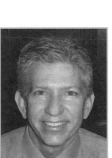

Dr. Jeffrey Shaw has been a neuropsychologist with Evergreen Hospital/ Booth Gardner Parkinson's Care Center in Kirkland, WA since 2001. He works with individuals diagnosed with Parkinson's disease, multiple sclerosis, Huntington disease, strokes and varied neurological difficulties. Although Dr. Shaw specializes in the field of neuropsychology (thorough evaluation of thinking skills), he also provides counseling and psychotherapy services.

He has taught at the graduate psychology program at Seattle Pacific University and the University of Missouri School of Medicine. Dr. Shaw earned his bachelor's in psychology from the University of Georgia and his master's in counseling from Georgia State University, and doctorate in Clinical Psychology at the American School of Professional Psychology in Atlanta. He is board certified in clinical neuropsychology and enjoys collaborating with his Parkinson's disease men's group in Seattle, Washington.

JESSICA SHURER, LCSW (p. 267, 293)

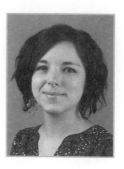

Jessica Shurer is a licensed clinical social worker and the center coordinator of the National Parkinson Foundation Center of Excellence at UNC Chapel Hill. She graduated from Penn State University with a BA in psychology and minors in human development & family studies and gerontology. She received her master of social work from UNC Chapel Hill in 2012, where she also obtained a certificate in aging and was a participant in the Hartford Partnership Program for Aging Education.

In her clinical role, Ms. Shurer is available to assess and support the psychosocial needs of patients and care partners, and provides connections to community resources and counseling as needed. She also has a strong focus on community education, outreach and advocacy through her organization of educational programs for Parkinson's families, the development of Parkinson's trainings for rehabilitation professionals and growth of the "ParkNC" referral network of Parkinson's-trained clinicians in North Carolina. In addition, she manages a specialty interdisciplinary Parkinson's clinic, helps to coordinate qualitative research projects and facilitates two monthly support groups: one for Parkinson's disease and one for Atypical Parkinsonism disorders. She also serves as a member of the Davis Phinney Foundation Science Advisory Board, National Parkinson Foundation's Center Coordinator Mentoring & Networking Task Force and planning committee for Moving Day® NC Triangle Walk for Parkinson's.

EVAN SIDDALL (p. 203)

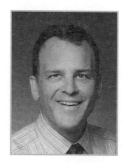

Evan is president and CEO of Canada Mortgage & Housing Corp, Canada's housing agency. CMHC is a Cdn $250 billion government-owned company spanning mortgage insurance, securitization, assisted housing and market analysis and research. Prior to entering public service with a senior posting at the Bank of Canada, Evan had a 20-year career in general management and investment banking with Lazard, Goldman Sachs and BMO Nesbitt Burns. He has degrees in law and management economics and has served on several corporate and charitable boards.

An active cyclist, Evan was introduced to the Davis Phinney Foundation after he was diagnosed with Parkinson's in early 2015. Immediately taken by the mission to "live well today," Evan and a group of close friends founded the Growling Beaver Brevet (GBB) to benefit the Davis Phinney Foundation. In two years, the GBB has become a core supporter of the Foundation and aided with the expansion of the Foundation's work to help Canadians with Parkinson's.

MIKE STUDER, PT, MHS, NCS, CEEAA, CWT, CSST (p. 238)

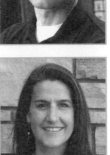

Mike is the owner of and full-time practicing clinician at Northwest Rehabilitation Associates in Salem, Oregon. He was awarded the "Clinical Excellence" award in 2011, by the Academy of Neurologic Physical Therapy and was awarded the same honor by the Academy of Geriatric Physical Therapy in 2014. He LOVES to help people with Parkinson's.

MICHELLE UNDERHILL, MA, CCC-SLP (p. 246)

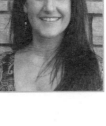

Michelle Underhill is a speech-language pathologist and the owner of Northern Colorado Therapy Services, a multidisciplinary private practice specializing in the care of people living with Parkinson's. She has extensive experience in evaluating and treating individuals with Parkinson's at all stages, and is a certified clinician in LSVT LOUD. She is passionate about the positive impact of therapy on daily functioning, and has focused her career on sharing hope and power within life's various circumstances.

Ms. Underhill completed a bachelor's degree in communication disorders from Colorado State University and a master's degree in speech-language pathology from University of Northern Colorado. She lives in Fort Collins with her husband, Jason, and two teenage children.

ROBERT VILLA (p. 287)

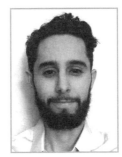

Robert was born and raised in Phoenix, Arizona. As the son of immigrant parents, he worked hard in school to make them proud. After graduating salutatorian of his high school class in 2011, Robert received a handsome set of scholarships to attend Arizona State University. At ASU, he majored in history and received two minors in philosophy and art history.

Directly after finishing his undergraduate studies, Robert went on to chase his dream of attending law school and is currently enrolled at the University of California, Berkeley School of Law.

CAROLYN ALLEN ZEIGER, PhD (p. 271)

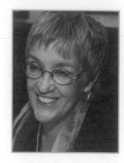

Dr. Carolyn Zeiger is a Parkinson's care partner for her husband, brother, sister, aunt and some close friends. In 2006, she co-founded a Parkinson's care partners' support group in Denver, Colorado, and for many years assisted her husband Paul in teaching yoga to people with Parkinson's.

Now retired, she was a clinical and health psychologist, and Jin Shin Jyutsu practitioner. From this multi-role perspective, she and her husband continue to speak to university classes and conferences about living with Parkinson's.

THE JEFF AND DIANE ROSS MOVEMENT DISORDERS CLINIC IN TORONTO, ONTARIO (p. 234)

The Assistive Technology Clinic (ATC) is a service dedicated to improving the quality of life for people with neurological and neurodegenerative conditions through rehabilitation and technology. The ATC clinical teams are comprised of physicians, nurses, occupational, physical and speech therapists, dietitians, biomedical engineers, social services and support staff.

ATC programs offer medical and rehabilitation management as well as leading edge assistive technology in the areas of mobility aids, communication, advance computer technology, specialized seating and positioning, environmental controls and home modifications. The ATC's goal is to provide the highest standards of patient-centered care by offering a broad spectrum of resources to help each person function at their optimum level of ability throughout the continuum of care. For more information, visit: assistivetechnologyclinic.ca.

EVERY VICTORY COUNTS.

Essential Information and Inspiration for a Lifetime of Wellness with Parkinson's Disease

■ PARKINSON'S: AN OVERVIEW

"You have Parkinson's disease…" For some people, hearing these words is a relief: *Finally there's a name for the symptoms I've been feeling.* For others, they trigger shock and disbelief: *How could this happen to me?* After a diagnosis of Parkinson's, you and your family will have many questions about the disease and the life challenges ahead. Yet, you may also feel overwhelmed by the sheer volume of information available to you.

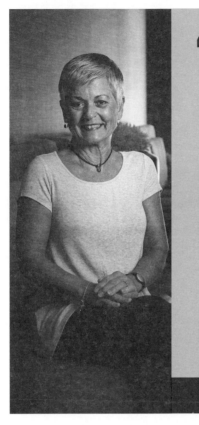

> " *Looking back, I was in a pity party for about a year after I was diagnosed. I didn't spend the whole year huddled in a corner feeling sorry for myself, but I went through the motions with no drive, no goals, no purpose. I felt empty and alone. Even though I had the support of a lot of family and friends, none of them could truly understand what I was dealing with. Finally I went to a local support group meeting and there was a person in the group who recognized my struggle. She'd been living with Parkinson's for about 8 years and said something very profound to me. She said, 'Look, these are the cards you've been dealt. Play your cards, and play to win.' That's when it clicked that living well was up to me. Nobody could fix me, but I could make it better.*"
>
> — EDIE

This chapter is designed to be a starting point for anyone recently diagnosed with Parkinson's. It answers some of the most common questions asked by people within the first year after diagnosis. It also provides some adaptive strategies to help set you on the best path for living well with Parkinson's, including staying engaged and informed about your health and about the things you can do to improve your quality of life. When you are ready to explore the rest of the contents of this manual, you will find many practical tools and approaches to do just that.

WHAT IS PARKINSON'S?

Parkinson's is a progressive, chronic, neurodegenerative disorder associated with damage to and loss of dopamine-producing nerve cells (neurons) deep in the brain. Dopamine is a chemical that helps regulate your body's movement. Less dopamine leads to less mobility and less control over your movements. In fact, Parkinson's is officially classified as a movement disorder because it involves damage to the areas of the brain that affect the speed, quality, fluency and ease of movement. Current medications for Parkinson's replace or enhance lost dopamine.

*By Steve Emerson, MA, person
living with Parkinson's*

It is indeed the rare and/or unusual human being who has not experienced shame at various points in their life. More often than not, shame manifests itself as feeling "less than" or embarrassed as a result of an event or action, usually in a social or interpersonal context. For example, one might legitimately feel shame in their community should they be caught shoplifting and it is made public. Other forms of shame are not necessarily illegitimate, but are the result of the fear of being perceived as unable to meet certain expectations. This is precisely the type of shame people living with Parkinson's are likely to experience.

CAUSES OF SHAME

As someone living with Parkinson's, feelings of shame can be common. You may find yourself fumbling for your wallet in a busy checkout line or having difficulty handling utensils in an upscale restaurant. You may be unable to enunciate your words with friends in a conversation. Maybe you used to excel on the golf course and now can no longer achieve the balance necessary to even stand over the golf ball. You may have been the primary breadwinner for your family and are now unable to work in your chosen profession due to debilitating fatigue or other Parkinson's symptoms. Your difficulty with

The more visible physical symptoms of Parkinson's are called motor symptoms, and include tremors, slowness or stiffness. These start in most people after 60-80% of the dopamine-producing nerve cells are damaged or die off. As dopamine decreases, routine everyday activities like walking and balance are affected. While the effects of Parkinson's on movement are often the most visible symptoms, other impacts of Parkinson's not related to movement can sometimes have an even greater impact on your quality of life. We will discuss these non-motor symptoms in greater detail later in this section.

BE INFORMED: *No two people living with Parkinson's will experience symptoms or progression of the disease in the exact same way.*

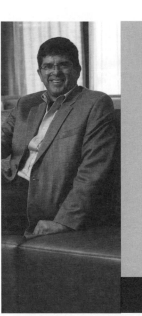

> *You know what they say: if you've seen one person with Parkinson's, you've seen one person with Parkinson's. Nothing that we do to manage it works for everyone, because it's an individual disease."*
>
> — COREY

Just because something is listed as a symptom of Parkinson's does not mean you will experience that symptom. There are also many actions you can take that will change how you feel and how your Parkinson's changes over time — everything from physical activity, to diet, to emotional wellness, to choosing the best wellness team for your needs. This manual outlines many treatment and lifestyle changes that you can make that will improve your symptoms and potentially slow future progression.

No one can predict how your Parkinson's will progress, and evidence is emerging that shows progression can be affected by many factors. Just a decade ago, researchers, clinicians and people living with Parkinson's alike did not stress the importance of exercise, stress management, diet and other positive life choices on Parkinson's. Today, we know that your experience with Parkinson's can be influenced in a positive way by your choices and actions.

By reading this manual, you're taking an important step toward learning how to be proactive, participate in your own care and shape your future. Hear how Linda is working to change the negative perceptions about Parkinson's: 🎥 **dpf.org/linda**.

HOW IS PARKINSON'S DIAGNOSED?

Parkinson's can be difficult to diagnose because there isn't one specific test that confirms the diagnosis. A diagnosis can be especially challenging for individuals who do not display the characteristic tremor.

BE INFORMED: *Getting a second opinion to confirm your diagnosis can provide peace of mind. Your doctor may encourage it and even be able to provide you with a referral to a neurologist who specializes in the treatment of movement disorders.*

Your doctor will determine you have Parkinson's after reviewing your medical history, self-reported symptoms and conducting a clinical examination.

physical movement may force you to change how you engage in intimacy with your spouse or partner.

To be perfectly honest, I've experienced shame in every single one of these situations after being diagnosed with Parkinson's ten years ago. Even after spending years as a professional counselor with a deep working knowledge about shame, I wasn't prepared for how once shame sets in, my stress level skyrockets and the very Parkinson's symptoms causing me shame in the first place go from bad to worse. As you can see from these examples and likely your own experience, shame can occur among strangers as well as at the most personal levels of our lives.

The good news is that I can assure you, and am in fact living testimony, that shame can be made fleeting and insignificant. And this isn't only for those of us living with Parkinson's, but for anyone experiencing embarrassment or other stress-producing emotions simply because of how we believe we are being perceived. You see, the common thread always present when shame rears its ugly head is fear. And fear can only survive in an environment of silence. Fear-based shame is rarely discussed in an open, candid and authentic setting. But when it is, something magical happens. The monster under the bed gets exposed and we experience freedom. This is the primary reason I almost never miss an opportunity to let people know I am living with Parkinson's and offer to answer any questions they may have. Almost immediately, I feel something that is quite the opposite of shame, and that feeling is empowerment.

MOVING FROM SHAME TO EMPOWERMENT

There are many tools available that can help change shame to empowerment. These include: support groups, self-education, having open conversations with loved ones or volunteering for an organization devoted to helping folks with Parkinson's live great lives like the Davis Phinney Foundation. Look, I get it, for many of us, these require action and aren't necessarily easy to do. But if the goal is to end silence, then noise needs to be made! For some of us, it may be speaking in front of a large group at a conference. For others, it may be a quiet conversation with your spouse. Even your choice to read this *Every Victory Counts* manual is a start. This book is literally crammed with tools to convert shame to empowerment. If a 1000-mile journey starts with a single step, then it is a good step to take. Take yours now.

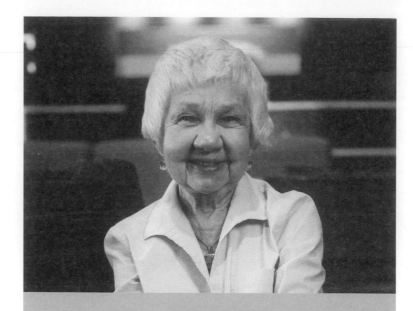

> **"** *I was officially diagnosed at 72, but I started noticing changes when I was trekking in the Himalayas at 70. I would stumble on hikes or struggle to get my leg over the crossbar during a long bike ride. I made up all kinds of excuses until one day I collapsed on the trail and was taken to the hospital. It took a year before I saw a movement disorder specialist and was officially diagnosed with Parkinson's."*

— BRENDA

A Parkinson's diagnosis requires you have two out of three primary motor symptoms:

- Tremor (shaking, usually of the arm, leg or chin, while at rest)
- Rigidity (stiffness)
- Bradykinesia (slow movement)

To support the diagnosis, your doctor will also look for other symptoms:

- Micrographia (small handwriting)
- Facial masking (reduced facial expression)
- Decreased arm swing or leg drag on one side of the body while walking

Your doctor will also test your responsiveness to levodopa, a medication that boosts dopamine in the brain and improves motor symptoms. However, your response to this medication alone cannot ensure an accurate diagnosis. Other conditions can improve with levodopa, and a placebo effect can occur in some people.

There are no definitive blood tests or brain scans that can positively identify Parkinson's with certainty, except during an autopsy. In some cases, brain MRIs or CAT scans are performed to rule out a stroke or other condition, but neither of these tests reveal Parkinson's. The DaTSCAN is a diagnostic test that measures levels of dopamine nerve cells in the basal ganglia structures of the brain. It was approved by the FDA in 2011 to help differentiate a Parkinson's tremor from other types of tremor, namely Familial or Essential Tremor.

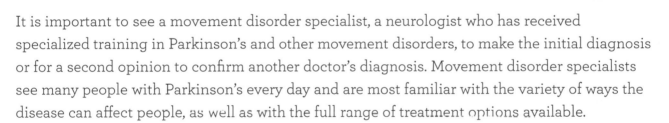

" Originally, I was diagnosed by a general neurologist. He was a great doctor, but what he did initially...it was a little haphazard, to tell you the truth. Part of my diagnosis was a drug challenge – and he used the wrong meds, in the wrong dosage and the wrong order to come to the conclusion that I wasn't responding to meds. Then I went to a movement disorder specialist, and he put together a drug challenge that was clinically effective and found that I did respond to the medication after all and had young onset Parkinson's. One of the benefits to me was a whole lot less mental anguish going to someone who had specific experience with movement disorders."

— COREY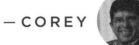

47

It is important to see a movement disorder specialist, a neurologist who has received specialized training in Parkinson's and other movement disorders, to make the initial diagnosis or for a second opinion to confirm another doctor's diagnosis. Movement disorder specialists see many people with Parkinson's every day and are most familiar with the variety of ways the disease can affect people, as well as with the full range of treatment options available.

Even if you don't have a movement disorder specialist close by, you may benefit by seeing one periodically, at least once a year between your primary care or general neurology appointments. Listen to Linda describe her experience being diagnosed with Parkinson's: ■ dpf.org/linda.

WHAT CAUSES PARKINSON'S?

The complexity of the brain has made the search for the underlying causes of Parkinson's challenging. While there is currently no known single cause of Parkinson's or predictor of who will get it, scientists and researchers believe a unique combination of genetics, environment, lifestyle and other factors are at play for each person who develops the disease. Some people with Parkinson's have been exposed to specific environmental elements, such as pesticides, or have experienced lifestyle factors, like head trauma, that may have influenced the development of the disease.

GENETIC FACTORS

In January 1999, *Journal of the American Medical Association* researchers first concluded that genetic factors play a role of varying degrees in the development of Parkinson's. In October 2003, scientists at the National Institutes of Health discovered that mutations in the alpha-synuclein gene could cause Parkinson's. These findings suggest that genetic components could play a more significant role in Parkinson's than originally thought. Abnormal genes have been identified in some people with Parkinson's, especially younger individuals and those with gene mutations whose Parkinson's "runs in the family." However, no single genetic abnormality has been found for the majority of people with Parkinson's. In fact, researchers have now identified more than a dozen gene abnormalities associated with Parkinson's.[1] Unlike the alpha-synuclein gene mutation, most of these genes are what is referred to as "susceptibility genes," meaning that they do not necessarily cause Parkinson's, but they do increase the risk of developing the disease. According to the National Institutes of Health, inherited cases of Parkinson's disease are caused by mutations in the LRRK2, DJ-1, PINK1 or SNCA genes, or by mutations in genes that have not yet been identified.

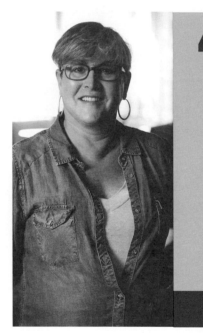

" *My mom and my sister both have Parkinson's — we have the LRRK2 gene — so when I was diagnosed, I understood what it meant. I'm not a doctor, but with my family experience and doing my own reading, I knew this was a progressive disease that doesn't get better. I didn't know what our future would hold, but I knew things were not ever going back to 'normal.' That said, not being 'normal' is a gift in itself! The Mack truck has hit us. The worst has already happened. Parkinson's has forced my family and I to make so many changes for the better.*"

— JILL

After receiving a diagnosis of Parkinson's, many people are concerned about passing the disease to their children. Remember that genetic factors play a role in only a small number of cases, and even if your children inherit an abnormal gene from you, they won't automatically develop Parkinson's. While genetic testing is available, it doesn't offer satisfying answers for most people. If you have a family history that includes many people with Parkinson's, you may wish to talk with your doctor about testing. If you decide to be tested, it's important to see a genetic counselor before and after receiving the results. These specialized counselors, available in many large medical centers and university programs, will help you understand

---

1   Hardy, John. Genetic analysis of pathways to PD. (2010, Oct 21). *Neuron*, 68(2): 201-206.

the results, their potential impact on your family, and how they may influence insurance qualification and other issues you may not have considered.

ENVIRONMENTAL FACTORS

Epidemiological studies based on large populations of individuals suggest that there are certain toxins that increase the risk of developing Parkinson's. For instance, there is an increased risk for people living in a rural community or who drink well water. This may be due to ingestion of or exposure to certain pesticides proven in the laboratory to be toxic to dopamine neurons. Other chemicals, such as solvents used in the industrial dry cleaning industry have been implicated, suggesting that certain environmental toxins increase the risk of developing Parkinson's.

Environmental Threats to Healthy Aging, in a report co-authored by the Science and Environmental Health Network consortium of advocacy groups based in Iowa, included a summary of 31 population studies examining the possible connection between pesticide exposure and Parkinson's. According to the report, twenty-four of those studies found a positive association, and in 12 cases, the association was statistically significant. In some studies, the group found there was *as much as a sevenfold greater risk* of Parkinson's in people exposed to pesticides than those who were not. In addition, scientists at the University of California Los Angeles published a provocative study in April 2009 connecting Parkinson's not only to occupational pesticide exposure, but also to living in homes or going to schools that were close to a pesticide-treated field.[2]

Despite this evidence, a January 2009 consensus statement from Collaborative Health and the Environment, working together with Parkinson's advocacy groups, found that there was "limited suggestive evidence of an association" between pesticides and Parkinson's and between farming or agricultural work and Parkinson's. This discrepancy highlights the fact that the search for a cause is extremely complex. Current conventional wisdom points to a combination of genetics, environment, lifestyle and other unknown factors.

LIFESTYLE FACTORS

A study published in 2015 identified possible factors that may positively or negatively influence the risk of developing Parkinson's. This list included habits like smoking, drinking alcohol, coffee or green tea, environmental factors such as well-water ingestion, exposure to anesthesia, maganese, solvents and farming chemicals, as well as exercise levels and certain vitamins and foods.[3]

2   Bronstein, Jeff, Carvey, Paul, Chen, Honglei, Cory-Slecta, Deborah, Dimonte, Donato, et. al. Meeting Report: Consensus Statement–Parkinson's Disease and the Environment: Collaborative on Health and the Environment and the Parkinson's Action Network (CHE PAN) Conference 26 – 28 June 2007. (January 2009). *Environmental Health Perspectives*, 117(1): 117-121.
3   Zeynep, S. Agim and Cannon, Jason R. (2015). Dietary Factors in the Etiology of Parkinson's Disease. *Biomed Res Int.*

A September 2016 analysis conducted by the *Journal of the American Medical Association*[4] of three major studies that used autopsy data to examine the association between traumatic brain injury (TBI) and neurodegenerative diseases found that TBI with loss of consciousness is associated with increased risk for Lewy body accumulation, progression of parkinsonism and development of Parkinson's. While important information highlighting the need for head injury prevention, this research supports one potential lifestyle factor cause, and does not explain how people who have never experienced TBI (or have the aforementioned genetic or environmental factors) develop Parkinson's.

WHO GETS PARKINSON'S?

Parkinson's is second only to Alzheimer's as the most common neurodegenerative disease in the US, affecting between 1 million to 1.5 million Americans. Between 7 and 10 million people are estimated to be living with Parkinson's around the world. There are more people living with Parkinson's in the US than the number of people living with multiple sclerosis, muscular dystrophy and Lou Gehrig's disease (ALS) combined.

Parkinson's affects men and women, and according to the National Institutes of Health, Parkinson's affects about 50% more men than women. About 1.5-2% of people over the age of 60 (the average age of onset) have Parkinson's, while there are fewer than 1 in 1,000 people under the age of 50 living with Parkinson's. It is estimated that 4% of people with Parkinson's are younger than age 50. Typically, those individuals are referred to as having early onset or young onset Parkinson's disease (YOPD).

> **"** *Life is incurable, life is progressive, life is degenerative, and all of us have to come to terms with that and live life to the fullest anyway. I don't feel like I'm any different than anybody else, I just have more insight into my challenges."*
>
> **— COREY**

WHEN DOES PARKINSON'S START?

Many people live with Parkinson's for years before an official diagnosis is made. Looking back after diagnosis, some people can pinpoint the onset of their disease, recognizing symptoms which make sense only in retrospect. Foot cramping is very common in the early stages of Parkinson's. Other symptoms, such as small handwriting, decreased arm swing on one side when walking, shoulder pain, depression, sleep problems, constipation and loss of sense of smell can begin before clinically-evident motor symptoms emerge. Since symptoms like these can be subtle at first, they are not always evident or meaningful prior to diagnosis.

4   Crane, Paul K., Gibbons, Laura E., and Dams-O'Connor, Kristen. (2016). Association of Traumatic Brain Injury With Late-Life Neurodegenerative Conditions and Neuropathologic Findings. *JAMA Neurol*, 73(9): 1062-1069.

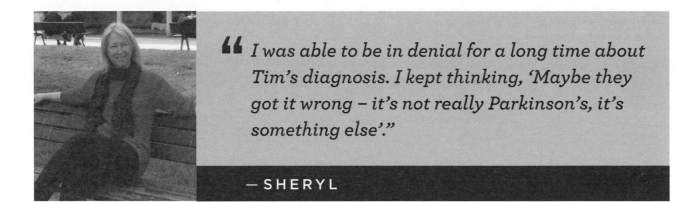

WHAT PREMOTOR SYMPTOMS MAY OCCUR?

The diagnosis of Parkinson's has traditionally focused on the well-known, characteristic motor symptoms of tremor, slowness and stiffness. Medical researchers are hopeful that identifying the early signs of Parkinson's, called premotor symptoms, will help doctors diagnose Parkinson's before there is extensive loss of dopamine-producing nerve cells that cause motor symptoms to appear. Premotor symptoms include:

- **REM Sleep Behavior Disorder (RBD)** – may occur 15–50 years before motor symptoms
- **Constipation** – may occur 10–20 years before motor symptoms
- **Depression and anxiety** – may occur up to 20 years before motor symptoms
- **Loss of smell** – may occur several years before motor symptoms

The earlier the diagnosis, the more clues may be discovered about why dopamine nerve cells experience decline. More knowledge about how the disease evolves over the years may also enable researchers to focus on slowing progression, developing disease-modifying therapies or even preventing the onset of motor symptoms. The challenge that researchers face is identifying the presence of premotor symptoms (which are often common in the general population) and being able to articulate who is indeed at risk of developing Parkinson's.

A current focus of ongoing research is discovering biomarkers of Parkinson's, biological characteristics that can predict if someone will develop a certain condition, such as Parkinson's.

WHAT MOTOR SYMPTOMS MAY OCCUR?

Motor symptoms, which we'll discuss in greater detail in the "Core Parkinson's Symptoms" chapter of this section, are those that impact movement. Primary motor symptoms include:

- **Tremor:** a rhythmic shaking in your arms, legs or chin. Tremor is not present in all people living with Parkinson's. About 80% of individuals with Parkinson's experience tremor at some time, although most people who experience tremor observe that it is worse when relaxing and resting. This type of tremor is called rest tremor. Others experience action tremor, which means shaking gets worse when trying to do

51

EARLY SYMPTOMS OF PARKINSON'S

By Peter A. LeWitt, MD, MMedSc

A mainstay of crime mysteries is the insignificant clue tying the story together, and that's the current situation for Parkinson's. In recent years, clues unrelated to the motor symptoms of Parkinson's have given insights for understanding how this disorder develops. Although the motor symptoms of Parkinson's often get the most attention and treatment, researchers estimate motor symptoms don't actually appear in most people until around 60–80% of the nerve cells in the brain that make dopamine have stopped working because of Parkinson's. Often, non-motor symptoms of Parkinson's begin long before the more visible physical symptoms. Sometimes these non-motor symptoms are called "premotor symptoms," because they come before the motor symptoms surface. Symptoms such as loss of smell, depression and constipation may appear years before your actual diagnosis. Like motor impairments, most of these premotor symptoms come from a damaged protein called alpha-synuclein that kills nerve cells in the brain and elsewhere.

Many people living with Parkinson's experience reduced sense of smell (olfaction), sometimes years before any other Parkinson's symptoms. This deficit is explained by the progressive loss of nerve cells in

something, like drinking out of a cup or eating with a spoon.

- **Rigidity:** painful or non-painful stiffness, often in your arms, legs, neck or back muscles.

- **Akinesia, Bradykinesia, Hypokinesia:** Akinesia means lack of movement, bradykinesia means slowness of movement and hypokinesia means small movements. Often people living with Parkinson's will experience aspects of all three of these. For example, the small, cramped handwriting (micrographia) some people with Parkinson's have is thought to be a combination of bradykinesia and hypokinesia.

- **Balance difficulties and problems walking:** such as stooped posture, decreased natural arm swing and shuffling steps.

Early motor symptoms can also include a mask-like face or loss of facial expression. Listen to Tufts researcher Linda Tickle-Degnen discuss facial masking research: 🔊**dpf.org/mask**. Some people may complain of a heaviness feeling, dragging or lack of use of one side or cramping in certain muscles.

Later in the progression of Parkinson's, soft or slurred speech, difficulty swallowing and walking and balance issues can become more problematic. Walking can change from shuffling steps to festination, or a tendency toward smaller, faster steps that pitch you forward. Freezing is a term used to define problems with initiating movements and is often described as feeling like your feet are glued to the floor. Freezing often occurs when you first begin to walk, turn and in tight or crowded spaces. Postural instability causes trouble with keeping your center of balance upright. This is called retropulsion if there is a tendency to fall backward.

Other motor symptoms include:

- Reduced manual dexterity
- Severe muscle cramping
- Pain without obvious cause

WHAT NON-MOTOR SYMPTOMS MAY OCCUR?

Although Parkinson's is officially classified as a movement disorder, Parkinson's can also cause problems not related to movement. These non-motor symptoms, which we'll discuss in greater detail in the "Core Parkinson's Symptoms" chapter of this section, may actually outnumber motor symptoms and can appear years before motor symptoms.

Non-motor symptoms include:

- Cognitive challenges
- Memory problems
- Feeling tongue-tied
- Fatigue
- Sleep problems
- Anxiety and depression
- Loss of confidence, initiative or apathy
- Loss of smell
- Numbness or tingling

Some of the non-motor symptoms of Parkinson's are connected to the effects Parkinson's has on the autonomic nervous system, which regulates functions your body "automatically" does, like controlling blood pressure, sweating and temperature management, digestion and heart rate.

the brain region devoted to odor recognition. Why this occurs so early in the progression of the disease is not understood, but perhaps it's a clue that brain involvement starts through the nasal passages.

Another non-motor feature that often precedes the development of Parkinson's motor symptoms is a particular sleep disturbance with vivid dreaming, often with speaking or physical enactment of dreams. Vivid dreaming occurs during a sleep stage associated with rapid eye movements, so this particular sleep disturbance is called rapid eye movement sleep behavior disorder (RBD). A sleep laboratory study often is needed for an accurate diagnosis. Medications can treat this problem. The brain origin of this sleep disturbance is not well defined, but likely represents additional regions where nerve cells are damaged by abnormal alpha-synuclein accumulation. The combination of RBD and impaired ability to smell signals a strong risk for eventually developing Parkinson's.

53

Non-motor symptoms of Parkinson's that can be caused by changes and impairment to the autonomic nervous system include:

- Constipation
- Frequent need to urinate that can develop into incontinence
- Lightheadedness, especially when getting up in the morning or rising from a chair or couch
- Sexual dysfunction, especially erectile dysfunction
- Excessive salivation (drooling)
- Excessive perspiration

HOW DOES PARKINSON'S CHANGE OVER TIME?

Everyone's experience with Parkinson's is different, so much so that anticipating its progression can be terribly frustrating. Doctors simply cannot tell you what will happen next or how severe or mild your symptoms will be. Each person's symptoms change at different rates and present different variations. Sometimes things change for the better in one area, but then a new symptom will crop up elsewhere. Age and health also can also influence the progression of Parkinson's.

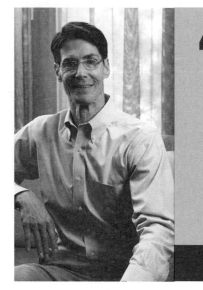

" *In the beginning, I really didn't have a whole lot of challenges. Now, a decade into this disease, I have to be really cognizant of sleep, schedule and medicine. If I'm not, I might be okay today, but I'll have an off day tomorrow. I need to manage Parkinson's more hands-on and consciously.*"

— STEVE

That said, there are similarities most people with Parkinson's experience over time. Symptoms typically evolve slowly. Many times, you may not be aware of a change in mobility or other symptom until someone else points it out. In the beginning stages of Parkinson's, symptoms such as tremor, slowness and rigidity typically begin on one side of the body and spread to the other side over time. Walking, speech or swallowing problems can occur, though these symptoms progress slowly over many years, as Parkinson's advances. For most people, balance problems occur in later stages, leading to concerns about falls and serious injuries. **Figure 1** (following this page) outlines common Parkinson's symptoms. Learn how Linda stays positive throughout all the changes Parkinson's brings: 🎥 **dpf.org/linda**.

54

PARKINSON'S **IS** DIFFERENT FOR EVERYONE

After "why me?" usually the next questions include: "What does the progression look like? What can I expect?" It's tou[...]
times. There are, however, some similarities in experiences over time and this manual provides suggestions and resou[...]
something is a symptom of Parkinson's does not mean you necessarily will experience it.

CHANGE IN FACIAL EXPRESSION

" *My facial expression was lost. My students thought I was always sad. I'm brighter now since DBS. I smile at myself in the mirror.*"

— CONNIE

Speech & Swallowing

ARM DOESN'T SWING

" *I have always been very active in various sports and assumed the gradual loss of arm swing was from two torn rotator cuff injuries to my shoulder. I even went to an orthopedic surgeon to check it out.*"

— STEVE

SHOULDER PAIN

SEXUAL DYSFUNCTION

Bradykinesia

FREEZING

SLEEP PROBLEMS

" *I have trouble falling and staying asleep because my tremors make it difficult. I drink an herbal tea before bed, and it helps me fall asleep.*"

— TIM

LIGHTHEADEDNESS OR DIZZINESS

Diminished Sense of Sm[...]

DEPRESSION

" *I talk to people in my support group[...] relate and understand. It's good to [...] something to think about besides th[...] – music, friends or whatever else yo[...]*

— NORMA

CONSTIPAT[...]

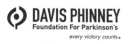

gh to get an answer because Parkinson's disease affects people differently and at different
ces to help you address the various symptoms you may have. Remember, simply because

LEG CRAMPING,
NUMBNESS

FALLING
Dyskinesia

INCONTINENCE

LOSS OF DEXTERITY

" *My writing has become very small and hard to read. Maybe I should have gone to medical school.*"

— DOROTHY

REDUCED MOBILITY & GAIT

" *Now I have to really focus on walking, picking up and putting one foot in front of the other.*"

— PAT

ell FATIGUE

RIGIDITY

Anxiety

who can
nd
e Parkinson's
u enjoy."

MEDS
WEARING
OFF

MEMORY & COGNITION

" *I lose track of the topic and go off on tangents. The short-term memory loss can be a struggle.*"

— MIKE

ION Tremor

APATHY

Figure 1.

AFTER DIAGNOSIS, THE FIRST QUESTION PEOPLE ASK IS: "WHAT CAN I EXPECT?"

EARLY STAGE

- Symptoms on one side of the body

- Decreased arm swing on one side when walking

- Decreased stride length or dragging your foot while walking

- Scuffing your toes, especially when tired

- Change in leg coordination when cycling or running

- Sense of muscle fatigue or heaviness in your arm or leg on one side of the body

- Difficulty completing repetitive movements due to sense of muscle fatigue

- Trouble with hand coordination, especially on one side. This is often apparent doing tasks that use both hands, like shampooing your hair

- Reduced range of motion in your shoulder, shoulder pain or frozen shoulder

- Mask-like face or change in facial expression called hypomimia

- Decreased or small handwriting called micrographia

MID STAGE

- Symptoms on both sides of the body

- Soft speech called hypophonia

- Mild swallowing problems, such as difficulty swallowing pills

- Flexed or bent posture and shuffling gait

- Motor fluctuations and dyskinesia

LATE STAGE

- Postural instability with balance problems and falls

- Walking problems, with increased shuffling, freezing of gait and festination

- Significant speech and swallowing problems

- Drooling

- Rigidity in the neck and trunk parts of the body

Some people find joining a Parkinson's support group helpful, in part because it provides an opportunity to learn how the disease looks and progresses in a variety of people and tips to manage its impact.

55

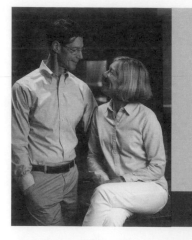

> **"** *We live in the moment, trying not to think too far into the future. Because Parkinson's progresses slowly, we can make changes as time goes on. We try to live day by day, knowing that yes — there will be changes."*
>
> **— NANCY**

An exercise program that includes balance, strengthening and posture exercises *as early after diagnosis as possible* is highly recommended to combat problems in these areas. A physical therapist with experience in Parkinson's can help you set up an exercise program if you do not know how or need help getting started. A speech therapist with experience in Parkinson's can prescribe speech exercises to keep speech loud and clear. By working on problems such as speech and balance early, you can reduce their impact later. That said, if you've been living with Parkinson's for some time, it's never too late to make positive changes. Start now!

BE ACTIVE: *There's no better time than today to commit to living well with Parkinson's.*

AFTER DIAGNOSIS

" *When I got the diagnosis, it wasn't like when I was diagnosed with breast cancer. Nobody said, 'We can fix this.' There is an action plan, it's just different. You don't focus on fixing Parkinson's. You focus on how to live with it so you can enjoy life.*"

— EDIE

ASSEMBLING YOUR WELLNESS TEAM

WHAT TYPE OF DOCTOR SHOULD I SEE?

Your health and wellness also depend on getting the best quality medical care available to you. A neurologist is a medical doctor who specializes in conditions of the nervous system (the brain and the spinal cord). He or she can confirm your diagnosis and establish an appropriate treatment plan. A movement disorder specialist is a neurologist with additional training in movement disorders. Movement disorder specialists are more familiar with Parkinson's and may be able to make a diagnosis sooner. They may also be more familiar with current research and treatment options and recognize when to refer you to an interdisciplinary team.

If you don't have a movement disorder specialist close to home, seek out an empathetic doctor who will listen to you and your family, work with you to define your needs and goals and be open to your suggestions and ideas as an active participant in your own treatment plan. If your local wellness team doesn't include a movement disorder specialist but you are able to travel occasionally to see one in another city, your movement disorder specialist and local neurologist can

VIRTUAL HOUSE CALLS: THE PROMISE OF TELEMEDICINE FOR HIGH-QUALITY PARKINSON'S CARE

By Ray Dorsey, MD, MBA

The way in which we deliver care to individuals with chronic conditions like Parkinson's is fundamentally flawed. We ask people with Parkinson's to travel, often with significant difficulty and at great physical and financial expense, to meet with clinicians on *their* terms — their office, their location, their hours. Instead, we should be thinking about ways clinicians could respond to the needs of people with Parkinson's on their terms. Factor in transportation times (sometimes, to distant locations that require an overnight stay), limited mobility and clinic wait times, and too often, 15 minutes of face time with a doctor involves an hours-long ordeal. For people living with Parkinson's, the need to travel long distances or into difficult-to-navigate urban centers with mobility barriers is a worst-case scenario that can discourage regular interaction with their Parkinson's specialist.

People with Parkinson's are often limited in their care by what I call the three D's: distance, disability and the distribution of doctors. Fortunately, thanks to the advances of technology in the early twenty-first century, things are beginning to change.

57

Telemedicine, the use of the Internet to provide care to patients who are separated geographically from clinicians, is rapidly reshaping healthcare.

If, for example, an individual has a stroke in a rural area, he is connected remotely from the emergency room of a rural hospital to a stroke neurologist for evaluation and management. If a child has a fever and sore throat at 11:00 p.m., her parents can connect with a board certified pediatrician for evaluation without having to go to an emergency room, urgent care center or wait in a room full of other sick children for care on the following day.

Thanks to research funding from the Davis Phinney Foundation and other Parkinson's organizations, telemedicine is now even testing healthcare delivery models that bring expert Parkinson's care to people in their own homes.

WHAT WE'VE LEARNED ABOUT THE POWER OF TELEMEDICINE

In one study funded by the Davis Phinney Foundation, more than 250 individuals with Parkinson's from five different states were connected to one of 11 Parkinson's specialists at the University of California San Francisco, the University of Florida or the University of Rochester for a one-time consultation. Rather than having to drive to see the specialist, individuals with Parkinson's could see the specialist from the comfort of their homes. Study participants received a web camera (if they did not already have one) and an email link to secure video conferencing software (such as Skype™) to download. They could then consult remotely with a Parkinson's specialist, with no concern for geographic proximity.

The telemedicine visits included a personal health history, Parkinson's-specific examination and time for consultation. Based on the virtual visit, the specialist frequently recommended an exercise program (88% of the time) or a change to their Parkinson's medications (76%). Satisfaction with these visits was high among participants (94% satisfied or very satisfied), and almost three quarters were interested in receiving such care in the future.

A more recent randomized, controlled trial (funded by the Patient-Centered Outcomes Research Institute) of virtual visits versus the usual, community-based care for Parkinson's was conducted nationally. Nearly 1,000 individuals with Parkinson's expressed interest in participating in the 200-person study. Each virtual house call, which included a video visit between a Parkinson's specialist at centers like Duke University, Johns Hopkins University and University of Pennsylvania and a person living with Parkinson's in their own home, **saved people with Parkinson's and their care partners, on average, about 100 miles of travel and three hours of time.** In addition, 97% of people who participated reported feeling satisfied or very satisfied with their care. More people with Parkinson's preferred their visits with the virtual doctor, compared to their in-person doctor on every domain measured, including the quality of the personal connection.

Based on these efforts and the generous support of foundations, my team and I launched Parkinson's Disease Care New York (PDCNY), which enables any New Yorker with Parkinson's to receive care in his or her home remotely from a Parkinson's specialist for at least a year, for free. Any New Yorker with Parkinson's can receive care in their home via telemedicine for free by simply visiting ⌃**pdcny.org**. We are hopeful this will be a model for other states and conditions.

BARRIERS TO TELEMEDICINE

With results like these and the growing number of individuals living with Parkinson's and advanced stage Parkinson's, it's becoming clear that care needs to be brought to the home. However, the biggest barrier to the widespread use of telemedicine for Parkinson's in the US is Medicare and its reimbursement policies.

Currently, Medicare only covers telemedicine services that are provided in health professional shortage areas and only then, in clinical settings, like hospitals and doctor's offices. Medicare does not cover any telemedicine care into the home. The result is that over 40% of older Americans with Parkinson's cannot or do not access appropriate neurological care, despite the fact that those who don't are more likely to die prematurely.

In contrast, another federal health program, the Veterans Health Administration (VA) covers telehealth extensively. Last year, the VA had over two million telehealth visits for a wide range of conditions, including Parkinson's. In 2015, Medicare spent less than 0.01% of its budget on telehealth services. Moreover, the VA allows veterans to receive care from any VA clinician while Medicare only allows Medicare beneficiaries to receive care from Medicare providers licensed to practice in their state. The result is that those with the greatest need, such as an individual with advanced Parkinson's in remote areas like Maine or Montana, often have the least access to care.

TELEMEDICINE: WHERE TO START?

We know now that the care of those with Parkinson's is improved via telemedicine. If you're interested in trying telemedicine, there are an increasing number of Parkinson's specialists seeing patients this way. Consider asking your current clinician if you can have follow-up visits performed via telemedicine. By now, most will have heard of it and may even consider it.

The equipment you'll need for telemedicine is minimal:

- An internet-enabled device, such as a smartphone, tablet, laptop or desktop computer with a web camera

- HIPAA-compliant video conferencing software (your telemedicine clinician will help you download this readily available software).

Telemedicine won't entirely replace your in-person doctor visits. Care is typically delivered through a combination of virtual and local providers.

Although my team has remotely diagnosed hundreds of people with Parkinson's, in some cases, remote diagnosis can be difficult and may require an in-person evaluation. Surgical treatments like deep brain stimulation generally require an in-person evaluation, in addition to the surgery and follow-up adjustments. My team and others believe in the near future DBS adjustments, for example, also could be done remotely.

INSURANCE COVERAGE

Telemedicine is widely available in Canada and in at least 29 states in the US. Private insurers must cover telemedicine services to the extent they cover in-person care; however, coverage for care provided into the home still very much depends on your situation and your insurance.

As described above, the VA provides extensive coverage for telehealth, although, Medicare only covers telemedicine services provided in health professional shortage areas and then, only in clinical settings. Medicare does not cover any care provided by telemedicine into the home. Medicare Advantage programs may also offer telemedicine coverage as part of the 21st Century Cures Act. The best advice is to check your policy and contact your insurer if you have questions.

59

- **You.** It may seem odd to include yourself, but you are the most important member of the team. Think about the role you want to play as the primary team member. Be an active participant in managing your condition. Being engaged and empowered in your own care gets results. Use this manual to learn what you can do to partner with your wellness team and how you can keep yourself on track.

- **Family and/or friends.** Your family is also living with Parkinson's and can be involved with your treatment. Talk about how you will work together to keep track of therapies and outcomes. Look to your friends, community and church or spiritual community as sources of healthy social connectivity and for support when needed.

- **Primary care provider (PCP).** Every person with Parkinson's should have a primary care provider. A doctor, physician assistant or nurse practitioner can fill this role. Ask about their familiarity with Parkinson's and discuss whether they would be open to receiving literature from you and your neurologist about Parkinson's. You can request an extra copy of this *Every Victory Counts* manual to give to your PCP (visit dpf.org/evc).

60

work together to address your needs. You may also be able to utilize telemedicine, the ability to meet with a movement disorder specialist remotely.

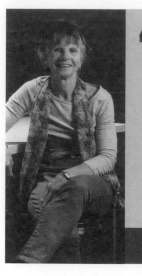

> " *A movement disorder specialist knows more about all the symptoms of Parkinson's, especially the non-motor stuff. They also know more about the medications and the disease in general.*"
>
> — LINDA

Common in many parts of Canada, this way of connecting can save time and hassle of driving long distances to see a specialist. In the event your movement disorder specialist is not located near you, you'll want to be organized and prepared to advocate for the treatment and services you need.

> " *Telemedicine has saved me many miles and stresses and does 90% of the things I need. I do about one appointment in person per year and I can meet with my own doctor via telemedicine the rest of the time. The local clinic technician can track my weight, assess movement, etc.*"
>
> — RYAN

- **Neurologist.** A neurologist or movement disorder specialist (a neurologist who has additional training in treating Parkinson's and other movement disorders) will manage your Parkinson's. Your primary care provider and neurologist will work together to treat your symptoms, especially non-motor ones.

- **Rehabilitation specialist(s).** Physical therapists, occupational therapists and speech therapists help diagnose and treat the physical challenges related to Parkinson's. Ask for a referral to a rehabilitation specialist who works with people with Parkinson's right away so that you can work on prevention from the start.

- **Mental health provider.** Psychological counselors, social workers and psychiatrists provide emotional health support, especially if you are having trouble with depression, anxiety or are experiencing fears and having difficulty adjusting to your diagnosis. A psychiatrist can help if your symptoms require medical treatment.

- **Community.** Support groups, senior and community centers, personal trainers, yoga, boxing and dance instructors are just some of the groups and individuals that you can lean on to keep you active, engaged and on track.

- **Spiritual advisors.** If faith is part of your life, a pastor, chaplain, rabbi or other spiritual advisor can help you find peace, bring meaning and accept life changes within the comfort and context of your beliefs. Many people, whether within the construct of traditional religions or through other forms of spiritual expression, rely on these advisors to help provide the support and hope they need to embrace the future.

BE ENGAGED: *Ask your doctor for a referral to a movement disorder specialist.*

Before you see your doctor, review the **Worksheets and Resources** in this manual designed to help you prepare to get the most out of your appointment and make sure that you communicate effectively. The **Goal Summary for Doctor Visits** and **Parkinson's Care Questionnaire** can help you record important information to make your time with your doctor more productive. Hear how Edie partners with her doctor and wellness team: ■◀ **dpf.org/edie**.

❝ *I love the worksheets in this manual because now I never go to an appointment and just say, 'Oh, I'm fine'.”*

— JILL

PALLIATIVE OR SUPPORTIVE CARE AND PARKINSON'S

By Janis M. Miyasaki, MD, MEd, FRCPC, FAAN

The term, *palliative care*, was coined by Dr. Balmont, a surgeon in Montreal, Canada meaning "to relieve symptoms" for those with prostate cancer. These days, palliative care is widely used in reference to care that encompasses a holistic, team-based approach that shifts the focus of care from an individual patient to the patient and their family together.[5] At its best, palliative care "provides relief from pain and other distressing symptoms, affirms life and regards dying as a normal process, intends neither to hasten nor postpone death, integrates the psychological and spiritual aspects of patient care, offers a support system to help the family cope during the patient's illness and their own bereavement, uses a team-based approach, will enhance quality of life and is applicable early in the course of illness, including when life-sustaining therapies are used."

For people living with Parkinson's, there are many moments when palliative care can be applicable. If palliative care resources were readily available, people with Parkinson's could access them at the time of diagnosis to address existential suffering; that is, to answer questions such as, "Why

In addition to your movement disorder specialist or neurologist, your primary care physician (PCP) will also be very important over the coming years. He or she will help you stay healthy with regular check-ups and will complement your neurologist in treating your non-motor symptoms. Remember, not all problems are related to Parkinson's. For example, fatigue is a common Parkinson's symptom but can also be caused by thyroid disease, anemia, vitamin deficiency, malnutrition, diabetes, heart and lung disease, to name a few. Your PCP can check for these and other conditions during your evaluation.

WHO ELSE SHOULD BE ON MY WELLNESS TEAM?

There are many ways to treat the symptoms of Parkinson's. Your neurologist or movement disorder specialist typically will manage your medications and refer you to additional healthcare professionals as needed for your situation. Establishing an integrative wellness team early will build a network of specialists who will become familiar with you and your symptoms and be able to work together to achieve the best outcome for you. With many medical problems, treatment occurs as symptoms emerge, but with Parkinson's, prevention is extremely important. Doctors can't predict how fast your disease will progress, but they know generally what to expect over time. Connecting with rehabilitation specialists, such as physical therapists, speech therapists and occupational therapists, will be essential at all stages of Parkinson's, even early on when symptoms are mild. These healthcare professionals can help prevent or delay problems, minimize the impact of symptoms and help you maintain function. Listen to Liz explain the importance of functional medicine for her wellness: ◼️ dpf.org/liz.

5   www.who.int/cancer/palliative/definition/en/

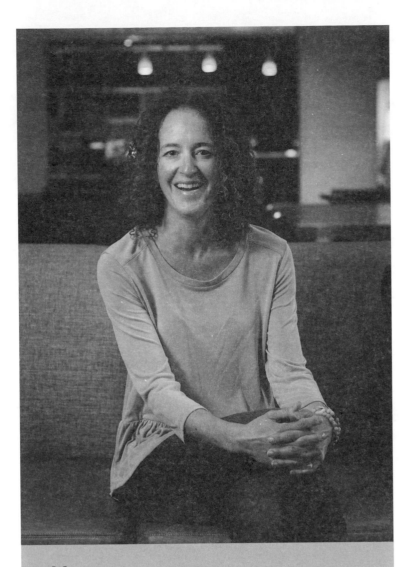

> **"** *My doctor said to me early on: 'Not everything is Parkinson's.' It's easy to fall into the trap of 'oh, this hurts,' and think it's directly related and feel like a victim. But it's not always Parkinson's fault. I recently had surgery that had absolutely nothing to do with Parkinson's, and it has been a welcome relief from the everyday grind of battling the disease."*

— LIZ

has this happened to me?", "How can I be hopeful?", "How can I go forward from this diagnosis?"

Currently, however, palliative care resources are finite, and many would contend, inadequate to meet the needs of the imminently dying, let alone to meet the needs of those living with a chronic condition. As a result, many specialists are adopting a palliative approach or seeking formal training to better meet the needs of people with Parkinson's throughout the course of their progress. The following applies to the US healthcare system, although many of the features are consistent with the Canadian system, as well.

WHAT IS THE DIFFERENCE BETWEEN HOSPICE AND PALLIATIVE CARE?

There is a saying: "All hospice is palliative care, but not all palliative care is hospice." In the US, *hospice* refers to care provided either in home or in day programs for those in the last six months of life. A hospice has a medical director, who is a palliative care specialist, and will work with nurses, physical therapists, occupational therapists, speech language pathologists, respiratory therapists and others to provide supportive care in the home or in supportive living. People may remain enrolled past the six-month duration, but the expectation is that those enrolled in hospice are imminently dying.

In contrast, *palliative care* is provided throughout the course of an illness or chronic condition. A study of palliative care for those with metastatic cancer found that those enrolled in palliative care survived longer than those not;[6] thus, it's natural for those with a complex, chronic disease, such as Parkinson's, to be referred to palliative care. Various stages have been proposed for referral, including unresolved symptoms, caregiver burnout, need for coordinated care, existential suffering and complex neuropsychiatric complications of illness, such as psychosis (hallucinations or delusions) or severe anxiety.

The first dedicated palliative care clinic for Parkinson's was established in 2007 at the University of Toronto, Canada. Using a multidisciplinary approach (including a pastoral counselor, palliative care physician, movement disorders neurologist, nurse and care coordinator), the clinic demonstrated that people with Parkinson's had a symptom burden similar to those with metastatic cancer and responded similarly favorably to interventions.[7] The most improved symptoms as measured by this study were constipation, dysphagia (difficulty swallowing), anxiety, pain and drowsiness.

WHEN SHOULD I BE REFERRED TO A PALLIATIVE CARE SPECIALIST?

You may be referred to a palliative care specialist if there are ambulatory services or a movement disorders program offering palliative care for Parkinson's in your community and if you are experiencing unresolved symptoms, existential distress, caregiver burnout or hallucinations, delusions or anxiety. Reluctance to refer people to palliative care persists, even among healthcare providers, so many palliative care programs have opted to use other names, such as Supportive Care, Comfort Care and Complex Neurologic Symptoms.

WHAT SHOULD I EXPECT AT A PALLIATIVE CARE CLINIC?

A well-developed palliative care program should consist of a multidisciplinary team, typically some combination of a neurologist, palliative care physician, social worker, pastoral counselor, nurse, physiotherapist, occupational therapist, speech language pathologist, respiratory therapist and nutritionist. Be aware that these resources are expensive, and therefore, not every service will be available, even in excellent palliative care programs. The program may elect to have you and your family be seen by all providers at once, or by all providers rotating through the clinic room. The latter approach is more efficient for the clinic staff, however, this can result in a long day for people and families and can generate many individual lists of follow-up tasks.

The objective of the palliative care clinic is to relieve unaddressed symptoms. For many, treating pain effectively by modifying medication schedules, using botulinum toxin or physical methods is possible.[8] You might also find it necessary to adjust your goals. Early in the course of Parkinson's, the primary objective is to optimize motor control. As the disease becomes advanced, and cognitive and behavior issues become challenging, reducing medications or changing medications may reduce mobility, yet improve overall cognition and result in better quality of life.

Supporting families during the long journey of Parkinson's is crucial. Spouses, in particular, express uncertainty that what they are doing is correct; after all, Parkinson's care is so complex. Providing families with options for approaching challenging situations is part of the team's role. The team can also affirm that the family's instincts are correct in dealing with a situation or gently steer them in the right direction. This can reduce the natural guilt and stress that may be associated with watching a loved one struggle with Parkinson's.

Addressing existential distress is an important role for the palliative care team. Although in very advanced stages of Parkinson's (those who are wheelchair-bound), there can be significant suffering,

6   Zimmermann C, Swami N, Krzyzanowska M, Hannon B, Leighl N, Oza A, et al. Early palliative care for patients with advanced cancer: a cluster-randomised controlled trial. *Lancet* 2014 May 17;383(9930):1721-1730.
7   Miyasaki JM, Long J, Mancini D, Moro E, Fox SH, Lang AE, et al. Palliative care for advanced Parkinson disease: an interdisciplinary clinic and new scale, the ESAS-PD. *Parkinsonism Relat Disord* 2012 Dec;18 Suppl 3:S6-9.
8   Bruno V.A., Fox S.H., Mancini D., Miyasaki JM. Botulinum Toxin Use in Refractory Pain and Other Symptoms in Parkinsonism. *Canadian Journal of Neurological Sciences* 2016 01 Sep 2016;43(5):697-702.

there are also many moments of beauty, happiness and connection. The palliative care team needs to impart this message of hope to people living with Parkinson's and their families, since many people I see in my clinic are concerned about "being a burden." Indeed, most caregiving literature speaks of "caregiver or care partner burden." The reality is that caregiving can also be a gift: to gracefully accept help and by doing so, allow those around you to serve and to experience selflessness. And for the care partner, doing this hard work can be one of the most rewarding things you do in life, to care for your loved one with patience and empathy.

Helping people with Parkinson's and their families build a web of support in the community should be a palliative care team's role, as well. Your palliative care team should be familiar with local resources, their suitability and cost to help you navigate this complex healthcare system. Although this may be the first time you and your family are facing this condition, the clinic faces this scenario daily, and they are well prepared to guide you. You are not alone.

Discussing uncomfortable topics, such as advance care directives or physicians' orders for life-sustaining therapies should occur with your physician or with your palliative care team. You should have this conversation while you and your care partner are able to understand the information presented in terms of outcomes for you in various medical scenarios and to compare this information with your values and experiences to make a choice that is best for you and your family. As a physician who also provides hospital care, the most challenging time for a family is when they find themselves in the Intensive Care Unit and are unsure of their loved one's wishes, because frank and detailed discussions did not occur in advance. I encourage everyone to have this discussion with their family and their doctor. Although lawyers often help people complete these forms, a lawyer cannot explain the possible outcomes to you or answer your questions about what happens with different levels of care. Individuals with cognitive concerns ("I'm not as sharp as I used to be") but NOT with dementia, can sometimes have problems understanding and reasoning to support a decision for their advance directives.

If such a time comes, your palliative care team should also offer support and care for those who are imminently dying. Particularly in the US, ambulatory palliative care teams coordinate with the local hospice for those that are ready to receive to hospice care.

Palliative care for Parkinson's is expanding in North America and throughout the world. Dedicated teams are recognizing the burden that Parkinson's can be for people living with it as well as their families and providing holistic and practical care throughout the long journey of living with this chronic condition. Many people and families living with Parkinson's share that the palliative care clinic is "THE most care" they have ever received. Pursuing a referral to a palliative care team may be your first step in addressing the complexities associated with Parkinson's care.

Because Parkinson's also affects emotional health, healthcare professionals who focus on it and on well-being can be very beneficial to your care. Counselors, social workers and psychologists are trained to assess emotional health and to work with you and your doctor to promote mental wellness. They can support you as you adjust to your diagnosis and provide support and guidance for you and your family when difficult times come. As we'll discuss in greater detail later, depression and anxiety are common symptoms of Parkinson's, and they are treatable. Furthermore, stress for any reason can aggravate many Parkinson's symptoms and cause additional strain on you and your family. Managing that stress is important, and these specialists can help you with strategies to cope and stay positive. They can guide you in responding with resilience to changes you hadn't anticipated.

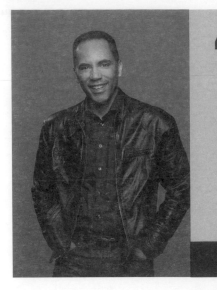

> " *If I was having a heart attack and didn't consult a cardiologist, people would think I was crazy. If I knew I had Parkinson's and didn't consult a neurologist, you'd think I was crazy. If I'm having mental health issues and don't consult an psychologist or psychiatrist, is that wise? No. We'll seek health for just about anything else, which tells me that we have a poor response to our own mental health, because it's terrifying.* "

— **TIM**

Turn to the "Complementary Therapies" chapter in the **Living Well Now** section to learn more about what an integrative care approach can do for you. If your doctor is familiar with the benefits of rehabilitative therapies for Parkinson's, you will probably be referred to one of these healthcare professionals early in the course of your disease. If not, don't be afraid to be your own advocate and ask for a referral. The **My Symptoms** worksheet in the **Worksheets and Resources** section will help you identify and capture problems you may be experiencing. Complete the worksheet to help you prepare for your next medical appointment. It will help guide your discussion with your doctor about what rehabilitation specialists may play a role in your treatment.

BE CONNECTED: *Find your community support network, or create your own. There are no right or wrong ways to be connected, but staying socially engaged is important for living well.*

> " *The friends I've made in the Parkinson's community are very aware of what I deal with every day. It's nice to have people understand that in a social setting.* "

— **BRENDA**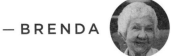

TAKE CONTROL

Parkinson's is a lifelong condition that will change over time. It's important to learn about the disease, to understand what to expect and to know what you can do to feel better today while preventing problems tomorrow.

WHAT CAN I DO TO TAKE ACTION?

" *If you focus on Parkinson's, then you will be depressed, anxious, apathetic. If you focus on what you can do to live well and be happy, that changes things. You've got to think about what makes you happy and then go make that happen. You have to be the one who initiates the action.*"

— EDIE

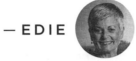

Below are some strategies to help you live better with Parkinson's. Remember to set priorities for yourself and try to balance life so that Parkinson's doesn't become your only focus. Learn what works for you, and over time you'll begin to recognize when your condition deserves your committed focus and when you can set it on the back burner.

- **Be Prepared.** Organize your healthcare documents and other information important to your medical team. Stay focused by organizing your thoughts and preparing a concise, direct summary for your doctor. Prepare for your medical appointments so that you get the best results from your time together. The **Worksheets and Resources** section of this manual contains self-assessments and other tools that will help you clearly review, prioritize and communicate symptoms and problems related to Parkinson's.

- **Be Engaged.** Advocate for yourself and your treatment. Ask for a referral to a rehabilitation therapist if you haven't received one. Talk with your wellness team about your goals and concerns. Make them aware of areas you want to improve. For instance, if using a keyboard has become difficult, ask your doctor about strategies to improve hand function or adaptive technologies that could help you type. If you

THE IMPORTANCE OF SELF-EFFICACY

By Diane G. Cook, person living with Parkinson's

Self-efficacy is the belief that we can achieve influence over the conditions that affect our lives. It is a concept increasingly used with people living with Parkinson's as a way to assist us in taking a proactive role in the management of our disease. Research shows that people who are able to exert some control over their lives fare better and experience a better quality of life. Virtually everyone has some degree of self-efficacy. The challenge for people like me and you, who are living with Parkinson's, is to strengthen our self-efficacy and focus it in ways that help us better cope.

HOW SELF-EFFICACY CAN HELP

Building belief in our own capabilities increases our level of self-efficacy and influences what we are able to do. This increasing belief in our own power to effect change is a catalyst for a range of new, healthy behavior patterns. For example, we are able to maintain a more positive attitude that in turn positively impacts our emotional state and level of motivation. We are better able to find the strength from within to accept setbacks as challenges and to more easily persevere in the face of difficulties. For instance, while exercise may be more difficult for us (and in some cases, it may seem entirely too hard) by applying self-efficacy principles we can, particularly with the help of others, reinvigorate our exercise regimen and gain the quality of life and symptom improvement exercise can bring.

ENHANCING YOUR SELF-EFFICACY

A scientifically-based process for enhancing self-efficacy was developed by renowned psychologist, Dr. Albert Bandura, of Stanford University. The first step is to set a series of ever more difficult goals; the accomplishment of each enhances the belief that we can achieve the next. This creates an **experience of mastery**, which is the foundation of a strong sense of self-belief. The second step is to **identify a model** to which we aspire, such as one or more people living with Parkinson's who are managing their Parkinson's well. Seeing others in a similar situation succeed through their own determined efforts raises the belief that we, too, can overcome the specific challenges we face. The third step is to seek out **positive reinforcement and encouragement**, which strengthens our belief that we have what it takes to succeed. This approach is being used in the Parkinson's Self-Efficacy Learning Forum (PD SELF) programs now being conducted in ten different metropolitan areas in the US.

WHAT IS YOUR CURRENT STATE OF PARKINSON'S-RELATED SELF-EFFICACY?

The questionnaire below can help you determine the extent to which you are currently

seek treatment early and are specific about bothersome symptoms or problems, you'll help your doctor tailor the most effective treatment plan for you.

- **Be Active.** Learn how personal and lifestyle habits can impact the symptoms of Parkinson's. The more you know, the more empowered you'll feel to form useful habits to combat your symptoms. For instance, physical activity is important at all stages of Parkinson's. However, a regular exercise program will take time and energy from other aspects of your life. Knowing which activities to keep or eliminate will maximize the positive impact of the choices you can control.

- **Be Focused.** Prioritize symptoms and problems that you can modify and/or prevent. This means taking medications on time to limit symptoms and may include beginning rehabilitative therapy to improve posture or speech volume. It may mean exercising to improve your fitness, or changing your lifestyle to promote overall health by losing weight, stopping smoking and eating a healthy diet.

- **Be Flexible.** Learn positive ways to adapt and work with symptoms that you cannot change. For instance, if a bothersome tremor doesn't always respond to medications, try reducing the anxiety that can feed the tremor by practicing deep breathing relaxation techniques, rather than isolating yourself from others by limiting your social activities.

- **Be Connected.** Seek out support from people with whom you feel most comfortable sharing your thoughts and concerns. Your support network may include people you trust, such as specific family members, friends or individuals from community activities or work. Formal support groups can be helpful, but may not provide the personal focus you may need during your first years with Parkinson's.

exhibiting self-efficacy as it relates to managing your Parkinson's, and it can give you some sense of where you could improve those behaviors to better support your efforts in managing your disease.

On a scale of 1 to 5, rate your current level of confidence that you can perform the activity described, where 1 = "not at all confident," 3 = "adequate" and 5 = "very confident."

Develop Knowledge about Parkinson's and Its Treatment

____ I can accurately describe my Parkinson's in-depth.

____ I can describe in detail my specific motor and non-motor symptoms.

____ I keep a complete and updated list of my medications and dosages.

____ I know and follow the nutritional guidelines for Parkinson's.

____ I understand the precautions and interactions of my medications and supplements.

____ I know the range of available complementary treatments.

____ I know techniques to address my stress and anxiety.

Create Critical Partnerships

____ I have a strong and supportive relationship with my care partner.

____ I have discussed my support needs with my family.

____ I have established an open and trusting relationship with my doctor.

____ I have sought out other healthcare specialists to assist, as needed.

____ I know where to go for help.

____ I am aware of national and community Parkinson's resources.

____ I attend a Parkinson's support group or similar group.

Proactively Manage My Parkinson's

____ I accept responsibility as the manager of my own well-being.

____ I set increasingly difficult goals and make progress toward them.

____ I actively replace any unhealthy habits with healthy ones.

____ I track all my symptoms on a regular basis.

____ I keep thorough and up-to-date healthcare records.

____ I prepare for appointments with my doctors.

____ I communicate my concerns openly with my wellness team.

____ I advocate for myself rather than letting others speak for me.

____ I follow a regular Parkinson's-specific exercise regime.

Maintain a Self-Efficacious Attitude

____ I stay firm in the belief that I can positively influence my disease.

____ I focus on possibility rather than loss.

____ I practice evaluating available options in order to solve problems.

____ I put setbacks in perspective.

____ I reframe to help manage any negative emotions.

____ I persevere in the face of difficulties.

____ I remain hopeful and focus on the positive.

The resulting snapshot from the survey should give you a sense of where you are on the Self-Efficacy for Parkinson's Scale. If you have any 1s or 2s, these are areas to focus on. If you have 5s, give yourself credit and build on this success in the areas you need to strengthen. For example, if you gave yourself a low score on setting increasingly difficult goals, but had a high score on attending a support group, you could ask the leader of the group to incorporate some regular goal-setting activity into the meetings. If you gave yourself a low score on understanding the precautions and interactions of your medications, but a high score on seeking healthcare specialists to assist, you could use that skill to find a pharmacologist with whom to consult.

As you build your level of self-efficacy, you will find a renewed focus and energy to support you in achieving your goals and positively impacting the course of your disease.

69

THE PROCESS OF RESEARCH IN PARKINSON'S: A LONG AND WINDING ROAD

By Tim Collier, PhD

As a research scientist working on Parkinson's, the process of moving a discovery from the laboratory to practical use that could make a difference in people's lives feels painfully long. I can only imagine how long it seems for people living with Parkinson's.

WHY DOES IT TAKE SO LONG?

The short answer is that the process of research has many steps and there are few, if any, acceptable shortcuts. Reviewing recent publications that study the lag time between discovery and application, the Medical Research Council of Britain concludes that the average time between the discovery of a new treatment and its widespread availability is 17 years...and that may be optimistic.

The process begins with "basic" research done in the laboratory, using model systems relevant to one or more features of Parkinson's, which may or may not directly connect to a discovery that will be useful as a therapy. Even in the best scenario, this phase of the process includes unpredictable periods of time spent applying for funding for the project (which is uncertain at best and often requires multiple, 9-month cycles of application, review and re-application), conducting the experiments, revising the

- **Be Positive.** A positive outlook and environment is very important for anyone living with a chronic condition. Being positive keeps the focus on what you can do, not what you can't. A positive attitude fosters hope. Don't be too hard on yourself if you're having a bad day. Remember that tomorrow will bring another opportunity to take action.

- **Be Informed.** Regularly learn about Parkinson's, consulting accurate information from reputable sources (major research outlets and institutions, such as the National Institutes of Health or the Mayo Clinic, as well as respected national and local Parkinson's organizations) about advances in Parkinson's treatments and knowledge. Additionally, learn about offerings in your local area for people with Parkinson's, whether it is an educational event or a weekly yoga class. Steve's wife, Nancy, explains how she stays grounded in the midst of the information overload that can come with Parkinson's: 🎥 **dpf.org/nancy**.

Hear from veteran Parkinson's nurse practitioner, Susan Imke, about her philosophy of improving "just one little thing:" 🎥 **dpf.org/jolt**.

> **"** *I often meet other people living with Parkinson's who are lost in themselves, which is hard. I can show you what I do and encourage you to take action for yourself, but I can't make it happen for you."*
>
> **— EDIE**

HOW CAN I GET INVOLVED IN RESEARCH?

Less than 1% of people with Parkinson's participate in research studies. Those who do participate in research do so for various reasons: the hope of finding a new direction of experimentation based on results and once convinced of a finding, replicating it. For most research findings, the process ends here.

For the lucky ones that advance, the difficulties associated with funding basic research are magnified in the second phase of the process, known as "clinical" research. In this phase, the basic research finding is translated to testing in humans as a clinical trial. For testing a drug for a condition like Parkinson's, the 2014 report of the US Department of Health and Human Services estimates the average cost of a clinical trial is $40 million.

A clinical trial is divided into four phases of increasing complexity and numbers of participants, each with specific goals in mind:

Phase I: assess safety and optimal dosing of a treatment, often in volunteers who don't have Parkinson's

Phase II: assess effectiveness of the treatment, as compared to a placebo in people with Parkinson's

Phase III: compare the new treatment to the best current treatment in a larger population of people with Parkinson's

Phase IV: obtain approval of the therapy by the Food and Drug Administration (FDA)

Failure to meet these goals at any stage halts the process.

If everything goes smoothly, additional time and resources are devoted to creating informative materials that describe how to use the medication and possible side effects, as well marketing, distribution and ultimately, acceptance by practicing physicians and incorporation into their treatment approach. Arguably, the delay from discovery to application in the treatment of the condition is necessary to ensure safety and efficacy of a treatment for the majority of people, but that's why it takes so long.

WHY HAS RESEARCH PRODUCED SO LITTLE FOR PEOPLE LIVING WITH PARKINSON'S?

The short answer is: it's not for lack of trying. At the present time, there have been no major advances in therapy for Parkinson's since the discovery of levodopa and the development of deep brain stimulation (DBS). Unfortunately, this leads to impatience in the Parkinson's community, a perception that clinical trials routinely fail and a sense that participation in clinical trials is a waste of time and effort.

Not so. The truth is that fascinating research is being done on Parkinson's in hundreds of research laboratories around the world, but as you can see, the process is detailed and arduous. For Parkinson's clinical trials, several barriers to progress complicate the process. Chief among these is that our increasing understanding of the condition reveals the complexity of Parkinson's. The combination of multiple genetic, environmental and biological factors at work in producing the symptoms does not lend itself to a "silver bullet" approach to treatment.

Indeed, it is likely that each person living with Parkinson's arrived at their condition in unique and individual ways. If that hypothesis proves true, clinical trials participants will present an unpredictable mixture of specific types of Parkinson's. Any given treatment is likely to be effective in some, but not all, leading to the perception of failure when it is in fact a mistake to believe that any treatment can ever be "one size fits all."

In addition, the majority of people living with Parkinson's choose not to participate in clinical trials, particularly newly diagnosed individuals that feel relatively well. It is absolutely clear to scientists that treating people early in their history of Parkinson's, before many years of damage have occurred, offers the best opportunity for success. It is impossible to preserve what has already been lost.

It is natural for people with Parkinson's and their care partners to be highly invested in a "cure." But this leads to unrealistic high expectations, and often, repeated disappointment. As a scientist working in this area, I believe that a realistic and attainable goal is to discover interventions that slow, or halt, progression of Parkinson's making it a manageable, chronic condition that individuals can live with and live with well, similar to other chronic conditions like diabetes.

Finally, people living with Parkinson's have access to a massive volume of information regarding research. However, more information does not *necessarily* equal good information. If a research finding appears in the press, be cautious about the conclusions drawn. The press is in the "news business" and needs your attention, whether or not the information is completely accurate. Also, consider the source. A report from a person with an MD or PhD after their name does not make them an authority in all cases. Be discerning and give greater weight to information from academic institutions known for their research and neurologists certified as movement disorder specialists. Look for information provided by reliable sources: the National Institutes of Health, university websites, national Parkinson's foundations like the Davis Phinney Foundation, the Parkinson's Foundation and the Michael J. Fox Foundation, among others. Last, but not least, discuss research reports with your peers and doctors. It is likely that a combination of opinions will avoid "snap judgments" and come closer to the truth.

treatment for themselves or wanting to contribute to knowledge that will benefit others in the future.

You may be approached to participate in a research study, since many trials focus on people with early-stage Parkinson's who are not yet taking medication. This combination of factors allows scientists to study the effect of medication on early disease without the influence of other medications. Some studies also recruit people who do not have Parkinson's at all, so your care partner or others interested might be able to participate in a trial.

When deciding if enrolling in a research trial is right for you, it's important to understand that although everything is done to ensure the safety of research subjects, the full risks and benefits of experimental treatments being studied are not fully known. That said, without willing participants for clinical trials, important medical therapies would never become available. Every prescription drug used to treat Parkinson's (or any condition, for that matter) in the US has been tested in clinical trials prior to gaining approval by the Food and Drug Administration (FDA). Other countries have similar drug testing protocols to ensure safety.

A potential medication or therapy must clear many hurdles before being approved for use by the public. It must first undergo rigorous testing for safety and benefit in pre-clinical studies. These studies involve animals or take place in laboratory settings. If a compound shows promise in the laboratory, its effect is next examined in people. Human clinical trials have four phases, which progress from the earliest stage of discovery to testing potential medications or therapies on just a few people to extensive testing in large groups.

The FDA serves as the governing body in the US that approves a treatment if efficacy and safety outcomes are reached in Phase III trials.

BENEFITS OF PLACEBO-CONTROLLED TRIALS

- **Open label** studies measure the effect of a treatment, but do not compare its effect or outcome against a placebo. These studies can help determine if a treatment has possible merit. They cannot determine whether a treatment's benefit (or negative effect) is real or due to a more general, nonspecific effect (called a placebo). A strong placebo effect is well-documented in Parkinson's studies. Simply expecting or hoping that a medication will help can increase the chance that participants will experience an improvement in their symptoms. Placebo-controlled trials help ensure that any benefits experienced are the result of the medication or treatment being tested, rather than the influence of positive expectations.

- **A randomized controlled trial** randomly assigns participants to one treatment versus a second treatment or placebo. Since the assignment is random and not based on other individual factors, both treatment groups will be similar, which ensures that the trial is controlled for individual influences that can affect outcome (age, gender, duration of disease).

- **A randomized placebo-controlled trial** assigns a placebo to one treatment group, while another receives the active treatment being studied. Participating in this type of trial means that you might not be given the active medication, but will instead receive a placebo, an inactive pill or treatment. These studies are necessary because it's important for researchers to be sure that a benefit is not due to the placebo effect.

- **A double-blind study** is conducted with neither the researcher nor the volunteer knowing whether or not the active pill or treatment has been administered. **A double-blind randomized placebo-controlled trial** combines these features, and is the gold standard by which new medications are evaluated and approved

- **An extension study** is usually an extension of a clinical trial, allowing participants in a formal study to continue receiving the research treatment while it is awaiting FDA approval. This allows for ongoing monitoring of participants and evaluation of symptoms and side effects of the experimental treatment.

Research trials are not for everyone. They do offer an opportunity to become involved in the advancement of treatment in a careful and controlled manner. It is important to know your rights as a research participant before you participate in any research.

YOUR RIGHTS AS A RESEARCH PARTICIPANT

Biomedical research ethics have greatly evolved over the past 60 years, with the primary goal of protecting study subjects. The Nuremberg Code, established in 1948, defined the importance of voluntary participation in research and the requirement of informed consent. The doctor or researcher prepares an informed consent document for the volunteer, which defines the purpose of the research and its potential benefits and risks, using simple, understandable language. An informed consent document must be read, understood and signed before any

73

By Israel Robledo, person living with Parkinson's

Clinical trials are studies conducted at research sites that are designed to test the safety and effectiveness of compounds (medications) in order to determine if they can be prescribed to the general population. These are considered to be the best way to find out if the compound is actually working on a specific target, thereby alleviating symptoms.

Participation in clinical trials is extremely important. The medications currently available to us are on the market thanks to people who participated in prior clinical trials and gave researchers necessary data regarding safety and effectiveness.

Involvement in clinical trials for those with Parkinson's (and in some trials that may require a control group of people without Parkinson's) starts with researchers defining the type of participant sought for a clinical trial. In essence, specific types of people with Parkinson's are sought for each trial, and certain criteria allows someone to be included or excluded. Protocols include the rights, responsibilities and expectations of those participating and set out the proposed timeline for the trials, including how the active compound vs. a placebo will be assigned to the participants,

research can begin. Participants may be asked to sign another informed consent document if any details about the study have changed. Good clinical practice stipulates that research participants should be given a reasonable amount of time to review the document and should have a detailed discussion with the doctor or researcher prior to signing. Informed consents should contain several sections, including:

- Title of the study and names of the lead researcher and sponsor

- The rationale for the study and type of research to be conducted

- Information about the study drug, therapeutic method and use of placebo

- Selection criteria for participation

- Exact expectations during the study, including procedures and protocols and study duration

- Review of potential benefits, side effects and risks

- Alternatives if you do not participate

- Reimbursements, if any

- How confidentiality is protected

- The right to withdraw or refuse to participate

- How and with whom results will be shared

- Who to call if you have questions or adverse reactions to the therapy

In 1962, the US Congress passed the Kefauver Amendment, which required the FDA to ensure that drugs are effective and safe before releasing them to the public. In 1964, the World Medical Association set rules for doctors offering biomedical research to patients. These rules are known as the Declaration of Helsinki. They focus on both clinical and non-therapeutic research and form the backbone of the Good Clinical Practices guidelines used today. Congress passed the National Research Act in 1974, creating the National Commission for the Protection

how the effectiveness will be measured, how many follow-up visits to the site are necessary to check this, etc.

What you'll be asked to do during a clinical trial depends on the type of trial. Some require minimal involvement over a few months. Often, this involves return trips to a clinic for testing, scoring, etc. Others may take place over a longer duration, all the while making sure that the compound is continuing to prove safe over time. Most clinical trials are set up as "double-blind, placebo-controlled," which means that neither the investigator nor the participant know who is taking the active compound and who is taking the placebo. This is designed so that the results that are sought are not subjective and the effectiveness is only known after the results are evaluated when the trial is completed.

A common concern while participating in a clinical trial is whether you'll receive the active compound or the placebo. In my work as an advocate, I often hear from participants that through volunteering, they feel that they are on the cutting-edge of research, which often is the case when trialing compounds before they reach the market.

You may wonder whether or not clinical trial-related expenses incurred are reimbursable. Most clinical sites have funding for specific, reimbursable expenses. Each site has their own guidelines, and it is within your rights as a potential volunteer to ask for which reimbursements you'll qualify for during the trial. The research team should be happy to answer any questions.

To find clinical trials in your area, you can contact local medical research centers or ask your movement disorder specialist if they know of any clinical trials for which you might qualify. Any information that is provided is held in the strictest confidence by secure messaging. The only time that any researcher/coordinator is aware of your personal information is when you give consent to be contacted about participating in a clinical trial.

Any of us who have benefited from Parkinson's medications have others in the Parkinson's community who took part in clinical trials to thank. I've often heard clinical trial participants say that the results may not benefit them directly at this point in time, but that the future value for so many others is immeasurable. Consider participating in a clinical trial, and help researchers continue their work to discover a breakthrough that could delay, slow or even reverse the effects of Parkinson's.

of Human Subjects of Biomedical and Behavioral Research. This commission produced the Belmont Report, which further defined and solidified ethical principles for research in the US involving humans. The Belmont Report identified three principles that remain in practice today:

- **Principle of respect for individuals**. All individuals have the right to information and the freedom to decide their treatment. In research, this is ensured by using the informed consent document that outlines the proposed treatment in very understandable terms, stating that the research is voluntary at all times. Individuals who cannot give consent must have a surrogate decision-maker who can best decide on their behalf.

- **Principle of beneficence.** Individuals must be protected from harm. Research should minimize risks and maximize benefits with a clear, understandable explanation in the informed-consent materials.

- **Principle of justice.** The selection of research subjects must be fair.

In 1991, the majority of federal agencies that sponsored human research adopted policies regarding the protection of human participants, known as the Common Rule. The Common Rule requires protection of vulnerable patients (i.e., prisoners, children, pregnant women), requires appropriate informed consent and sets standards for institutional review boards (IRBs), conduct of research institutions and record keeping. While researchers and doctors must conduct themselves ethically, patients must also follow through on their commitment to allow for the most accurate data collection when a new therapy is under consideration, in order to protect individuals who may use the therapy in the future.

These rules help ensure that research is conducted in a humane and respectful fashion and maintain the highest level of safety possible for participants of research trials.

There are many ways to learn about clinical trials, including through your doctor or wellness team. Another good resource is the Michael J. Fox Foundation's Fox Trial Finder tool (☞ **foxtrialfinder.michaeljfox.org**), which matches volunteers with research opportunities.

WHAT CAN I EXPECT IN THE FUTURE?

Parkinson's changes over time, and each person experiences the progression and types of symptoms uniquely. Individuals react differently to the evolution of Parkinson's, the rate of change over time and how they cope with these changes. For some, uncertainty and fear of the unknown is one of the most difficult challenges of living with Parkinson's. **Figure 1** in this **What You Need to Know About Parkinson's** section provides a snapshot of changes that can occur, and this section also discusses both motor and non-motor symptoms in detail. Learn how Brenda lives in the present, while still planning for the future: 🎥 **dpf.org/brenda**.

> ❝ *Our life today is pretty good, so I try not to borrow tomorrow's trouble today. I really wanted to not allow Tim's diagnosis to steal the joy from whatever would be in 5 or 10 years. I was a little scared and frustrated and worried abut the future, but I've mostly pushed that away and tried to be an optimist.*❞
>
> — SHERYL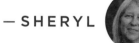

How you cope with changes emotionally will be an important factor in determining how you feel overall. Understanding that you'll have good days and not-so-good days will help you accept a bad day when it happens and remain hopeful for better days. Your reaction to the bad days is important, because the temptation to spend a lot of negative energy on them will take a toll on your well-being over time. Instead, try to devote your energy to being positive about the good days and as Davis Phinney suggests, being mindful of the days, the hours and celebrate those Moments of Victory® when Parkinson's is not in the forefront of your mind. Hear Davis describe his philosophy of celebrating Moments of Victory: 🎥 **dpf.org/davis**.

" When you don't accomplish one of your short-term goals, don't let that hold you back. Success is measured by the fact that you get back up and try again. You only fail if you stay down."

— EDIE

MANAGING EMOTIONS

Some people find it helpful to seek out positive things in life to focus on, rather than letting the negative prevail. One easy way to improve mood and attitude is through a simple exercise in gratitude, focusing on what you have, instead of what you don't or on what you've lost. Your own gratitude exercise could be as simple as finding a few minutes every day or week to reflect on what or who makes you feel grateful. Some people find it helpful to write these thoughts in a gratitude journal and return to them when they need a lift.

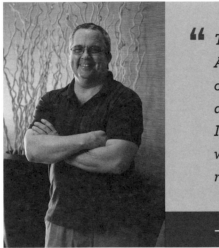

" There is always a choice, and that's where people struggle. Adversity hits and we think there's no way out, and get ourselves into a hole. I was so focused on what I couldn't do after I was diagnosed that I missed many of the things I could do. I wasn't finding the choices I have. Dealing with Parkinson's gets better when you understand the resources and the choices you have and take action."

— BRIAN

Early non-motor symptoms of Parkinson's can include anxiety, depression and insomnia. These symptoms can come, in part, from ineffective coping strategies and can lead to more stress or even to isolation. Talk to your doctor about these symptoms, even if you're not currently experiencing them. It's important to learn about the warning signs of emerging mood problems or inadequate coping strategies so that you can treat them and put your energy into what's most important in your life. Listen to Edie's husband, Scott, discuss Parkinson's-related emotional changes: ◼ **dpf.org/scott**.

Remember, you don't have to cope with Parkinson's alone. Younger people who've been recently diagnosed often don't tell family or friends. If you're inclined to keep your diagnosis private, consider confiding in at least one other individual. Have coffee with a friend or another person with Parkinson's, or share your thoughts with a loved one. Reading about the people featured in this manual, all of whom are living valiantly and graciously with Parkinson's, can be inspiring and empowering. Connect with a Davis Phinney Foundation ambassador at ↗ **dpf.org/ambassadors**. Their shared experiences and stories will assure you that you're not alone in what you're going through. Moreover, they can help reduce your learning curve by helping you identify issues, resources and strategies on a range of Parkinson's topics, saving you time and frustration.

You don't have to be clinically depressed to seek the help of a counselor or similar professional. They are there to help you (and your loved ones) understand your feelings, adjust to your diagnosis and take positive steps that will make a difference. Ask your doctor about a referral to a counselor.

INITIAL TREATMENT

WHEN SHOULD I START MEDICATION, AND WHICH ONE IS BEST?

The right medication, at the right time, in the right dosage is the best answer, but what does that mean for you? After initial diagnosis, some people want to start medication right away to eliminate all their symptoms. Others worry that medications are unnatural or toxic, and should be delayed until symptoms are more severe, focusing instead on exercise and other so-called "natural therapies," such as vitamins and supplements. You and your doctor should decide together when it's time for you to begin medication. There are some important factors to consider before and after you start medication:

- Over time, the motor problems associated with Parkinson's will affect the way you move and walk. Your pattern of muscle control will change, along with the fluidity, speed, precision and coordination of your movement. These changes will result in diminished movement or in altered patterns of movement that lead to further decline. Waiting to start medication can increase the impact of these motor problems. As your activity levels drop off, your strength and endurance will also decrease. You'll feel more tired and in need of assistance. Medication can help you maintain the control, coordination and speed necessary to walk, use your muscles and maintain a level of fitness that supports better quality of life.

- Medication can improve the neuroplastic benefits that occur with exercise. Neuroplasticity describes a change in brain function influenced by activity and experiences, so medication can improve how exercise and other activities may in fact affect the progression of your Parkinson's. This concept may also apply to the timing of medication. Medication can "normalize" altered patterns of movement, reinforcing positive brain changes that respond to enhanced motor fluidity, speed, precision and coordination.

- Research supports the early use of medication to treat Parkinson's motor symptoms. People participating in research have done better in the long term if they start the medication rasagiline early after diagnosis rather than delaying. Findings reinforce the hypothesis that timing in starting medication seems to impact motor function months later. Research has proven that medication reduces the accumulating health problems and disabilities associated with untreated Parkinson's.

- There are multiple medications for use in early stages of Parkinson's, including benztropine, trihexyphenidyl, carbidopa/levodopa, dopamine agonists, amantadine, selegiline and rasagiline. Which medication is best for you depends on many factors, including your age and the risk of side effects, and is best discussed with your doctor.

- The medication levodopa has been the gold standard for the treatment of Parkinson's since it was introduced in the 1960s, and it is still the most effective medication for the treatment of motor symptoms. Levodopa is most often found in combination with carbidopa, which reduces nausea caused by levodopa. As well, carbidopa increases the effectiveness of the levodopa, which means you need less levodopa to effectively treat the various symptoms levodopa helps manage.

- There are some misconceptions surrounding the use of levodopa. Contrary to what you might hear, levodopa does not stop working after five or six years of use. However, as your Parkinson's progresses, levodopa can wear off before your next dose, causing "on/off" fluctuations (read the chapter on "Medication" in the **Living Well Now** section for more information). There is a greater risk of dyskinesia (extraneous, uncontrollable movements) as dopamine neurons decline in mid-stage Parkinson's when levodopa is used at higher dosages. While fear of side effects like dyskinesia may lead some people to start with medications other than levodopa when they are initially diagnosed, levodopa may be the best first medication when side effect risk of the other medications options are high, such as in older individuals, people on many medications or those with more severe movement problems.

- Longer-acting medications, such as rasagiline and dopamine agonists, have a low risk of dyskinesia when used alone. Fear of levodopa side effects led to the common treatment approach of simply avoiding levodopa for as long as possible. This is not the best strategy for everyone. Other medications, such as dopamine agonists, have higher risks of serious side effects like confusion, hallucinations, dizziness, leg swelling and impulse control problems. Rasagiline has a lower side effect risk, but is often not strong enough to treat the movement symptoms as Parkinson's progresses, so treatment must be customized. A "levodopa-sparing strategy" can be used in younger people with less risk, which means using dopamine agonists or rasagiline together with levodopa to improve motor symptoms, while limiting side effect risks posed when individual medications are used at higher doses.

Talk to your doctor about which medication is best for you. Be sure to ask how side-effect risk and long-term complications, such as dyskinesia, influence this choice.

79

WHAT ABOUT COMPLEMENTARY AND ALTERNATIVE THERAPIES AND SUPPLEMENTS?

Complementary and alternative medicine (CAM) is a growing field in healthcare. It addresses many of the non-medical therapies that offer symptom relief. Complementary therapies such as physical therapy, occupational therapy and speech therapy are additional, important companions to medication. They can treat or prevent many symptoms affecting movement, speech and your ability to perform daily life and work activities. The **Living Well Now** section is devoted to living well with Parkinson's today and includes detailed information and tips on staying physically active, eating a well-balanced, nutrient-rich diet and tending to your emotional, creative and spiritual needs.

Vitamins, massage therapy and acupuncture are common alternative therapies used by people with Parkinson's. Research studies analyzing the effect of these therapies are limited and seldom control for the placebo effect. It's important to understand this, since some complementary and alternative therapies are helpful *only* by the placebo effect: that is, if you expect and believe that they will help, they will. Such therapies often rely on anecdotal stories from individuals touting their benefit.

> " *I don't see any alternative therapies as a cure, but I view them as a complement to the traditional medications I take. I use medical marijuana edibles for anxiety that are the same formulation they give children with epilepsy, and have a transdermal cream that I rub into my muscles when I get bad cramps. Nothing is a cure-all, but the cream relieves cramping at night so I can sleep.*"

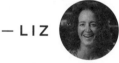

— LIZ

To date, no vitamin or supplement has been shown to help or delay the changes associated with Parkinson's, yet more and more people seek out vitamins and supplements for their health. Some people wish to boost their health with products more "natural" and "less toxic" than they perceive conventional medications to be. Others feel a greater sense of control when taking supplements they believe are good for their bodies. Still others feel that these natural chemicals may improve the body's intrinsic healing abilities. Watch Dr. Benzi Kluger discuss complementary and alternative therapies, including the research and possible side effects of medical marijuana: **dpf.org/alternative-therapies**.

Nevertheless, alternative therapies are gaining popularity and can be helpful. Be sure to talk with your doctor before beginning any therapy, including vitamins or supplements.

Some important information to consider:

- Vitamins and supplements are marketed and sold for their wellness and disease-fighting potential. Research shows that vitamins are only helpful if you have a deficiency in that particular vitamin. Amino acid therapy, Coenzyme Q10, glutathione, citicholine, NADH, N-acetyl cysteine, turmeric and fish pills are just a few of the supplements taken by people with Parkinson's, despite a lack of hard, scientific evidence for their benefit. Yet many people still take vitamin B12 for energy, vitamin C for immune health and vitamin E for potential antioxidant effects. Note that high dose vitamin E and use of calcium supplements is associated with early mortality and heart disease in some studies, showing that even vitamins have risk.

- Many people with Parkinson's have low levels of vitamin D, which can negatively impact bone strength, thinking and even the risk of falling. Before taking vitamin D, it's important to understand that it is a fat-soluble vitamin, meaning that high doses will be stored cumulatively in fat tissue. Therefore, taking too much vitamin D can be toxic and supplementation should be guided by your doctor. Dose range varies significantly, so a simple blood test is recommended to detect whether you have a deficiency and the degree of its severity. The results of your blood test will determine how much vitamin D you should take in order to avoid toxicity. Be sure to get your blood levels rechecked a few months after starting vitamin D to ensure treatment is effective.

- A nutritious diet is much tastier and easier to stomach than a pill, especially considering the cost of supplements. Vitamins and supplements are expensive and should never take the focus away from healthier eating. Nutrients in food are associated with health promoting effects, but this is not always the case when the same nutrient is taken in pill form. Increasingly, researchers are finding direct correlations between health risk, disease and the typical American diet high in red meat, processed and fatty foods. A healthier alternative is a Mediterranean diet, low in saturated fats from red meat, but high in good fats (olive oil, avocado and nuts), whole grains and powerful, antioxidant-rich fruits and vegetables. The many benefits of this type of diet include anti-inflammatory effects and cardiovascular health. One study linked a Mediterranean diet to a 48% reduction in the risk of developing Parkinson's.

- Acupuncture, massage and energy medicine, such as Reiki therapy or therapeutic touch, are not proven therapies in the treatment of Parkinson's; however, they can improve well-being for many. These and other relaxation therapies can decrease stress, and stress negatively affects the motor symptoms of Parkinson's. These alternative therapies can be helpful, but you'll need to engage them regularly to derive the most benefit.

- Mindfulness meditation is an effective way to manage stress, fear and uncertainty about the future. Mindfulness is a technique in which one brings their full attention to the moment without judgment. Simply bringing awareness to the moment helps you control the "mind-chatter" or negative reactions and emotions that can accompany your symptoms.

81

- A quick-fix in a pill is likely too good to be true. Better, lifelong strategies for living your best with Parkinson's include improving your lifestyle through diet and physical activity and focusing on emotional health and stress reduction. More information on vitamins, supplements and living better through lifestyle change is available in the "Diet and Nutrition" chapter in the **Living Well Now** section.

- Be aware of the potential extended side effects of taking supplements. These include the financial costs, as well as the limitations you might place on your well-being if you neglect your exercise routine or diet in the hope that a supplement will compensate for insufficient attention to these healthy behaviors.

- When searching for a vitamin or supplement, look for products tested for purity, potency and bioavailability (how the vitamin or supplement is absorbed by the body) by an independent laboratory that tests the purity, potency and bioavailability of products and ensures that what is claimed on the label is an accurate description of purity and strength of the substance.

Discuss CAM therapies with your doctor to weigh the risk versus benefit for you, being sure to consider the cost of the therapy as you make your decision.

82

❝ *I didn't know what to expect before I started taking medical marijuana. It felt like a real counter-culture that I didn't see myself fitting into, but now that I've tried it, I think differently and it's made me more open to alternative therapies. I do discuss using medical marijuana with my doctor. She believes that there hasn't been substantial research on the effects of marijuana, especially in conjunction with all of my other medications. So while she doesn't necessarily recommend it, she's open to keeping it in the mix if it seems to be working for me.*❞

— LIZ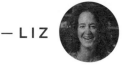

FAMILY, RELATIONSHIPS AND WORK

You may wonder how your diagnosis will change you, your relationships and your family. As you read the many personal accounts of people living well with Parkinson's throughout this manual, you'll notice a common thread: Parkinson's can change relationships over time. However, you may be surprised to learn that for some couples, these changes can be positive ones. Couples who cope most successfully tend to understand and prepare together for the challenges of Parkinson's. They prioritize their time with one another, reconnect and strengthen relationships with family members.

HOW WILL MY PERSONAL RELATIONSHIPS CHANGE?

Your spouse or partner and family members are dealing with the diagnosis of Parkinson's in the best way that they can. Some people take on the role of care partner, seeking to do as much as possible. They may deal with the uncertainty of diagnosis by taking control of medical appointments, treatment decisions and lifestyle changes. They may be vigilant about monitoring your movements, carefully noting any changes from day to day. If the focus on your Parkinson's is too great, it may cause anxiety and tension in your relationship. Some partners choose to deal differently with the uncertainty and fear accompanying diagnosis. They distance themselves and avoid getting involved with medical appointments or treatment decisions. Others take a middle-of-the-road approach, balancing their involvement in a way that allows the person with Parkinson's to remain in primary control. Hear how Linda's husband, Mike, helps her as her care partner: ■**dpf.org/linda**.

> " *The biggest thing is to not forget that we are a couple, and that doesn't change. We just have to problem-solve together whatever life is giving us today. Sometimes he has to hold me up, and he rises to the challenge. We play that role for each other.*"
>
> — SHERYL

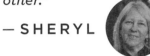

There is no right or wrong approach. Over time, reactions to your Parkinson's will evolve. Of course, those reactions depend on the personalities of both people in the relationship. Your own response to your diagnosis will inevitably affect your partner and his or her response. Talk about your concerns and how you would like to handle Parkinson's together. Decide the extent to which you want your care partner involved in your treatment. Read the **Parkinson's and the Family** section for additional perspectives from spouses and children of people living with Parkinson's.

> " *I've grown to recognize how protective Lily is of me and my energy, but for a long time, I felt like I was being treated like a child and it created conflict. After I became a care partner for Lily when she was battling breast cancer, I finally understood the tremendous amount of anxiety that comes when you're worried about your partner. Now if I get upset with Lily about something, I sit back and wonder what I would do if I was in her shoes.*"
>
> — BRIAN

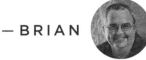

Coming together in times of adversity can sometimes strengthen relationships, and this can certainly be true after the diagnosis of Parkinson's. Take this moment as an opportunity to examine your life and decide what's most important to you. Prioritizing your close relationships can be important for the whole family during times of change and uncertainty. Listen to Steve discuss how he and his wife manage Parkinson's together: ■**dpf.org/steve**.

> *I was head-down focused on my job all the time, and the energy I had left, I spent at home – not volunteering. It took Parkinson's to shake me out of my complacency. The things I think are important and the way I choose to spend my time have changed. I don't think Parkinson's is a gift, but it's made me focus more on things that are important as opposed to things that are urgent and demanding my attention."*

— COREY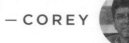

Communication is an important part of any relationship, and this is especially true when dealing with a chronic condition like Parkinson's. If you're suffering from depression or apathy, it may appear to others that you just don't care. Parkinson's can also blunt your facial expression, a condition referred to as facial masking, and cause softer, more monotone speech. Friends and family may assume that you're uninterested or not invested in what's going on around you. A speech therapist can help you manage these symptoms, and letting people know that some of what they're seeing is symptomatic of Parkinson's will foster greater understanding. Learn more about how facial masking influences perception and relationships: 🔊 dpf.org/mask.

> *I have to bite my tongue sometimes because my husband doesn't understand all that I'm dealing with. He's learning, but he's on his own journey. We give each other space when things get crazy."*

— EDIE

WILL PARKINSON'S AFFECT MY SEX LIFE?

Later in this section, we'll discuss sexual function and intimacy for people with Parkinson's in general. If you've just been diagnosed, however, you may also experience changes in sexual function or intimacy for many reasons other than Parkinson's or the side effects of your medication. The emotional impact of the diagnosis can interfere with your desire for sexual intimacy, and you may be too distracted to initiate sex or participate with any interest.

In its early stages, Parkinson's can drain you emotionally, leaving little energy for other people. Discussing emotions isn't always easy, and it may simply take time to adjust and adapt to the idea of living with Parkinson's. On the other hand, some people experience an enhanced sex drive after being diagnosed. This may be a reaction to the unknown future, or it may also be a side effect of certain medication, especially dopamine agonists.

You may find the topic of sexual dysfunction gets little to no priority during medical visits, even though it may be high on your list. If your concerns aren't getting enough attention, ask your doctor who is best suited to address them. Sexual dysfunction is a pervasive problem in Parkinson's, and it may take a multidisciplinary approach to achieve the best outcome for you and your partner. Medical problems such as diabetes, hypertension, heart disease and the side effects of some medications can also affect sexual performance. Specialists who can help include gynecologists, urologists, sex therapists, counselors or a primary care physician.

> *I have a lot of pain because of Parkinson's that gets worse at night, which has limited some of our intimacy. At the same time, my wife and I have a very rich connection and intimacy in our conversation that is better than it's ever been. We're more emotionally intimate as well as more aware of gentle, tender touching."*
>
> — BRIAN

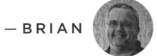

If you're concerned about sexual intimacy, talk about it with your spouse or partner. This might be an opportunity for you to connect on an emotional level. Make time for this discussion, and remember that intimacy is an important part of your relationship. A counselor can help you and your partner navigate these relationship changes.

WHOM SHOULD I TELL ABOUT MY PARKINSON'S?

With whom and when you should share your diagnosis is a very personal decision, and it depends on many different factors. Before talking openly about their diagnosis, many people worry about:

- The added stress on their children
- Not being able to explain the many unknowns about Parkinson's
- Being treated differently by family, friends and peers
- Receiving too much attention due to the Parkinson's
- Losing a job or friendships
- Being misunderstood or left out
- Feeling vulnerable
- Talking about the diagnosis makes it real

Ask your doctor to refer you to a social worker or other professional with whom you can discuss your fears or worries. You may feel less anxiety if you learn how to begin talking about Parkinson's with your family and friends without fully revealing your diagnosis. The more you know about Parkinson's, the easier it will be to talk with others and alleviate their fears on your behalf.

> *You have to get people on board with you. I used to be embarrassed when my husband would tell people I had Parkinson's. Now, I ask the gal next to me at Bible study to encourage me to write with intent."*
>
> — LINDA

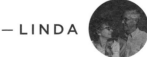

WORKPLACE ISSUES

The average age of onset for Parkinson's is 60 years of age, so many people won't reach retirement age until years after diagnosis. Young onset individuals may just be hitting the peak of their careers or still raising young children. No matter when the diagnosis hits, the financial implications are real and concerning. Hear more about Jill's experience running a business with Parkinson's and her choice to retire: 🎥 **dpf.org/jill**.

> *" Be sure you've taken steps to make a deliberate, well-informed decision about when to stop working. We all have to think about when to retire, whether or not we have Parkinson's. I don't think you should just wake up one day and say, 'I think I'll retire'."*

— **COREY**

SHOULD I TELL MY COWORKERS I HAVE PARKINSON'S?

There are pros and cons to informing your employer and colleagues about your diagnosis. In an ideal workplace situation, you won't have to spend much energy hiding your symptoms or worrying about being found out. You may find support, camaraderie and genuine kindness from your coworkers. Your positive, take-charge attitude will be a source of inspiration and admiration for your peers. Your boss and coworkers may work with you to find new ways to achieve your goals, perform difficult tasks and get the job done.

> *" My physical symptoms and inability to concentrate during meetings became so obvious that I was afraid I'd lose my job – I would have lost all my insurance, which would have been devastating to my family. So I trusted my boss, and told him."*

— **COREY**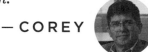

Conversely, revealing your diagnosis could have very different consequences. Your boss and coworkers might be inflexible and unaccommodating to your situation. They might show little or no commitment to making work a positive experience for you, or even possible.

Before you decide whether or not to be open at work about Parkinson's, think about your job, coworkers and the people in positions of authority in your workplace. Is there a history of trust, a culture of flexibility and innovation, camaraderie and teamwork? What is the economic and financial situation of your company? Do your unique skills and experience make you irreplaceable? Are there protections that will prevent you from being pushed out? Do you have disability insurance?

These are tough questions that deserve serious consideration. Many organizations offer confidential counseling through employee-assistance programs. Seek counseling outside the workplace if you're uncomfortable bringing up the diagnosis with your employer. The decision about whether to be open at work is an individual one, and learning your options will help you in your deliberations. Know your rights, and consult with an attorney who specializes in disability, discrimination or workplace issues. He or she can help you decide how much and how soon you want to disclose at work, as well as to understand what may be covered under disability.

> " *I looked normal, I wasn't shaking or walking funny. People probably wondered why I was retiring, but I started to feel the effects of Parkinson's and thought I'd cut bait and get the most out of life while I still could. We went on cycling trips to Europe and really took advantage of spending a lot more time with my family.* "
>
> — S T E V E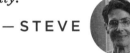

Workplace issues are some of the more stressful topics that people with Parkinson's confront. Financial circumstances are often the overriding concerns when making this decision. It's important to talk with your doctor about these issues, as the added stress is likely to worsen your symptoms. Once the decision is made, many people find that their symptoms improve.

WHAT STEPS CAN I TAKE TO ENSURE I CAN WORK AS LONG AS POSSIBLE?

Make a list of the duties that your job requires today and may require in the future. The following list of questions to ask yourself is not complete, but illustrates duties and skills to include:

- Is the job physical, requiring a good deal of mobility or stamina, or is balance needed to climb ladders, etc.?

- Do you primarily have a desk job that requires you to multitask and be cognitively sharp throughout the day?

- Do you use the computer?

- Is driving required for work?

DISABILITY OPTIONS FOR PEOPLE WITH PARKINSON'S

By Deanna Power

You and your doctor have talked about the progressive nature of Parkinson's. You probably feel some uncertainty about the future, knowing that your symptoms will eventually worsen, making it difficult or impossible for you to keep working. If you are like most people living with Parkinson's, considering how your health will eventually affect your financial security can cause some degree of anxiety or panic to set in. Questions may race through your mind:

- What if I have to stop working before I'm able to retire?

- How will I get by without a paycheck?

- What am I going to do about health insurance?

- How will I pay the bills?

- What if I can't afford to go to the doctor or get my prescriptions?

- Am I going to qualify for disability?

- Where can I get help?

Thinking about the uncertainty of it all can be scary, so you probably try not to focus too much on what might happen and when. Instead, you try to stay positive, do what you can to manage symptoms and go on with your life.

87

Still, you also know that just like everybody else, you do have to plan for the future, and as a person with Parkinson's, that means facing those nagging, anxiety-inducing questions head on.

WHO QUALIFIES FOR DISABILITY WITH PARKINSON'S?

Given what you know about Parkinson's and how it progresses, it may surprise you to learn that not everyone that applies for disability is approved. Sometimes people are denied because they apply too soon, before they meet the medical eligibility rules. Others simply don't qualify for a particular disability program, and to make things even more confusing, eligibility requirements vary by location.

Knowing whether you'll qualify for disability means digging deep into the program rules that apply where you live:

- In the US, disability benefits are managed by the Social Security Administration (SSA), and the specific requirements for qualifying are detailed in the Blue Book (⌨ **ssa.gov**), which we'll discuss in more detail below.

- In Canada, provincial and territorial governments administer some disability programs, while the national government is responsible for others, such as the Canadian Pension Program (Visit ⌨ **canada.ca** and search "Canada Pension Plan Disability Benefit - Overview"), the Registered Disability Savings Plan (Visit ⌨ **canada.ca** and search "Registered Disability Savings Plan") and the Disabled Tax Credit (Visit ⌨ **cra-arc.gc.ca** and search "Disability Tax Credit"). Canadians should explore these programs to learn more.

- Throughout the European continent, social insurance is common, including some form of disability benefits or disability pension for qualified individuals. As a European, you should consult the social insurance, disability or welfare section of your local, regional or national government's website to learn more.

WHAT ARE THE SSA'S DISABILITY PROGRAMS?

Americans that receive Social Security disability benefits may include people with disabilities and, sometimes, their children and spouses, as well. Benefits may be paid through Social Security Disability Insurance (SSDI) and/or Supplemental Security Income (SSI). Each program has its own technical eligibility rules:

- SSDI is a program for disabled workers. It requires you have worked in the last 10 years and that you have sufficient work credits accumulated from your previous employment (learn more at ⌨ **disabilitybenefitscenter.org**). Credits are earned through the payment of Social Security taxes and usually build at the rate of four per year of employment. Fortunately, the vast majority of people with Parkinson's will qualify for SSDI benefits. You will only need to have earned about $5,000 per year to qualify.

- SSI is a program with no work history requirement, but strict financial qualification rules since it is need-based. Before approving an SSI application, the SSA must review all of your income and assets in addition to those of your spouse or possibly others in your household.

MEETING THE SSA'S PARKINSON'S DISABILITY LISTING

Although Parkinson's is an eligible medical condition under SSA guidelines, you'll only qualify for benefits if your current medical status meets the severity levels described in the Blue Book Parkinson's disability listing (found at ⌨ **ssa.gov/disability/professionals/bluebook**). Specifically, your medical records must show your that symptoms remain uncontrolled, despite following prescribed treatments for at least three months. Your symptoms must additionally include at least one of the following:

- Disorganized motor function in two extremities, making it extremely difficult or impossible for you to do at least one of the following:

  - Rise to your feet from a seated position without assistance
  - Balance when walking or standing, again, without assistance
  - Use your shoulders, arms or hands to reach, push, pull or perform other actions

OR

- Pronounced limitations in functioning physically, along with at least one of the following mental limitations:

  - Comprehending, recalling or processing information
  - Interacting with other people
  - Completing tasks at a reasonable pace due to persistence or concentration issues
  - Adapting to new situations or circumstances

HOW DO YOU KNOW WHEN TO APPLY FOR DISABILITY FROM THE SSA?

Remaining in the workforce for as long as possible may reflect a desire for personal and financial independence that you're not ready to give up just yet. If your symptoms worsen though, you might not have a choice and will need to consider disability. The thought may worry you from the perspective that continued employment gives you consistent income, access to medical insurance and other benefits.

Disability benefits also afford you consistent income, and if you receive SSDI, you'll be eligible for Medicare coverage in two years. In the meantime, you may qualify for Medicaid, particularly if you also receive disability payments through the SSI program, since the need-based measures for these two programs are quite similar.

Providing for your healthcare needs is a major concern, but an employer-sponsored medical plan is only one way to maintain insurance. There are other methods for ensuring you have what you need while you wait for a disability decision or while waiting for Medicare eligibility to kick in after you start receiving disability benefits. Options include:

- COBRA coverage through your former employer
- Income-based, state-sponsored insurance plans, if available in your home state
- Benefits through your spouse's insurance plan
- Coverage for yourself purchased through an independent plan or the Healthcare Marketplace (**healthcare.gov**)

It's also important to note that Medicaid coverage is offered in several states to individuals that receive disability benefits, even if they don't get SSI. In other words, you may be eligible for Medicaid immediately after SSDI approval, even if you aren't sure you'll meet the income-based eligibility requirements for also getting benefits through SSI.

You'll need to consider other options for providing for your medical and general financial needs too, especially since a disability application can sometimes take weeks or months to go through the SSA's review processes:

- You may decide to borrow money from a retirement or life insurance plan
- You can draw from or cash out a 401k or other savings or retirement account

Other social assistance programs can also help ease financial concerns, and you may qualify for support through county, state or federal programs. A social worker with the department or bureau of family and social services in your home state can help you investigate available programs and apply for assistance through those for which you may qualify. You can also investigate some of your options independently, via the US government's website (**benefits.gov**), which provides links to various assistance programs for people with disabilities.

PREPARING TO SUBMIT A DISABILITY CLAIM

Before applying for disability, you'll want to review the SSA's Adult Disability Starter Kit (found at ⌖ **ssa.gov/disability**). This kit will give you a better understanding of the application process and the kinds of information you'll need to gather for completing disability claim forms. It also contains some forms you'll complete in advance that are then used throughout the application process as "cheat sheets," if you will. These cheat sheets are important because answering questions consistently in the disability application can help you avoid unnecessary delays in the review of your claim.

Timing a disability application appropriately can mean the difference between a quick review resulting in approval for benefits, or a denial notice from the SSA. The potential that you could be denied may make you hesitant to submit a claim, and some people wait until their situation is quite desperate before they start the process. Waiting too long can put you in dire straits financially, so it's important to consider all your options and ideally, begin your application before your circumstances enter the critical stage.

A disability attorney or advocate can advise you on the right time to start your application and can even manage your claim throughout the review and appeals processes, if an appeal hearing is necessary in your case. If you're worried about how you'll afford legal help, you should know that disability attorneys offer free, initial consultations and then work on contingency, meaning they only get paid if you get approved for disability benefits.

SUBMITTING AN APPLICATION ON BEHALF OF SOMEONE WITH PARKINSON'S

The first step in filing a claim for disability is to complete the SSA's application. This can be done online (⌖ **ssa.gov/disabilityssi**) or in person at your local SSA office.

- Filing online is often the fastest way to initiate a claim, and a disability attorney, advocate, social worker, or a friend or family member can help you file, if you need assistance.

- If you decide to apply in person, an SSA representative can assist you. You also can have someone else attend the application appointment along with you, like a friend, family member or attorney.

- If necessary, someone else can even apply for benefits on your behalf, though you will still need to sign off on the application forms before your claim commences through the review process.

Some people living with Parkinson's don't automatically qualify under the standard disability listing from the Blue Book but may be eligible for benefits nonetheless. Arguing eligibility in cases like this usually requires an appeal hearing (learn about an appeal hearing at ⌖ **disabilitybenefitscenter.org**). Winning benefits at a hearing often means tapping into the experience and knowledge or a disability attorney. In fact, a legal advocate can significantly increase the chances of approval due to the fact attorneys know what evidence or arguments are needed to win a claim in front of a judge, which makes hiring a disability attorney even more crucial to consider. If you are consider hiring an advocate or attorney for help, keep in mind that your attorney is also not paid unless you win, so there will not be any steep out-of-pocket costs. If you do choose to find legal assistance, a great resource to start looking for Social Security attorneys is your state bar association's website.

The most important component of any claim is making sure you carefully fill out your application. If the SSA cannot find your medical records, your claim will not be approved. The average claim takes approximately five months to be approved, but some applicants could receive benefits even sooner.

- Do you rely on specific talents, such as drawing?

- Do you manage people or events?

- Do you enjoy your job, does it add a sense of self-worth or value to life, and does this override the stressors that come with work? Is the opposite true?

Put a plan in place to help you stay on top of your job requirements now and in the future. Assemble your team (remember the importance of teamwork described earlier!). Talk to your doctor about medications, especially if they are not controlling your movement symptoms, they are wearing "off" during certain periods of the day or if you're experiencing side effects that can affect your job performance (sedation, thinking changes and impulsivity control).

An occupational therapist can help you with time and organizational management, as well as setting up an efficient and ergonomic workstation. He or she can also recommend adaptive aids and computerized gadgets to help you get the job done. A physical therapist can help if your job requires physical strength, stamina or balance. A neuropsychology evaluation is useful if you're experiencing changes in attention and concentration, multitasking, planning or completing a task. Rehabilitation specialists are integral to helping you manage the demands of work.

> **"** *When I sold the business, I stayed involved, maybe 30 hours per week the first year. Before Parkinson's, I enjoyed working 55-60 hours per week, but that 30 hours per week felt like I was on vacation and made a huge difference in my stress level and how I felt."*

— STEVE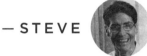

Depending on the symptoms that you experience, workers in the US may be protected under the Americans with Disabilities Act (ADA). While specific conditions, including Parkinson's, are not covered under the act, as of 2014, the ADA provides a general definition of disability (⊂ **ada.gov**) that each person must meet in order to be protected. It is important to note that because Parkinson's is different for everyone, you might not fit the ADA definition of disability; however, if you do, your employer is required to provide you with reasonable accommodations to ensure that you can perform the essential functions of the job, as long as it does not cause an "undue hardship" for the company. Your human resources department can help you determine what accommodations your employer can make if you wish to continue working. Some examples of reasonable accommodations are using assistive technology, telecommuting or creating a flexible work schedule. Your employer may offer an Employee Assistance Program (EAP), a voluntary, confidential program that helps employees navigate various life challenges that may affect their health, job performance and personal well-being through counseling and support. EAPs are often offered in conjunction with your employer's health insurance plan, but depend on the company. Check what options are available at your place of work. An important difference between consulting your human resources department and

LEGAL ISSUES WITH RESPECT TO EMPLOYMENT: WHAT TO CONSIDER WHEN YOU'VE BEEN DIAGNOSED WITH PARKINSON'S

By John Baumann, JD, person living with Parkinson's

In a strange twist of fate, when I was diagnosed with Parkinson's, I was an employment lawyer defending employers against allegations of disability discrimination. I was just 41 years old and in shock when I heard the words, "You have Parkinson's disease." I believe many, if not all, people with Parkinson's who are still in the workforce don't know what to consider with respect to informing their employer.

There are so many things that you feel that you have to deal with first, following diagnosis. Add to your list one more task: identify an employment attorney before informing your employer of your diagnosis.

Telling your employer you have Parkinson's brings many concerns, including potential impacts this could have on your career. In the US, there are two primary legal statutes to be aware of that will impact your work as someone living with Parkinson's. The first is the Family & Medical Leave Act (FMLA), which requires covered employers to provide employees with job-protected and unpaid leave for qualified medical and family reasons. The second is the Americans with Disabilities Act (ADA), a civil rights law prohibiting discrimination against individuals with disabilities in all areas of public life.

Your Parkinson's may qualify you (and possibly, your care partner) for FMLA benefits. FMLA time off includes intermittent leave. That is important because most of us living with Parkinson's suffer from fatigue, and intermittent leave can be taken in small increments, allowing you to take periodic leave when you are suffering from any manifestation of Parkinson's that prevents you from working for a period of time.

The ADA is violated if an employer negatively considers your disability in not hiring you, not promoting you, disciplining you, demoting you, firing you, etc. Further, the employer must provide any "reasonable accommodation" needed. While this is the employer's responsibility, it is in your best interest to involve yourself in the process. Take charge. Provide input. You know how you are affected by your disability better than anyone. If you want to reduce the chance that you will be provided with an unacceptable or less favorable accommodation, you need to offer an accommodation that works best for you. At the very least, you are on record of providing an accommodation. **Remember to put everything in writing.**

It can be very difficult to prove that an employer violated the ADA. To help determine if an employer has violated the ADA, the courts have developed a 3-step analysis:

First, the individual must prove that they suffered an adverse employment action and that they are a member of a protected class (in the case of Parkinson's, a disability). You clearly are a protected class, as long as you have notified our employer that you have Parkinson's.

Second, the employer must simply "articulate" a non-discriminatory reason for the employment decision.

Finally, the individual has the burden of proving that the reason given is a "pretext" — that not only is the reason given by the employer not the real reason, but also, that the real reason is because of your disability. So, you could prove that the employer is lying about the reason provided, yet fail to **prove** that the real reason is your disability and lose the case.

It is unlikely that you will find a "smoking gun" email stating, "We should fire Joe Smith because he has Parkinson's." It's more likely that to uncover a pattern of discrimination (i.e., everyone living with a disability is disciplined, demoted, not promoted or fired). My advice is to bend over backwards to **not** give your employer any reason to discharge you.

If you are seeking employment and feel that a company violated the ADA by not hiring you because of your disability, you have a much more difficult hill to climb. You must prove that the companies you applied to for a position **did not hire you due to your disability**. If you secure an interview and you decide to disclose that you have Parkinson's (for instance, when your hand tremors while you're answering questions), the potential employer will be on notice of your disability and, if they don't hire you, be subject to the above 3-step analysis. There is usually some objective component to the hiring process, so you would have to obtain access to the results for you and the candidate or candidates hired. This is not easy to do. Furthermore, if there is a subjective component to the hiring process, it becomes even more difficult to prove pretext, or that the reason the prospective employer had for not hiring you was not what they've stated, but instead solely the fact that you have Parkinson's. Finally, before filing a lawsuit under the ADA, you must file a complaint with the Equal Employment Opportunity Commission (EEOC). The EEOC may be able to assist in obtaining the necessary records to build your case.

All this said, you should be encouraged that some employers have seen the light and are making changes, such as adopting a "Workplace Proactive Prevention Culture Program" to teach management how to comply with the law.

Just as Parkinson's is different for all of us, each job situation is unique. The best approach is to take the time to pause and consult with an employment attorney before you find yourself in an adverse situation. It's important to note that many companies really do want to do right by their employees. Unfortunately, you might not know for sure which side your employer is on until you're in the situation of disclosing your Parkinson's. When the time comes to have that conversation, you want to have the peace of mind that comes from knowing your rights under the law and being ready to speak with confidence, prepared to advocate for yourself as necessary.

an Employee Assistance Program is that EAPs are employee benefits designed to help during stressful events and are required to keep all conversations confidential.

If you need to take time off from employment for reasons related to Parkinson's (while adjusting to medication, for surgery, etc.) you might qualify for medical leave under the Family and Medical Leave Act (FMLA). This act entitles employees to an unpaid, extended leave of absence for specified family and medical reasons. It also ensures that your employer provided health insurance continues during your leave. There are specific criteria that must be met in order to qualify for FMLA, so be sure to check with your employer to verify your eligibility before you schedule a leave. You can find more information about FMLA at the Department of Labor (dol.gov). If you live outside of the US, see what similar protections may exist in your country.

" *I felt like I needed to explain it, rather than just saying, 'I have to retire.' Once I went on long-term disability, I knew I wasn't going back to work ever again. I felt guilty, embarrassed and ashamed."*

— COREY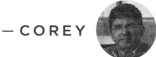

It's impossible to overstate the impact of stress on you and your symptoms; if you are uncomfortable in the situation and feeling anxious, your symptoms will be aggravated, which will only make you feel more stressed. Until you have established a plan to help yourself be effective at work, the worry and stress of job-related concerns can be overwhelming, making it more difficult to focus at work. Making a plan and enlisting the help of an attorney, financial planner or other advisor knowledgeable about these things can provide the peace of mind that you need to reduce your stressful feelings. Additionally, many stress-management techniques may fit your lifestyle; some serve a dual purpose, such as yoga for relaxation, strength and balance, or meditation for stress management, emotional well-being and clarity of thought.

HOW CAN I PREPARE FOR RETIREMENT?

Review all of your insurance policies (life, long-term care and disability). Evaluate whether they are adequate to protect you and your family or whether your coverage should be increased. Insurance policies can be obtained after you have been diagnosed, but may be much more expensive. A financial planner or accountant can help you analyze the costs and benefits of increasing or adding insurance policies. Organizations such as the American Association of Retired People (aarp.org) can also provide good information as you review your options.

> " *My Parkinson's encouraged my husband to retire earlier to spend time with and take care of me. He was working all day and then coming home to take care of both me and the kids, which was a lot. He does the laundry, the housework, the finances. Like many husbands, he's always done some of those, but now it's on a totally different level. When I do help, it's not with the same energy at the same level I used to."*
>
> — JILL

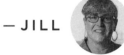

If you're just nearing retirement at the time of diagnosis, you have an opportunity to make this time fulfilling for yourself while enjoying the flexibility to proactively manage your schedule to keep you feeling your best. Commit to focusing on positive lifestyle changes and social engagement. People often experience a loss of self or identity when they retire from a life of working. Resist the temptation to replace work with passive time in front of the television. Instead, add purpose, meaning and value to these years by volunteering, taking up a hobby, getting involved in the community, joining an exercise class or club, engaging in spiritual activities and supporting others.

WHAT ABOUT LONG-TERM CARE PLANNING?

Long-term care planning is a task that resembles the other proactive strategies reviewed in this manual. Being proactive and discussing the situations you may face in the future is a positive endeavor and will help you avoid a crisis later on. Ask your wellness team about their experience with people with Parkinson's who find they need long-term care. Their insights will help guide your thoughts about possible future needs and how to plan ahead. For instance, when falling becomes one of your mobility challenges, living in a multi-story home adds to the risk. For this reason, many people with Parkinson's decide to transition to a one-story home before it becomes necessary. This way, making a move can be about simplifying life and the positive experience of creating a new home, rather than a negative reaction to a crisis or to a forced move due to safety concerns. Some people find that they prefer to live closer to metropolitan areas in order to reduce the distance they have to drive and for easier access to medical services, municipal services and activities. While moving may not be the right solution for you, talking through the issues related to Parkinson's before problems occur gives you and your family time to think without the added stress of urgency.

" *When my husband semi-retired, we built a house with a lot of adjustments to help me down the road. I didn't need all of them at the time we moved in, but I wanted them there for when I need them in the future.*"

— LINDA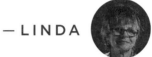

It's impossible to predict exactly when you will need more advanced care. Parkinson's is a slow-progressing condition, so there will be time to make preparations. Most people will have a decade or more to prepare for the unknown.

Getting your health-related documents in order is another aspect of long-term care planning. This is a simple task, and once the documents are completed, they will be there when you need them. The following are typically included in long-term healthcare planning:

- **Durable Power of Attorney.** A legal document allowing you to give someone else the authority to make financial and legal decisions for you in the event that you are incapacitated.

- **Medical Power of Attorney.** A legal document designating a person who will have the right to make healthcare decisions for you if you are incapacitated by illness or accident and unable to do so for yourself.

- **Advanced Care Directive.** A document prepared in advance, giving specific instructions about your healthcare wishes in the event that you are unable to give those instructions yourself.

Talk with your partner or family member about your end-of-life wishes so that they are known. The Family Caregiver Alliance offers additional information and guidance on these topics at **caregiver.org**.

For more detailed information about long-term care planning, see the **Parkinson's and the Family** section of this manual.

95

■ CORE PARKINSON'S SYMPTOMS

MOTOR SYMPTOMS

TREMOR

Tremors are involuntary shaking movements and often the most visible symptom of Parkinson's. As dopamine cells disappear because of Parkinson's, a neurotransmitter called acetylcholine becomes overexpressed and this excess results in involuntary shaking. Parkinson's-related tremors usually start on one side of the body, often in the hand or foot.

Most people with Parkinson's experience resting tremor, occurring when the body part is not actively being used. This is different than an action tremor, which happens during an activity, such as a bringing a cup of coffee to your mouth.

BE INFORMED: *Handling a drinking glass can be made easier by winding several thick rubber bands around the glass.*

Some people with Parkinson's report having internal tremors that may feel like an episode of anxiety or nervousness. While internal tremors can be extremely difficult to identify, they often respond to medications in a similar way to external tremors.

Over time, tremor can spread to affect both sides of the body, including arms and legs. As with all motor and non-motor symptoms of Parkinson's, the rate of how a tremor may progress can vary from person to person.

Tremor can draw unwanted attention and make once routine daily activities like getting dressed, using the computer or even taking medications challenging and tiring. Early in the progression of Parkinson's, tremor can often be managed by moving the affected body part or even simply bringing your attention to it. Over time though, tremors may become more severe or less able to be controlled by medications.

Strategies to help manage tremor include:

- **Take your medication on time!** This helps minimize "off" times that can make tremor worse.

- **Streamline your focus to reduce multitasking.** Rest your elbow on the table when taking a drink to stabilize yourself or sit down when you button your shirt to concentrate more intently on the task at hand.

- **Reduce stress.** Nerves and stress in general can make tremor worse, as can fatigue.

- **Consider adaptive technologies and products.** These are designed to make everyday tasks easier, such as specially-designed razors, pens, keyboards, utensils, cups and dishes.

RIGIDITY

Rigidity refers to muscle stiffness and tightness associated with Parkinson's. Like tremor, rigidity usually appears first on one side of the body and spreads to both sides over time. Occasionally, rigidity can go unrecognized as a symptom of Parkinson's, instead being attributed to past injuries or old age.

Muscle stiffness associated with Parkinson's can make movement difficult and can also impact how you walk (your gait). Stiff muscles combined with slowed, smaller movements particularly increase your risk of falling.

Rigidity usually responds well to Parkinson's medications, especially dopaminergic medications such as carbidopa/levodopa (Sinemet). Regular exercise, seeing a physical therapist and alternative therapies such as acupuncture and massage can all help manage rigidity.

BRADYKINESIA, AKINESIA AND HYPOKINESIA

Parkinson's tends to make movement slower, smaller and generally more difficult. Bradykinesia refers to the slowing of movement, while akinesia refers to the lack of movement that can be caused by Parkinson's. Hypokinesia refers to a loss of momentum or force in movement that can come with Parkinson's, usually in connection with akinesia, bradykinesia or both. People experiencing any of these have a hard time keeping up a normal pace and/or intensity of movement.

Although akinesia means lack of movement, people with Parkinson's typically can start activities with a normal range of motion. However, momentum decreases as the activity goes on. For instance, your handwriting might become smaller and more cramped as you progress across the page, your voice may become softer as you speak to someone and your steps may become smaller as you walk long distances.

Regular exercise as well as specific activities for the areas you are experiencing slower and smaller movements, like hand exercises or speech therapy, can be beneficial. Physical therapists, occupational therapists and speech therapists can all provide important instruction and tools to help you adapt and best manage the effects of akinesia, bradykinesia and hypokinesia.

GAIT AND BALANCE

Changes in walking or gait that occur over time might include shorter shuffling steps, fast or runaway steps (called festination), slow, cautious steps and gait freezing. Postural instability is a problem with keeping and correcting your center of balance upright and over your feet. Postural flexion, or bending forward at the neck, back, hips and knees, also leans the body and your center of mass ahead of your toes – compromising your base of support. These problems can lead to falls.

BALANCE: SO AUTOMATIC, SO VULNERABLE, SO RE-TRAINABLE

By Helen Bronte-Stewart, MD, MSE

Balance is a general term that refers to our ability to stay upright whether seated, standing or moving. If we can't balance, we fall. Imbalance is an inevitable complication in Parkinson's and leads to falls in more than 50% of people living with this disease. Falls may result in severe injuries and have a major impact on independent daily living activities.

People with Parkinson's fall most frequently when changing position, turning, moving in dim light and/or on an unstable surface. All of these movements challenge their dynamic balance control. Thus, activities like bending, coming up from a squat, going from a seated to a standing posture, moving on a thick carpet at night and walking on a rocky trail may lead to falls from imbalance.

Why does Parkinson's affect balance? It is thought that the brain has difficulty recruiting learned "templates" of how to maintain balance when incoming orientational sensory information is incongruent or absent. Another problem in Parkinson's that makes a fall more likely is that postural "righting reflexes," reaction time and movement speed are all delayed or slow. If the body sways off its base of support it might take too long to "right" and a fall may occur.

Walking problems do not always improve with medication, making physical therapy and exercise even more important. This is why you are encouraged to see a physical therapist who specializes in neurological conditions like Parkinson's to begin exercises for balance from the very beginning, rather than waiting until balance becomes a problem.

Freezing of gait is when your feet get stuck or feel glued to the floor. Freezing may be a problem if:

- You have trouble turning in small rooms, such as the kitchen, closet, bathroom or around corners.

- Your foot sticks to the floor or will not move when trying to sit in a chair, after standing up from a chair, when beginning to walk or when changing directions.

- You have difficulty walking through doorways, on and off carpets or over changes in floor surface, in cluttered rooms, in rooms with patterned wallpaper or clutter, in low-lit areas or when the floor is too shiny.

- Your feet freeze when you get anxious, nervous or feel like you need to move quickly.

Many factors can affect your walking, balance and tendency to freeze. Your medications, environment, posture, stamina and strength, energy levels, anxiety, blood pressure problems, dizziness or vertigo, heart and lung function, joint conditions, choice of footwear, circulation and sensations in your legs and feet are just a few of the areas you and your doctor can work on to improve health, walking and balance. Find tools to help freezing of gait: ■ **dpf.org/fog**.

Don't wait for your doctor to suggest occupational or physical therapy. Be proactive and ask for a referral. Occupational therapists can help with mobility in your home or in places around your community. If you are having trouble keeping up with earlier exercise recommendations, talk with your doctor and return to

RE-TRAINABLE BALANCE ISSUES

The key thing to understand about the balance system is that it is learned. If we hadn't spent our first year or two of life falling over and getting up again, we would not have been able to balance as we know it. Learning is constant in the balance system, but most of us don't even think about it as we challenge our balance every day by our activity. The hopeful aspect of this for people with imbalance is that it can get better with training.

TRAINING THE DEFICIT: THE ATHLETE MODEL FOR IMPROVING BALANCE IN PARKINSON'S

Balance is one of the most vulnerable, yet one of the most re-trainable mechanisms we have. If you don't use it, you lose it – familiar words by now if you are living with Parkinson's, but nevertheless true.

Consider athletes: Their static and/or dynamic balance are/is superior to what they need in daily life because they practice specific aspects of balance for their sport. Studies have shown that gymnasts have superior static balance; soccer players have better dynamic balance than swimmers; judo athletes have better static balance than ballet dancers (probably because they practice kicks and balance with their bodies at angles rather than only straight upright). Gymnasts practice on the balance beam, dancers do pointe classes, cyclists ride on rough ground at high speed and yoga participants practice one-legged balances. Football players do weight lifting while balancing on balance balls. These are just some of the focused balance exercises athletes do in addition to general conditioning and aerobic training.

It therefore makes sense for people with Parkinson's to "train up" imbalance by training into the deficit. The goal is to bring balance back to normal.

The first step is identifying your specific balance deficits. I recommend getting a comprehensive assessment of your static and dynamic balance. The sooner you know the problem the sooner you can start to fix it.

Once you know the specifics, you can work alone, with a physical therapist, with a personal trainer or with a sports or movement disorders neurologist to develop a focused training program to specifically address your balance deficits.

As with athletes, focused balance re-training should be one part of an overall wellness routine. You also need to maintain the health of other systems, like keeping muscles and bones strong, and your heart healthy.

MEASURING PROGRESS

An important component of balance training is measuring progress; the more specifically, the better. If you have access to a center with dynamic posturography and gait analysis technology, then by all means take advantage of it. If you don't have technology to help you, you can effectively measure your progress at home using a journal and charting specific observations.

The days of sitting on the couch and giving up because of imbalance are over. It's time to get out and practice balance. If you don't know where to start, just stand up. If that is easy, close your eyes. If that is still a simple task, make it a bit harder. Try putting a firm pillow on the floor beside a wall where you can hold on if necessary. Now stand on the pillow. You are on your way to training your balance.

Talk to your neurologist about getting a balance assessment and re-training program, and then do it every day. It works, it is usually free, it's fun and it has no side effects!

FALL PREVENTION IN PARKINSON'S DISEASE

By Jorik Nonnekes, MD, PhD and Bastiaan Bloem, MD, PhD

Falls are common and can be debilitating in people with Parkinson's disease. They can have devastating consequences, often leading to injuries, reduced mobility, loss of independence and a lower quality of life.

For the management of falls in Parkinson's, it is important to appreciate the complexity and the multiple factors which can contribute to their occurrence. Deficits in balance and gait disorders are common in Parkinson's and both can lead to falls. Environmental factors in your home and other places in your daily life can also lead to falls and include slippery floors, loose rugs, and poor lighting and/or inadequate or inappropriate footwear. There is an increasing awareness in the healthcare community that freezing of gait is one of the leading causes of falls, presumably because freezing events typically occur suddenly and without warning. Recent research has underscored the additional importance of cognitive impairment (for example, difficulties with handling complex situations or sudden changes) as a key factor contributing to both falls and freezing.

Preventing falls might seem difficult, but it is not impossible. Given that there are so many factors that can contribute to falls, a multidisciplinary approach aimed at the specific factors in your situation is important. Crucial elements for minimizing falls include optimizing Parkinson's medication, stopping any sedative medications (such as sleeping pills or anxiety drugs) and tailoring physical therapy, based on evidence-based practice guidelines.

Fall prevention is possible when the solution is tailored to your unique situation and takes into account environmental, cognitive and physical factors.

INDIVIDUALIZED ASSESSMENT

Each person with Parkinson's deserves a careful and systematic approach to identify all factors contributing to falls. Your doctor should place particular emphasis on testing you for freezing of gait (rapid turning on the spot is the best test for this). You should also tell your doctor if you feel afraid of falling again, which is common. Fear of falling is not only a risk factor for falling again; it can also lead to decreased mobility. Balance and gait training to improve confidence might be an option for you if you experience these fears. Preventing osteoporosis through exercise, diet and/or medication also reduces the chance of fracture if a fall does occur.

OPTIMIZING MEDICATION

Most balance deficits are not improved with dopaminergic medication; however, some gait problems – including freezing – can improve. Higher or more frequent doses than those typically needed to increase hand functioning might be required. Again, sedative drugs should be stopped whenever possible.

PHYSICAL THERAPY

The evidence-based guidelines on physical therapy for Parkinson's were recently updated, providing a menu of treatment options designed to improve mobility and reduce falls. Designing and implementing specific interventions requires the expertise of a trained physical therapist that can tailor the approach to your unique situation and needs. Examples of evidence-based physical therapy strategies include cueing techniques, cognitive movement strategies and the use of exercise. Rhythmic auditory or visual cues can improve gait and freezing difficulties. New, inventive cueing approaches include "walking glasses" with different patterns of visual and auditory stimulation (not yet available for the general market) and mentally "singing" to yourself while walking. Listening to music with a strong beat and appropriate tempo can also be helpful for improving gait.

Another promising approach, especially for people experiencing freezing of gait, is through cycling, a skill that can be remarkably preserved in some people with Parkinson's, even when gait has become very difficult. If outdoor cycling has become too difficult or if your climate or geography aren't conducive, you can still benefit by riding a stationary bicycle at home. Various other exercise programs – walking, tai chi and dancing – can clearly improve strength, endurance and balance, and several controlled trials have shown a significant reduction in falling.

Physical therapists can also teach people to make safer transitions (e.g., from sitting to standing or rolling over in bed) and to increase overall fitness (with an individually tailored exercise program).

Promoting the use of walking aids also deserves specific attention. Many people do not use them, either because their doctor has not recommended that they do so or because they are ashamed or embarrassed. This is unfortunate, because for those who cannot improve their stability adequately through physical therapy alone, the benefits of regained confidence, mobility and independence that walking aids can provide far outweigh the cons.

Individually tailored exercises, visual and auditory cueing and training for making safer transitions between sitting and standing or rolling over in bed can help prevent falls. For some, walking aids can also provide welcome stability.

OCCUPATIONAL THERAPY

Home visits by occupational therapists can reduce hazards in your living space. In addition, an occupational therapist can screen for medical and behavioral risk during their visit, and can assess the appropriateness of your preferred footwear. Sometimes, people are reluctant to make changes to their homes or to their behaviors, or doubt that doing so will reduce their fall frequency; therefore, for any preventative measure to succeed, your cooperation and agreement to make changes is important.

Many people fall more often at night, when rooms are dark. Proper lighting should be installed if you frequently fall during nighttime visits to the toilet. A commode next to the bed (or a condom catheter for men) can provide peace of mind for those with limited mobility.

The key to successful preventative intervention is cooperation from the person living with Parkinson's.

IMPLICATIONS FOR CLINICAL PRACTICE

Your neurologist should ask you about falls and their impact on daily functioning as a standard part of their medical evaluation. As a person living with Parkinson's (or as a care partner), you can also initiate the conversation by asking your doctor to build a multidisciplinary team approach to tackle the vexing problem of falls.

your physical therapist for a re-evaluation. If you are noticing new symptoms, ask for a referral again! If you are lacking the motivation to stick with an exercise program, look for a personal trainer or join a group exercise class to help keep you committed and accountable.

BE ACTIVE: *Remember, you are your own best advocate for your care.*

Learn how exercise can improve your balance: 🎥 **dpf.org/exercise-balance**. Review the **Gait, Balance and Freezing Worksheet** for more helpful tips.

NON-MOTOR SYMPTOMS

Although Parkinson's is considered a movement disorder, many problems not related to movement also occur. Identification and treatment of these non-motor symptoms can greatly enhance quality of life for you and your family. Recognizing your symptoms is the first step to getting the help you need. Symptoms can occur at any time, including when medications are too low and not working well. Symptoms can also occur as a result of medication side effects.

Take a look at the **My Symptoms Worksheet** as well as the **Current Symptoms Summary** in the **Worksheets and Resources** section. Use the **My Symptoms Worksheet** to identify your symptoms as a first step, then prioritize these symptoms to determine which ones you should focus on first. The **Current Symptoms Summary** offers a quick snapshot outlining your problems and concerns related to your Parkinson's. You can use this and the **My Symptoms Worksheet** to educate your wellness team about your concerns and help guide an integrated approach to care. Treatment serves you best when all your symptoms as well as your lifestyle are considered so that the approach is tailored to meet your needs.

COGNITIVE CHANGES

Changes in cognition or thinking abilities tend to occur with aging, but can happen at any time. The most common cognitive difficulties in Parkinson's can be classified as "executive function" challenges. Problems in this area of cognition include slowness in thought processing time, trouble with multitasking, getting confused during the middle of a task, problems switching from one task to another and problems with judgment and poor insight. Language and speech challenges include word-finding difficulties (trouble getting the right word out) and naming difficulties. Memory itself is usually not a problem until other thinking activities are impaired, and dementia is diagnosed only when cognitive problems are more advanced, impacting your daily functions, activities or independence.

Cognitive changes can manifest themselves in different ways and can vary greatly from person to person. Fatigue, depression, stress and sensory overload can all worsen cognitive function. Parkinson's medications can also impact thinking abilities. It's not unusual for someone taking Parkinson's medication to experience behavioral changes, behaving erratically, experiencing mood swings and exhibiting uncharacteristic behavior, such as impulse control disorders that can take the form of spending sprees, gambling, hypersexuality or other atypical, compulsive behaviors. Impulse control disorders are most often a side effect of certain Parkinson's medications and must be brought to the attention of your doctor immediately. Hear Brian talk about how he and his wife Lily addressed compulsive changes in his behavior: ◼ **dpf.org/brian**.

A diagnosis of thinking problems or dementia requires a thorough examination and often calls for specific tests such as a brain MRI or CT scan, vitamin B12, thyroid function, liver function, folate, blood count, kidney function, electrolytes and blood glucose levels to rule out other possible causes of cognitive impairment.

An evaluation by a neuropsychologist, a specialist trained in evaluating thinking and behavioral functions, can help diagnose cognitive difficulty or dementia. Neuropsychological testing measures thinking abilities such as concentration, attention, memory, language abilities, abstract thinking, spatial skills and executive functions. These tests can help your doctor determine the cause of thinking problems.

❝ *I went to a neuropsychologist about 8 or 9 years ago to have comprehensive tests after I was in a car accident that triggered my Parkinson's. She gave me brain games and other suggestions to challenge my brain because I do have cognitive deficits.*❞

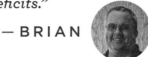

— BRIAN

103

Medications such as rivastigmine (Exelon), donepezil (Aricept), galantamine (Razadyne) and memantine (Namenda) can improve thinking functions associated with Parkinson's and other forms of dementia, such as Lewy body disease or Alzheimer's disease.

Just as physical exercise can improve movement and strength, brain exercises can help improve some aspects of cognitive function. The brain has specialized areas that control movement, language, memory, vision, planning, multitasking, problem solving, coordination, creativity, interpretation of our surroundings and visuospatial skills. Many types of puzzles, games (popular video game formats now offer brain teasers and games designed for brain fitness), art projects and music may enhance function in these specialized areas. Exercise caution if you find a program or website that offers brain exercises for a subscription service or high fee, or makes unsubstantiated claims about the effects of their service.

Cognitive challenges or brain puzzles are not the only exercises that help thinking functions. Physical exercise is proven to help not just the physical body, but also the mind and reduces the risk of dementia.

Diet is also important for cognitive health. Although the diet cannot reverse or slow memory loss, a poor diet and certain vitamin deficiencies can cause confusion, a sense of sluggishness and worsen fatigue. These can, in turn, affect your concentration and ability to keep your

PARKINSON'S PSYCHOSIS: THE ELEPHANT IN THE ROOM

By Cherian Karunapuzha, MD

Psychosis is a non-motor symptom of Parkinson's. Parkinson's psychosis manifests in different ways, such as **hallucinations**, seeing, hearing or feeling something that is not there, and **delusions**, irrational beliefs or convictions. People living with Parkinson's have a 50% risk of developing psychosis at some point during their disease. Psychosis can occur at all stages of the disease. In the later stages of Parkinson's, psychosis can be an integral feature of the Parkinson disease dementia. When psychosis occurs earlier in the course of Parkinson's, it is usually in relation to starting certain classes of medication or when pushing to higher doses. However, it can also occur without many provoking factors in the middle stages of the disease.

CAUSES OF PARKINSON'S PSYCHOSIS

The exact mechanism is not understood, but the circuits involved in psychosis seem to have an imbalance of dopamine and serotonin neurotransmitters. Some of the factors which would predispose one to getting psychosis include:

- Older age of onset of Parkinson's
- Longer duration with the disease
- Presence of mood disorders like depression and anxiety

SYMPTOMS OF PARKINSON'S PSYCHOSIS

The term psychosis encompasses several features including false sense of presence, illusions, hallucinations and delusions. **False sense of presence** is the feeling that someone is standing beside you or is in the room with you, but you turn around and no one is there. An **illusion** is a distortion or misinterpretation of something real that was sensed, like mistaking a belt for a snake. On the other hand, a **hallucination** is an imaginary sensation perceived without anything in the environment to provoke it, like seeing an imaginary dog in the corner of your room when there is nothing there. A **delusion** is a false, irrational belief which cannot be shaken despite being given evidence to the contrary.

Typically, psychotic symptoms are subtle when they first start. In the evenings, you may begin to see shadows fleeting by or hovering at the edge of your vision or a feeling that someone is standing behind you. Gradually objects at the corner of your vision start to look like something else, and the illusion goes away when you look straight towards it. Afterwards, the images at the edge of your vision may start to become vivid, distinct and stereotypical every time. For the most part, in the beginning you can distinguish these symptoms from reality. These subtle symptoms can persist for months or even a few years, but it is often unclear when these early symptoms get worse. Usually an infection or anesthesia from a surgical procedure can worsen it.

As these visions start to worsen, psychosis can occur more during the day and you lose your ability to distinguish what is actually happening. When these visions blend with reality, they start to become intrusive and, at times, scary. At this stage, more patterns of hallucinations can start, such as feeling things crawling on your skin, odd smells, hearing music, etc. along with delusions. Possible delusions include unshakeable feelings of being unduly persecuted by others or that one's spouse is cheating on them. Nights can become disruptive with paranoid thoughts of strangers in the house or backyard. Fearful hallucinations and delusions make it stressful even for care partners and may lead to ER visits, admissions to psychiatry units or even nursing home placements.

PROACTIVELY ADDRESSING PARKINSON'S PSYCHOSIS

Hallucinations, along with infections and physical complications like falls, are some of the most common reasons for hospitalizations in people living with Parkinson's. Almost inevitably, even a few days hospitalization makes Parkinson's worsen, and it is something physicians strive to proactively prevent through activities like speech therapy to prevent aspiration-related chest infections and physical therapy to prevent or reduce severe falls. In the same way, Parkinson's psychosis should be caught and addressed early before things spiral out of hand. However, physicians rely on you to bring up these symptoms, and only 10-20% of people experiencing Parkinson's psychosis proactively report it to their doctors. Psychotic symptoms have a negative connotation and many are fearful that they could be perceived as being crazy or be placed in a nursing home if they admit to these symptoms. Sometimes subtle early symptoms are simply misjudged or wrongly attributed to something else like poor vision, cataracts, hearing loss. Other times, there is not enough time to discuss or screen for symptoms of psychosis in a normal appointment, as most of the time is spent discussing motor symptoms or other more obvious non-motor symptoms, like depression and apathy.

The first step towards addressing Parkinson's psychosis is to understand and accept that this is a common non-motor symptom with Parkinson's. Report these symptoms early so your wellness team can keep track of them over time. Care partners, you can help tremendously by being supportive and vocal about these symptoms with your loved ones. You can also help your loved ones by bringing this up proactively with your wellness team if your loved one doesn't. Care partners can be very useful in clarifying symptoms that may be overlooked or normalized by the person living with Parkinson's.

TREATMENTS FOR PARKINSON'S PSYCHOSIS

There are several approaches to treating Parkinson's psychosis effectively. First, ensure that there is not a provoking factor, like a brewing infection or dehydration. Then, talk with your physician about removing anticholinergic medications or reducing dopaminergic medications, especially in the evening. This may appear counterintuitive, as one would think we need more dopaminergic medications as Parkinson's progresses. However, while dopamine is good for physical symptoms, it almost inevitably worsens confusion and psychosis, especially further along into the disease. If there is also a thinking issue, starting dementia medications can help to an extent to improve thinking as well the features of psychosis. Finally, starting antipsychotic medications to treat the symptoms can also help. Traditionally physicians had to use off-label antipsychotics that were typically used in schizophrenia for Parkinson's psychosis. These medications often caused various side effects, including worsening physical symptoms, drops in blood pressure, excessive sedation and even worsening confusion. Understandably, these medications were typically used only when symptoms were greatly interfering with quality of life. In 2016, pimavanserin, the first FDA-approved anti-psychotic for Parkinson's psychosis, was released. It has fewer side effects, meaning it can be used much earlier in the course of Parkinson's without having to wait until the symptoms get severe.

Parkinson's psychosis can often feel like the figurative (or even literal) elephant in the room, but it is important to bring this aspect of Parkinson's to light. The earlier psychotic symptoms are noticed and addressed with your care team, the better they can be managed to give you the best possible quality of life.

attention sharp. Detailed information on nutrition and diet tips can be found in the "Diet and Nutrition" chapter in the **Living Well Now** section.

Sleep problems, anxiety and depression can also cause mental sluggishness, diminished attention and poor concentration to such a degree that a person can experience memory or thinking problems.

Visual hallucinations caused by a combination of changes in the brain associated with Parkinson's and dopaminergic medications are more common when thinking problems are present. These hallucinations are usually visual illusions of movement or well-formed objects, such as animals or people. Visual hallucinations are treated by addressing any underlying illness, such as a bladder infection, dehydration or infection, and if possible, by reducing medications that have cognitive side effects that cause thinking problems.

" *It was hard to talk about hallucinations with my family and friends because their immediate assumption was that I was losing my mind."*

— COREY

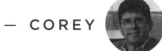

Listen to Corey discuss the hallucinations he experienced: ◼ **dpf.org/corey**.

It is sometimes necessary to use medications to treat hallucinations. The dementia medications rivastigmine (Exelon) or donepezil (Aricept), can improve thinking functions and mild hallucinations. If hallucinations are more significant, an antipsychotic medication, such as quetiapine (Seroquel) or clozapine (Clozaril) can be used. Use of these medications can be limited due to sedation and lightheadedness side effects. Recently, an antipsychotic medication, pimvanserin (Nuplazid), was introduced as a once-daily medication proven helpful for the treatment of Parkinson's disease psychosis and hallucinations with fewer side effects.

Refer to the list of medications people with Parkinson's should avoid in the "What To Know About Hospital Stays and Emergency Room Visits" chapter in the **Living Well Now** section. Common antipsychotic agents and other medications on this list should be avoided, as they can worsen motor symptoms.

See **Parkinson's Psychosis Self-Assessment** in the **Worksheets and Resources** section if you or your loved one may be experiencing hallucinations, delusions or other symptoms of Parkinson's psychosis.

FATIGUE

Fatigue is very common and can feel like a sense of tiredness, low energy, lethargy, sleepiness, weakness or a loss of stamina when active. When fatigue is a problem, things like everyday tasks, exercise and participation in family or social activities can be overwhelming.

Fatigue, low energy or early muscle exhaustion can worsen with Parkinson's movement problems, because movement control becomes less efficient and requires greater energy. For instance, a body that is slow or stiff requires more energy to move, and a body moving constantly (from involuntary movements, such as tremor or dyskinesia) will burn many more calories during the day, leaving you feeling tired in the afternoon and evening.

> **"** *Rest, absolutely rest. I now regularly take a short nap without fail, and I had to get to the point where I gave myself permission to do that."*
>
> — TIM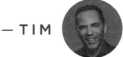

Taking your Parkinson's medications on time can reduce the stiffness, slowness, tremor or dyskinesia that otherwise worsens fatigue. In addition to movement problems, there are many other causes of fatigue. Fatigue occurs with sleep problems, restless legs syndrome, sleep apnea, depression, anxiety, diabetes, heart and lung disease, hypothyroidism, dehydration, anemia, malnutrition, decreased exercise endurance, poor dietary habits and obesity. Many of your Parkinson's medications can exacerbate daytime fatigue. This can be especially true for dopamine agonists. Be sure to review all medications with your doctor if you suffer from daytime fatigue or sleepiness. These tips may be helpful for reducing daytime fatigue:

- Pay attention to your diet. Eat smaller, more frequent meals rather than big heavy ones. Be sure your diet has enough protein, complex carbohydrates and fluids. Refer to the nutrition information in the "Diet and Nutrition" chapter in the **Living Well Now** section for a list of "energy foods."

- Caffeine in the late morning can decrease midday sleepiness. Use caution if anxiety is present and avoid caffeine after 3:00 p.m.

- Exercise can diminish fatigue by improving endurance, heart health, promoting wakefulness during the day, improving mood and decreasing insomnia. To reduce the effects of fatigue, plan your exercise when the medications are working and you are at your best. Refer to the "Exercise" chapter in the **Living Well Now** section for additional information on the benefits of regular exercise.

- Psychological stress causes fatigue. Pay attention to how you feel. Fatigue can be a sign that you feel overwhelmed or fearful, have little "down time" or time to relax.

See **Fatigue** in the **Worksheets and Resources** section for more helpful hints to improve your energy.

107

By Roseanne D. Dobkin, PhD

Although Parkinson's is defined by a triad of motor symptoms (tremor, rigidity and bradykinesia), the majority of individuals (about 80%) also experience non-motor complications, such as depression and anxiety. By many accounts, these emotional concerns are one of the biggest determinants of quality of life and overall well-being for both people living with Parkinson's and their care partners.

Depression is one of the most common non-motor symptom observed in Parkinson's, affecting up to 50% of people. The exact cause of depression in Parkinson's cannot be neatly pinpointed. However, the high incidence likely results from the combination of less dopamine and serotonin available to help regulate mood, as well as how people living with Parkinson's and their families think, feel and react to living with this medical condition. Depression may be characterized by any combination of the following symptoms: sad, low or irritable mood, feelings of guilt, agitation, helplessness, or hopelessness, loss of interest/enjoyment in activities or other people, decreased motivation to get things done, sleep problems, appetite changes, weight loss or gain, problems with memory and concentration, feelings of fatigue or low energy and most seriously, thoughts that life is not worth living. For some, these symptoms may be mild, come and go intermittently throughout the day or week, or be related to the timing or wearing "off" of their Parkinson's medication. For others, the symptoms of depression are more intense, continuous and unrelenting.

Anxiety commonly co-occurs with depression in Parkinson's. Although somewhat of an artificial distinction, depression is best characterized by low mood and loss of interest, while anxiety typically has its roots in worry, fear, panic, apprehension and avoidance behaviors (e.g., staying away from situations, such as social interactions, that may make you uncomfortable). Like depression, symptoms of anxiety may vary greatly from person to person. Anxiety may be persistent, episodic or both. It is also quite common for people living with Parkinson's to experience high levels of worry related to their medication wearing "off" or not working properly ("off anxiety"), as well as in response to upcoming events that they fear that they will lack the skills or resources to handle ("anticipatory anxiety").

While some may first experience emotional symptoms at any point during the course of their Parkinson's, it is not uncommon for people living with Parkinson's to report a history of depression or anxiety prior to their diagnosis. **Any and all combinations of mood symptoms are important and warrant attention.** Symptoms do not need to be "new" or "severe" or bear a resemblance to those portrayed on TV commercials in order to initiate discussion with your doctor. At times, people living with Parkinson's may be reluctant to inform their wellness team about their mood symptoms. While there may be many explanations for this hesitation, several common themes have been reported. Some have shared that they are so accustomed to feeling "below average" that it almost feels "normal" to them and thus, is not newsworthy. Others have noted difficulty describing their inner experiences (the symptoms of depression and anxiety outlined above should help) and/or have feared that there was no point in bringing up their emotional symptoms, as limited (if any), help was available (oh contraire!).

TREATMENT OF DEPRESSION AND ANXIETY

Both depression and anxiety in Parkinson's can be effectively treated. Successful treatment may enhance all aspects of Parkinson's care, like physical and cognitive health. So, if you feel something — anything — that you don't like, say something. It is very important to report any and all symptoms that are bothersome and/or affecting your relationships or daily activities. If you are unsure as to how best approach the topic with your doctor, it may be helpful to discuss your concerns and potential action plans with a family member or trusted confidant first. It may also be helpful to ask your care partner for

 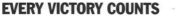

ANXIETY

Anxiety is experienced as nervousness, worrying, feeling jittery, having an unsettled mind or the inability to stop thoughts interfering with daily activities or sleep. Anxiety can result when changes take place in brain regions that influence mood. Anxiety can be present throughout the day, during medication "off" periods or can surface sporadically as a panic attack. Hear how Brian experiences anxiety: ◼️ **dpf.org/brian**.

Anxiety can be part of your worries about diagnosis, your future or other life concerns. In addition, anxiety can be a symptom of Parkinson's that can begin even before motor problems are noticed. It can be constant or vary with your changing motor symptoms. For example, feelings of anxiousness can occur when Parkinson's medications wear "off," usually prior to when the next dose is due. Certain motor symptoms can increase or worsen with anxiety, especially tremor, dyskinesia and freezing of gait. Motor challenges can worsen anxiety, which in turn, aggravates motor challenges. If you have tremor, chances are, you have observed the escalation and interaction of these two symptoms at certain times.

Anxiety can cause restlessness, sleeplessness, fatigue, pain, thinking problems and can even increase your sensitivity to medications and their side effects. Anxiety can rob you of much-needed energy.

❝ *For me, I get really hyper when I get anxious. I talk real fast and it can take me a lot longer to get ready. Anxiety wasn't always there for me with Parkinson's, it really started a couple of years ago when I had digestive issues.*❞

— LINDA

Mild anxiety can improve with relaxation, exercise, meditation and biofeedback techniques. Ask your doctor for a referral to a counselor for more information about these techniques. If anxiety is worse at the

their impressions of your mood and coping efforts. (Consider using the **Emotional Wellness: Depression** and/or **Emotional Wellness: Anxiety** worksheets to guide this discussion). It is not uncommon for loved ones to notice subtle (or not so subtle) changes that you are unaware of. "Minor" symptoms that go undetected or unreported can lead to "major" symptoms over time. As untreated mood symptoms have been linked with a faster progression of physical symptoms, greater cognitive decline and poorer quality of life for people with Parkinson's and their families, the timely recognition and treatment of these emotional concerns is key to optimizing health and quality of life in Parkinson's. Even if you are currently feeling at your best, it may be helpful to educate yourself about lifestyle strategies that may help to optimize your mood over time.

If you are a care partner or loved one of someone with Parkinson's that you believe may be experiencing depression and/or anxiety, speak directly to your loved one about your observations and concerns. Emphasize that your concerns are common in Parkinson's and effective treatments for both depression and anxiety are available as you collaboratively decide on the next best steps. If you are able, attend the next neurology appointment with your loved one and raise your concerns with the doctor and other appropriate medical professionals. This will start an important conversation and put mood changes on the doctor's radar to continue to monitor. While you're there, ask for appropriate suggestions and recommendations from your wellness team. Remember that healthy habits and lifestyle changes such as exercise and staying connected with others in your community can improve your mood and help with both depression and anxiety.

Cognitive-behavioral therapy (also known as CBT) is an example of one type of treatment that addresses behaviors and thought patterns that contribute to depression and anxiety. CBT is time-limited and skills-based and may be used alone or in combination with medication. It may be a particularly useful option for people living with Parkinson's who can't tolerate (i.e., had uncomfortable side effects), do not wish to take or have not been sufficiently helped by antidepressant or anti-anxiety medication. Several different CBT strategies can be used to help people living with Parkinson's cope more effectively with the numerous symptoms of depression and anxiety described above, as well as with the daily stress of living with Parkinson's. CBT is also very amenable to care partner involvement in the therapeutic process. Care partners may participate in treatment sessions and/or attend separate educational sessions that arm them with tools needed to support their loved ones in their daily practice of newly acquired coping skills. Care partner involvement in treatment is encouraged as it has been

end of medication doses, treatment for your "on/off" fluctuations may be needed. Moderate to severe anxiety may need medication. Selective serotonin reuptake inhibitors (common antidepressants) or a category of medications called benzodiazepines are examples of medications used to treat anxiety. See the **Emotional Wellness: Anxiety** tool in the **Worksheets and Resources** section for non-medication suggestions to help you manage anxiety.

DEPRESSION

Depression is reported to occur in about half of people diagnosed with Parkinson's.[9] Depression can begin before the motor symptoms become obvious. The cause of depression in Parkinson's is thought to occur from biochemical changes (particularly the chemicals serotonin, dopamine and norepinephrine) in brain regions that influence mood. Depression can also be caused by other circumstances such as a reaction to your Parkinson's diagnosis, life worries, social isolation or loneliness or even chronic frustrations when symptoms bring challenges with everyday tasks. A clinical definition of depression involves consistently feeling blue or down for a period of two straight weeks, although many people with Parkinson's will experience low moods that come with bad days or as Parkinson's medications wear "off."

One thing you need to know is that feeling depressed is not elective. You do not choose to be depressed. Depression is a weight that can really pull you down. Care partners and friends might be the ones who notice the changes in you and can help you rally to seek help.

Symptoms of depression include depressed mood, memory problems, fatigue, sleepiness and insomnia. Other symptoms of depression include irritability, poor concentration, loss of enjoyment in social activities

9   McDonald, William M., Richard, Irene H., and DeLong, Mahlon R. (2003). Prevalence, etiology, and treatment of depression in Parkinson's disease. *Biological Psychiatry*, 54(3): 363-375.

and hobbies, loss of appetite or increased appetite, feeling of hopelessness or guilt, excessive worrying, feeling of worthlessness or failure and suicidal thoughts. Apathy and anxiety can also occur with depression. Learn to recognize signs of depression: ◼️ **dpf.org/help-depression**.

> " *I'd always been able to juggle a lot of things at once and ideas about what I was doing next, but I became unable to cope with that volume of information after Parkinson's. Things came into my mind, very dark things. A lot of feelings of loss of control and feeling depressed, down, sad. A lot of days, I'd go to work and it was very difficult to concentrate or feel productive and to deal with the volume of work I had at the time.* "
>
> — TIM

Depression affects you and your family's well-being in many ways. It changes your perception of how well you are doing. For instance, you might feel that your movement problems are worse than they actually are, which can aggravate your frustrations and anxieties. Depression combined with movement problems further impacts your ability to do everyday activities. For this reason, it is very important to recognize symptoms of depression and honestly discuss these concerns with your doctor or another member of your wellness team. Remember: the better your mood, the more apt you are to tend to your health with exercise, a nutritious diet, adapt to your difficulties, problem-solving, action-taking and socializing with people important to you. Depression is treatable.

shown further bolster depression outcomes in Parkinson's.

In summary, your mood is a critical aspect of living with Parkinson's that you can control. **DON'T SUFFER IN SILENCE!** Effective treatments are available. Health insurance coverage for mental health services is commonly provided by most (if not all) plans, including Medicare. Importantly, unlike other Parkinson's specialty care such as physical therapy and speech language therapy, mental health services are not "capped" or "limited" in any way over the course of the calendar year. Referral information can be obtained from your personal physicians, insurance carrier, Parkinson's support group, all of the major Parkinson's organizations and your local psychological associations (each state has one). There are also several high-quality self-help resources available (books, relaxation/meditations soundtracks) in local bookstores and libraries. Depression and anxiety are common and nothing to feel embarrassed about. Seeking treatment is a positive step toward improving quality of life and part of proactive self-care.

111

> **BE ACTIVE:** *Keep doing the things that make you "you" and that lift your mood. Don't disengage from activities and interests that provide pleasure, mental or physical stimulation just because you have Parkinson's.*

Talk about it. Sharing your feelings with others is helpful, and a counselor can be a valuable resource. Support groups can also help you realize that you are not alone in your experience.

Exercise, and take care of yourself. Taking steps to reduce stress, improve your sleep, diet and exercise are also very important parts of treatment for depression. Vigorous cardiovascular exercise produces endorphins in the body and brain that can improve depression and your overall outlook.

Medications may have a role. Antidepressants can help and may be needed. Over-the-counter remedies, such as St. John's Wort, are used by some people, but are generally not recommended unless prescribed by your doctor. Inform your doctor if you start taking an herbal antidepressant remedy, since some ingredients can interact with prescription medications and increase the risk of bleeding. Always report a change in your mood to your doctor.

Although depression is common in Parkinson's, people who experience suicidal thoughts might not express them to family members or their doctor unless they are asked directly. Adjustment counseling, family support and medications are helpful, as is having honest conversations with your wellness team.

See the **Emotional Wellness: Depression** worksheet in the **Worksheets and Resources** section for more helpful hints to improve your mood.

APATHY

Apathy is a loss of motivation to participate in regular activities, socialize or express emotions. Apathy can take on multiple forms, including:

- **Physical apathy.** Loss of interest in physical activity, decreased appetite, increased sleep and decreased libido.

- **Cognitive apathy.** Lack of self-initiation or interest in pursuing new challenges or tasks.

- **Emotional apathy.** Disinterest or blunted emotions (positive or negative) to daily events and relationships. In other words, a person may seem like they just do not care.

> *I have times where I will wake up and for no apparent reason, have a bleak day. Sometimes I will come out of it in the afternoon, others it will last all day. I can't just 'cheer myself up'."*

— EDIE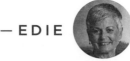

Apathy can be a primary and isolated symptom or can co-exist with other problems, like depression. When it is a symptom of depression, apathy is also associated with negative feelings, hopelessness, irritability, lack of enjoyment in pleasurable activities and sadness. Apathy can also be seen in people with cognitive difficulties, often manifesting as an increased level of disinterest in daily activities. Consulting with a neuropsychologist can help determine if you are suffering from apathy alone or if more significant cognitive problems are also present.

BE ENGAGED: *If you feel a lack of enjoyment or interest in activities you used to enjoy, it could be apathy. Talk with your wellness team and enlist the help of a professional to help you overcome it.*

Since body language and facial expression are important parts of communication, especially when it comes to the communication of emotions and interest, the loss of facial expression (called facial masking) and spontaneous body movement can be misinterpreted as apathy.

Apathy is difficult to treat. Antidepressants and counseling can help apathy when it's associated with underlying depression. Cognitive-enhancing medications, such as rivastigmine or donepezil, can help apathy when cognitive challenges are a primary problem.

Non-medical treatments are more effective if apathy is present without depressed mood. For many people living with Parkinson's and their loved ones, simply understanding that apathy can be a part of Parkinson's is helpful. An occupational therapist, recreational therapist or counselor can help you tackle apathy. These specialists help you and your loved ones prioritize your activities and develop routines and strategies to compensate for a loss of motivation, establish goals and schedule activities to combat apathy.

PHYSICAL SENSATIONS: TINGLING, ACHES AND PAIN

Parkinson's can bring a variety of new physical sensations, including pinched nerves, joint pain or even arthritis. Muscular and skeletal pain (such as back pain) can increase with stiffness, change in posture or muscle rigidity. Stiff muscles can feel like a spasm or dull ache. This can be worse on the side of your body where Parkinson's motor symptoms are more persistent.

Spasms, primarily in the feet and lower legs, are common and are also referred to as dystonia. Dystonia causes muscle contraction, pulling, flexing or bending at the joint (toe flexion, foot pointing or inversion, neck pulling). An example is painful early morning foot dystonia, with bending of the toes or foot (often associated with a medication wearing "off" state). In some cases, muscle spasm or dystonia can improve with a change in your Parkinson's medications. For some types of dystonia, botulinum toxin (Botox, Dysport, Xeomin or Myobloc) injected directly into the overactive muscle is helpful.

> " *When I walk my dog, Maggie, around the park, sometimes I get dystonia so badly that the only way I can get home is by walking backwards. I may look silly, but at least I'm getting out and walking.*"
>
> — LIZ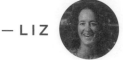

Some people with Parkinson's experience tingling sensations in their muscles or limbs, but this is less common than muscle spasms. Numbness and tingling sensations also can occur during "off" periods. Pain in the arms and legs, tingling sensations and numbness radiating down the leg can be due to other problems such as nerve damage from diabetes, sciatica (usually associated with low back pain), nerve compression, circulation and problems with blood clots. Shoulder pain is often present on the side where motor symptoms are worse and may precede the diagnosis of Parkinson's. Any new sensations should be reported to your doctor, who should search for other causes for pain to avoid misdiagnosing all pain as a symptom of Parkinson's. Regardless of the underlying cause, pain should be treated.

SLEEP PROBLEMS

Parkinson's can have many different effects on your sleep, including trouble falling or staying asleep, vivid dreams, waking up frequently during the night and excessive sleepiness during the day. Like other non-motor symptoms, sleep problems can appear before the motor symptoms.

Often people living with Parkinson's experience some combination of insomnia (trouble falling asleep) and sleep fragmentation (waking up frequently during the night). Studies have shown people with Parkinson's have different sleep patterns and that their deepest periods of sleep during the night are shorter and interrupted more often than people without Parkinson's. Often this is made worse by medications that may wear "off" in the night, causing tremor, painful stiffness or other symptoms to return and disrupt your sleep.

> *The pain associated with stiff muscles and rigidity interrupts sleep. I have difficulty turning over in bed. I typically don't sleep more than 3-4 hours at a time. I take a couple of naps during the day, and that gets me through. Exercise is about the only thing that works. I've tried medication, and I'm like a zombie."*

— COREY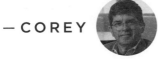

Anxiety, depression, nighttime sweating and trouble moving in bed are other Parkinson's symptoms that can make getting a good sleep difficult. Fragmented sleep is also exacerbated by how often some people with Parkinson's find themselves waking up often during the night to use the toilet because of bladder changes that can come with Parkinson's.

BE INFORMED: *Satin sheets or pajamas can make moving and turning over in bed easier.*

The medication selegeline, an MAO-B inhibitor that is used to treat Parkinson's motor symptoms, can cause problems falling asleep. Your medication dose timing may also impact time to fall asleep and should be reviewed with your doctor to avoid adding another medication to help you fall asleep. Occasionally, dopaminergic medications like carbidopa/levodopa (Sinemet) and select antidepressants, sleep aids and cognitive medications like donepezil (Aricept), can cause vivid dreams or nightmares and disrupt your sleep.

As unsettling as these dreams can be, they present serious concerns when combined with another sleep disturbance symptom of Parkinson's called rapid eye movement sleep behavior disorder (RBD). RBD causes people to physically act out their dreams, including yelling, thrashing, punching or even jumping out of bed. Even before being diagnosed with Parkinson's, many people experience RBD as a premotor symptom. Your doctor may diagnose RBD after reviewing your sleep patterns with your bed partner. A sleep study may be warranted to determine the most appropriate treatment. Learn more about RBD: 🔊 dpf.org/rbd.

Typically, people with RBD report that the dreams they act out are very vivid and that they do not feel rested in the morning. The bed partner often reports being the target of violent responses from the person with RBD, including being punched, bitten or kicked, while the person acting out the dream is unaware of this behavior. If you or your loved one is experiencing symptoms like these, discuss them with your doctor. There are medications that can help, as well as adaptations and modifications to beds and bedrooms to enhance the safety for the person with Parkinson's, as well as the partner. Some couples living with Parkinson's discover the safest and most effective way to ensure both partners sleep safely and as soundly as possible is to sleep in separate beds.

Restless legs syndrome (RLS) is common in people with Parkinson's and can present another interruption to a good night's sleep. RLS is characterized by unpleasant feelings in the legs when they are at rest that is usually relieved with movement. Because RLS worsens with relaxation, symptoms usually peak at night, making it difficult to fall asleep. They also can occur during periods of sitting, or when Parkinson's medications are low or wearing "off." Some people have a hard time describing the sensations and might only report trouble falling asleep to their doctor. RLS can result from medications and medical conditions other than Parkinson's, so discuss with your doctor if you are experiencing RLS. Some medications used for Parkinson's, such as ropinirole (Requip) and pramipexole (Mirapex), can also be used to treat RLS. Other treatments may include gabapentin (Neurontin).

Periodic limb movement disorder (PLMD) often occurs alongside RLS, but is a different sleep disorder altogether. PLMD involves repetitive movements, typically in the legs and feet, that occur about every 20-40 seconds and cluster into episodes lasting anywhere from a few minutes to several hours. These movements can be brief muscle twitches, jerking movements or an upward flexing of the feet.

While the exact cause of PLMD is unknown, scientists believe that the underlying mechanisms probably involve factors in the nervous system. PLMD is not considered medically serious, but can contribute to insomnia or daytime fatigue as these movements can cause you to wake up several times during the night. About three quarters of people with RLS have PLMD.

116

Sleep apnea is another sleep condition common in Parkinson's. While sleep apnea is not more prevalent in people living with Parkinson's, it does occur more frequently as adults age. Sleep apnea's characteristic symptoms are frequent awakening and aggressive snoring. Sleep partners may observe the person with sleep apnea's breathing patterns change with pauses and gasping for air during the night. Untreated sleep apnea can result in heart disease, memory decline, confusion, daytime sleepiness, fatigue and poor endurance. Diagnosis requires a sleep study that enables a sleep specialist to tailor treatment for each individual.

Anxiety and/or depression can cause sleep problems, including difficulty both falling asleep and staying asleep. Treating mood-related symptoms can be a good place to start, as doing so may eliminate the need to treat the sleep problems separately.

Many people with Parkinson's also experience excessive daytime sleepiness, which can be caused by the various effects of Parkinson's that interrupt sleep at night as well as from side effects of some Parkinson's medications.

Good sleep habits are important. This includes going to bed and getting up at the same time each day, and avoiding caffeine, alcohol and late-night heavy snacks. It is also recommended that you sleep in a room with limited distractions, such as TV or a computer. A dark room at night is important for falling and staying asleep and lights left on can disrupt sleep. However, turning a light on when waking during the night can help reduce the risk of falling, just be sure to turn lights off when you return to bed. Gentle stretching can also help sleep when done before bed. Discover more tips to improve your sleep at: **⟳ dpf.org/sleep-better**.

There are many healthcare professionals who can help you with sleep. Occupational therapists can review your sleep habits, physical challenges that affect sleep and recommend changes to improve bed and sleep comfort. Relaxation therapy and meditation can help sleep by reducing the cognitive "worries" that lead to insomnia.

A music therapist, massage therapist or counselor can help. Some find it helpful to play a relaxation soundtrack prior to sleep. Discuss your sleep problems with your doctor and wellness team to find a plan that works best for you.

See the **Insomnia and Sleep** worksheet in the **Worksheets and Resources** section for additional suggestions.

LIGHTHEADEDNESS AND DIZZINESS (BLOOD PRESSURE PROBLEMS)

Dizziness or lightheadedness can occur as a symptom of Parkinson's, as a side effect of medication, as a result of lifestyle habits such as not drinking enough fluids or restricting salt in your diet or as a symptom of other serious medical problems. A separate condition called neurogenic orthostatic hypotension that causes your blood pressure to drop when you stand up can also be present in people with Parkinson's. It is important to discuss lightheadedness or dizziness with your doctor to treat the problem, as well as to rule out heart problems or other issues. There are various medications outlined in the "Medications" chapter in the **Living Well Now** section that can help treat nOH.

There are also several non-medication ways to reduce lightheadedness. Rise slowly from seated to standing position, and use caution while walking or changing positions if you feel lightheaded or dizzy. Try not to stand still for long periods of time, and get regular exercise. Compression socks (available in different sizes and "strengths" of compression), elevating your legs when sitting, increasing fluids, increasing salt intake and elevating the head of your bed by 30° may be helpful. You can also try avoiding carbohydrate-heavy meals, caffeine and alcohol. Your physical therapist can show you exercises to reduce the problems of dizziness when you stand.

See the **Low Blood Pressure and Dizziness** worksheet in the **Worksheets and Resources** section for more helpful hints to improve dizziness and low blood pressure.

INTIMACY

Concerns related to intimacy and sexual relationships rank among the most difficult communication issues for couples. Our perceptions of masculinity and femininity and what we expect from our intimate relationships are as unique as our personalities. Self-concept, body image and self-esteem all impact the quality of our sexual relations. The physical challenges presented by Parkinson's also can have specific effects on sexual participation and satisfaction.

NEUROGENIC ORTHOSTATIC HYPOTENSION (nOH) IN PARKINSON'S

By Jose-Alberto Palma, MD, PhD and Horacio Kaufmann, MD

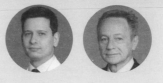

Neurogenic orthostatic hypotension (nOH) is a condition that is part of a larger category called orthostatic hypotension (OH), which is also known as postural hypotension. nOH is caused by dysfunction in the autonomic nervous system and causes people to feel faint when they stand or sit up.

WHAT IS ORTHOSTATIC HYPOTENSION (OH)?

OH is a sustained fall in blood pressure that happens within 3 minutes of standing. OH can reduce blood flow to organs above the heart, most notably the brain, and its symptoms can have a profound impact on your quality of life. OH is more common in the elderly, and certain medications, dehydration, varicose veins, severe anemia and conditions such as heart disease can lead to OH. OH can also be related to the nervous system. Parkinson's disease, pure autonomic failure, multiple system atrophy and other types of autonomic dysfunction can all cause OH.

OH can be caused by the body not releasing enough of the neurotransmitter, norepinephrine. When your body doesn't release enough norepinephrine, your blood vessels don't constrict when they need to, lowering your blood pressure and causing you to feel faint when you stand or sit up. When OH is caused by problems in the release of norepinephrine, it is referred to as neurogenic orthostatic hypotension (nOH).

HOW COMMON IS nOH IN PEOPLE WITH PARKINSON'S?

An estimated 30-50% of people with Parkinson's experience nOH. The prevalence of nOH in increases with both age and number of years of living with Parkinson's. Although nOH in Parkinson's is relatively common, not everyone will experience symptoms. For that reason, people with Parkinson's should be screened for nOH, even if they have no symptoms.

Conversely, nOH can be one of the earliest symptoms of Parkinson's and can appear several years — even decades — before the onset of motor problems like tremor or stiffness. Therefore, people who have nOH, but do not have any significant motor or cognitive symptoms, should also be monitored closely to watch for early signs or symptoms of Parkinson's.

WHAT ARE THE SYMPTOMS OF nOH?

nOH can appear with or without symptoms. The typical symptoms of nOH are lightheadedness, dizziness, blurry vision and, when there's a significant drop in blood upon standing up, fainting. Symptoms almost always occur when standing up, less frequently when moving from standing to sitting and abate when lying down. People with nOH may also experience weakness, fatigue, leg buckling, headaches, neck and shoulder discomfort and shortness of breath. Severity of symptoms varies from day to day and fluctuates throughout the day. Often, mornings tend to be most difficult, as nOH symptoms are aggravated by overnight urination, which is common in people with Parkinson's. Meals, particularly those rich in carbohydrates and sugars, also cause drops in blood pressure.

Not all people with nOH have symptoms. Symptoms emerge only when the blood pressure standing falls below a certain limit. In people living with Parkinson's, this usually occurs when your mean blood pressure upon standing falls below approximately 90/60 mmHg (systolic/diastolic) as measured with a blood pressure cuff on the arm. Symptoms of nOH typically disappear upon sitting or lying down, because gravity restores blood flow to the brain. Indeed, people with nOH are frequently able to tolerate wide swings in blood pressures and often remain conscious at pressures that would otherwise induce fainting in healthy people. Fainting can still occur, however, especially after a large meal, consuming alcohol, in very warm weather, if dehydrated or if taking medications to lower blood pressure.

In people with Parkinson's, symptoms of nOH can also be non-specific, including fatigue and difficulty concentrating, and may sometimes mimic a levodopa "off" state. It's easy to miss nOH unless your doctor measures your blood pressure while you are in a standing position. Conversely, it is important to realize people with Parkinson's can experience lightheadedness that mimics nOH, but may instead be caused by balance problems or other issues. For this reason, careful evaluation of your symptoms by a movement disorder specialist is strongly advised.

HOW IS nOH DIAGNOSED?

Diagnosis of nOH requires blood pressure readings taken while lying flat as well as while standing up. At least a 20 mmHg drop in your systolic blood pressure and a 10 mmHg drop in your diastolic blood pressure when you stand up is required to make the diagnosis.

Some people with Parkinson's don't experience a drop blood pressure every time they stand up. In these cases, a doctor may use a monitor to measure the person's blood pressure every 30 minutes for an entire day to assist in diagnosis and subsequent management of nOH.

HOW IS nOH TREATED?

The good news is that nOH is treatable. The goal of treatment is not to achieve normal blood pressure values, but rather, to reduce symptoms of nOH and improve your quality of life. Management of nOH includes three components: correcting aggravating factors, lifestyle changes and medication.

Correct aggravating factors

Stopping medications that can reduce blood pressure, such as diuretics, anti-hypertensives, some medications used for prostate and urinary symptoms, medications for erectile dysfunction, medications for angina and some antidepressants, is a first step. Levodopa (Sinemet) can lower blood pressure, and adjusting dosage may be necessary in people with Parkinson's and nOH. Anemia (a condition where you have low levels of hemoglobin, iron, in your blood) can aggravate nOH and should be investigated and treated accordingly.

Lifestyle changes

Symptoms of nOH can improve with time, patience and non-pharmacological changes. It is tempting to try to control nOH only with medications; however, this approach is less effective and may have adverse side effects. Treatment of nOH is more successful if lifestyle changes are also made.

Below are lifestyle steps you can take to improve symptoms of nOH. You can adopt all of them at the same time. If performed properly, these actions can lead to a dramatic improvement, even without medications.

1. **Increase water intake.** People with nOH need more water and should be drinking 3 quarts per day (~2.5 liters). Ideally, the best approach is to drink water and supplement it with salt (see Tip #2). Diet (sugar-free) beverages are also acceptable. Tea and coffee increase urine output, so they may worsen your symptoms. Sports drinks, juices and non-diet beverages are <u>not</u> recommended, due to their high-sugar content (see Tip #8).

2. **Increase salt intake.** Be sure to discuss adding salt to your food with your doctor, but increasing salt in your meals will help to increase your blood pressure. Most people do not need to take salt tablets, and in fact, salt tablets can cause abdominal discomfort in some people.

3. **Wear compression stockings (also known as TED stockings).** You can find compression stockings in medical supply stores. Wearing them will reduce the venous pooling that occurs when standing up and, therefore, will increase your blood pressure when standing. There are several "strengths" or "levels" of compression stockings. At first, you can try a medium strength (i.e, 20-30 mmHg). *To be useful, compression stockings should be worn up to the abdomen. Knee-high stockings are not effective.* You do not need to wear the stockings while sleeping.

119

4. **Wear an abdominal binder (i.e., a Velcro belt around your belly).** You can find this item in medical supply stores and it functions in a similar way to compression stockings. You do not need to wear this while you sleep.

5. **Sleep with the head of your bed raised by at least 30° (ideally 45-50°).** Elevating the head of your bed is useful because people with nOH frequently have supine hypertension (i.e., *high* blood pressure when lying down), too. To avoid supine hypertension, people should never lay completely flat. Sleeping with the head of the bed raised will also reduce urine output, causing fewer nighttime urinations and improved blood pressure in the morning. The best way to raise the head of the bed is to get an electric bed or an electric mattress. These are commercially available in several sizes. Other, less effective ways to increase the head of the bed are using a wedge, or just by putting some books/bricks under the upper feet of the bed.

6. **Drink 16 oz. of <u>cold</u> water 30 minutes before getting out of bed in the morning.** This will increase your blood pressure when you get up. Drinking 16 oz. of *cold* water at any time of day will also increase your blood pressure. You can do this on an as-needed basis, ensuring that you drink the recommended total (see #1) of about 3 quarts per day of liquids.

7. **Start a physical therapy program.** In people with nOH, physical exercise will decrease blood pressure; however, exercise is crucial to keep muscles active and for overall well-being. In order to avoid low blood pressure when exercising, your physical therapist can recommend recumbent exercises (e.g., recumbent bicycle, elastic bands, rowing machine, etc.). The best exercises, by far, which are safe for those with nOH, are those performed in a swimming pool. The hydrostatic pressure of the water will prevent your blood pressure from falling dramatically, even if you are standing, as long as most of your body is underwater (with your head out, of course, so that you continue to breathe). While you are in the water, you will feel much better and will be able to exercise with no significant symptoms. The better your baseline fitness, the less intense your symptoms of nOH will be. Therapies such as yoga and tai chi are also highly advisable.

8. **Avoid factors that decrease blood pressure and worsen nOH.** These include:

   a. Hot and humid temperatures

   b. Physical exercises which cause blood pressure drop (see Tip #7)

   c. Dehydration (see Tip #1)

   d. Alcohol

   e. High-glycemic index carbohydrates. Try to reduce high-glycemic carbohydrates in your meals. Try eating several, small meals (5-6) instead of the three traditional meals.

High-glycemic carbohydrates to reduce or avoid:

• Potatoes	• Corn	• Cereals (corn, flakes, etc.)	• Cookies	• Rye
• Yams	• Rice		• Ice cream	• Yogurt
• Candy	• Rice cakes	• Soft drinks	• Chocolate	• Corn syrup
• Bagels	• Oatmeal	• Bottled juice (orange, apple, etc.)	• Full fat milk	• Maple syrup
• White bread	• Wheat		• Watermelon	
• White pasta	• Grits		• Bananas	
• Pizza		• Cakes	• Grapes	

Low-glycemic index carbohydrates to include:

• Whole-wheat bread	• Reduced-fat yogurt	• Just-squeezed juice	• Peas	• Diet soda
• Whole-wheat pasta	• Apples	• Prunes	• Hummus	• Almonds
• Brown rice	• Grapefruits	• Beans	• Lentils	• Nuts
• Pearl barley	• Oranges	• Black-eyed peas	• Soybeans	• Quinoa
• Skim milk	• Pears	• Chickpeas	• Cashews	• Olives
	• Peaches		• Peanuts	
			• Carrots	

9. Be aware of your symptoms. If you experience symptoms of nOH, you will find relief by performing physical counter-maneuvers, such as making a fist, crossing your legs or clenching your buttocks, which increase your blood pressure when you are standing. If these counter-maneuvers are not enough, sit or lie down quickly to avoid fainting and injury.

Medication

While lifestyle changes can be very effective for nOH when performed properly, many people still require medication to manage symptoms. Two complementary strategies are used when it comes to medication: a) fludrocortisone for long-term increase in water and salt retention; and, b) midodrine or droxidopa for short-term increase in blood pressure.

All available drugs that raise blood pressure in the standing position also raise blood pressure while lying down, therefore increasing the risk or worsening hypertension while lying flat with your face up. Although there are no specific data on cardio- and cerebrovascular events induced by hypertension in the flat position, doctors treating people with nOH should be aware of this potential side effect. Before beginning treatment with any of the above medications, your doctor should carefully review your other medications.

Once Parkinson's is diagnosed, coping with the diagnosis and the evolving role from partner to care partner can impact the relationship in both positive and negative ways. Understanding how Parkinson's impacts intimacy, sexual function and desire as well as relationships is the first step in discussing the complicated and often avoided subject of sexual function and intimacy.

❝ *The honest way we can talk about sexual intimacy and sexual things helps us a lot."*

— BRIAN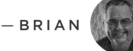

Often movement problems and medications are the primary focus during medical visits, and intimacy and sexual function become a lower priority. Doctors may be reluctant to discuss problems associated with intimacy. People may feel there isn't enough time during their appointment and feel too rushed to engage their doctor about their changing sexual function. However, sexual function and the importance of intimacy in your life can be one of the more important priorities for many at all stages of Parkinson's.

Changes in sexual function and desire can occur even before Parkinson's is diagnosed. The reason for these changes can be complex and vary from one individual to the next. Some people with Parkinson's experience anxiety, depression, insomnia, fatigue, restless legs, bladder problems, constipation and personality changes. All of these symptoms can impact intimacy and relationships. Identifying and understanding how symptoms of Parkinson's can impact your sexual life is the first step to combat changes and maximize intimacy in your relationship.

TALKING TO YOUR DOCTOR ABOUT SEX

By Jeffrey Shaw, PsyD, ABPP-CN

In my practice, I work with people who have been diagnosed with Parkinson's, MS, strokes and other neurological difficulties. People are sometimes hesitant to talk about intimacy and sexuality, or are not sure how to bring up the subject.

There are two important things to consider when you talk to your doctor about sex. First, realize that your doctor is also a sexual being and he or she has had, does now, and/ or will struggle with aspects of sexuality and sexual functioning. Second, although sex may seem to be relatively simple on the surface, it is actually quite complicated because it is intertwined with other aspects of your health. Complex things are much more prone to becoming problematic. If you have a significant medical issue such as Parkinson's, the connection between the physical, emotional and cognitive aspects, in addition to relationship and communication issues, cannot be separated and typically affects sexual interactions in one way or another.

Many individuals are afraid to discuss sexual factors because they are embarrassed that they will not appear normal, or believe that what they are experiencing is rare. This is simply not so. Avoiding candid discussions with your doctor or counselor is unfortunate,

Parkinson's can cause changes in the body and brain that lead to erectile dysfunction (ED), decreased libido and difficulty reaching orgasm. While it is not safe to use with certain heart conditions, it is generally safe to use ED medication in combination with Parkinson's medications. If you are experiencing ED, see a urologist to discuss the best medical approach to the problem.

On the other hand, select medications used to treat Parkinson's can cause an elevated libido or sex drive. Dopamine influences sexual desire and satisfaction and can contribute to impulse control problems including hypersexuality, which can be very disruptive in a couple's life. Dopamine agonists (ropinirole, pramipexole and rotigotine, the Neupro patch) are a type of Parkinson's medication that carries a high risk for increasing sexual drive. An increased or decreased libido, impulsivity or sexual dysfunction can all put a strain on a relationship.

Depression is common in people with Parkinson's and can decrease sexual desire and energy. In women, Parkinson's may affect libido more than performance. The onset of Parkinson's during the perimenopausal years of hormone fluctuations can be particularly challenging. It is recommended that women work with a gynecologist and a neurologist to choose how to manage and treat changes in sexual function or libido.

Additional possible causes of changes in sexual function and desire include other medical problems, stress, apathy, pain or inability to participate in physical intimacy due to movement problems. Heart disease, respiratory disease and the complications of diabetes are other common medical problems that can cause declines in sexual function. Some medications are known to interfere with sexual function, including narcotic pain medications, antipsychotics, allergy and blood pressure medications. Serotonin reuptake inhibitor antidepressant medications are associated with decreased libido, erectile difficulty, delayed ejaculation and difficulty with orgasm. Watch for tips to address intimacy concerns with your partner and wellness team: ◾ **dpf.org/intimacy**.

Your primary care provider may investigate hormonal changes that can influence sexual function, such as testosterone, estrogen and androgens. A referral to a gynecologist or urologist is helpful if further diagnostic testing is needed to determine all possible contributing factors when there is a change in sexual function. As with Parkinson's care in general, a team approach is needed to optimize sexual health.

Intimacy can be more complicated to discuss than the mechanics of sexual function. Intimacy is a very dynamic exchange between partners, ranging from feelings of closeness to physical pleasure. Intimacy also can take the forms of caring and empathy from a close friend or the emotional and physical connection you share with your partner or spouse. The impact of Parkinson's on relationships is as important for quality of life as mobility, communication, mood or cognition. The loss of intimacy endured by the partner or spouse may go unrecognized by the person with Parkinson's. A simple touch can be a very powerful source of intimacy, but may decrease in frequency for both the person living with Parkinson's and their partner as Parkinson's progresses. Speech problems and facial masking alter communication and can add to the challenges a couple might experience over time. Added to this challenge is the fatigue experienced by both partners, with little energy left to cultivate the relationship.

Intimacy can fluctuate over the course of Parkinson's. There will be changes over time in the roles of both the person living with Parkinson's and their partner or spouse. At times, more help or support will be needed from your partner, and the care partner status may come to the forefront. Couples should discuss this in order to negotiate how to manage the changing roles associated with care partner and intimate partner. The loss of intimacy is a loss that can be avoided.

because there are often effective interventions that can improve the situation. These improvements can in turn improve crucial aspects related to overall quality of life. Sexual interaction and intimacy can dramatically improve relationships through bonding, trust, richer communication and a sense of shared adventure that no other activity can replace. Problems with sexual interaction can be very destructive to these same relationship factors.

Rather than feel embarrassed about your questions related to sex, try to think of them as another important aspect of your overall health. Realize that whatever you are experiencing is likely something your doctor has seen before, and he or she will be ready to help you address your issues. Treat sexuality as you would any other aspect of your health and your commitment to take control of your Parkinson's and your own well-being.

123

> *" By the end of the day, we're both fairly wiped out. We manage to hug, kiss and talk for a few minutes every night and every morning. I'm very happy with our relationship."*

— LILY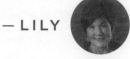

Positive steps are an important focus for couples and include being open and honestly sharing feelings. Identifying strengths in a relationship helps build the foundation for the best possible experience for a couple living with Parkinson's. Revisiting the memories that all couples share keeps both invested in creating new memories over their life together. Problems with intimacy can be very emotional and leave each partner feeling vulnerable. Talking about what is working, what is missing and what is needed in the relationship can be guided by neuropsychologists and counselors who are trained to help with coping strategies to maximize sexual health and can bridge the gap with medical providers. Primary care physicians also play an important role to optimize your general health for sexual activity. Communication is the key for emotional health, including intimacy and sexual relationships.

Couples may need to be creative about when and how they have sex. Although penetration provides pleasure and intimacy, other forms of touching can also provide sexual satisfaction that may downplay the presence of sexual dysfunctions. Foreplay and touching may become more important. Intimacy that once took place at night may be experienced in the morning. Satin sheets may help mobility.

Changes in sexuality need not lead to tension between couples. Although many people find it difficult to talk openly about their sexual concerns and problems, doing so is the key to maintaining a relationship in which respect, partnership, tenderness and love may be freely and warmly expressed.

Review the **Sexual Dysfunction** worksheet and the **Our Relationship Self-Assessment** in the **Worksheets and Resources** section for starting points to discuss changes and concerns related to intimacy with each other as well as your wellness team.

■ YOUNG ONSET PARKINSON'S

Although many people associate Parkinson's with the elderly, Parkinson's can affect people of all ages. While the definition varies from source to source, most refer to a diagnosis of Parkinson's before the age of 50 as young onset Parkinson's disease or YOPD. Estimates vary, but between 4% and 10% of people living with Parkinson's were diagnosed as young onset. Sometimes, people can get caught up in the YOPD label because the word "young" conjures attitudes and self-image issues, along with the diagnosis itself. For example, a fit and active person of 60 might identify more with the YOPD label, but medically speaking, he or she does not fit the classification. How a person feels about him or herself and how they approach the disease, regardless of their current age or age at diagnosis, must be distinguished from the medical aspects of YOPD.

There are some differences between young onset and older onset Parkinson's that are worth mentioning. Although the cause of Parkinson's is not known, research studies suggest that genetics may play a bigger role in young onset Parkinson's compared with older onset. For example, one gene abnormality, called PARK2 (Parkin gene), is found in up to 15% of younger individuals with Parkinson's. Despite this frequency, genetic testing is not routinely performed. While the presence of an abnormal gene may predispose someone to developing Parkinson's, it does not guarantee it.

" *I started having symptoms in my mid-thirties and they came back once I finished breastfeeding my second son. I was first diagnosed with so many other things because no one thought to look for Parkinson's that young. I had two little boys at the time and was untreated and unmedicated. I was a wreck."*

— LIZ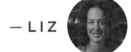

Young onset Parkinson's also differs slightly from older onset in the specific symptoms one might experience and in the response to medication. People with YOPD can have the same Parkinson's motor symptoms as older people, including tremor, rigidity and bradykinesia. Dystonia, a sustained involuntary, sometimes painful, contraction of the muscles that leads to twisting, pulling or bending across a joint, is a common early symptom in YOPD not typically present at time of diagnosis in older onset Parkinson's. This can be experienced as toe curling, foot inversion (turning in) or arm or hand flexion or cramping. Any young person with dystonia of the arms and legs should be evaluated for YOPD.

Motor symptoms of both young and older onset Parkinson's respond well to medication. Over time, motor complications such as end-of-dose wearing "off" and levodopa-induced dyskinesia can become a problem, leading to fluctuations in response to medications throughout the day. The combination of long-term treatment and disease progression lead to motor fluctuations and dyskinesia, collectively called motor complications. Both motor fluctuations and dyskinesia occur earlier in the disease progression and tend to be more severe in YOPD, compared to older onset Parkinson's.

Given the problem of earlier motor complications in YOPD, different medication strategies are often used to reduce or delay the onset of these problems for this group. One such strategy is a levodopa-conservative strategy. In this strategy, other medication, such as dopamine agonists or MAO-B inhibitors, are used as initial therapy; or added to levodopa when symptoms persist and progress despite other therapies. These other medications do have similar side effects to levodopa, but some are associated with more sedation, cognitive effects, hallucinations, lightheadedness and impulsivity control. Therefore, it is important to discuss the risk and benefit of these therapies, as well as the appropriate timing for levodopa use with your doctor to be sure you are treated with the combination that is right for you. Deep brain stimulation (DBS) is an effective surgical treatment in advancing YOPD, when motor fluctuations and dyskinesia are still problematic even with the best medication therapy.

Despite earlier problems with motor complications, young onset Parkinson's progresses more slowly and other problems, such as dementia, are less common in YOPD. People with YOPD will live with Parkinson's for many years and need to find ways to adapt to its effect on their lives. For some, this means adjusting to changes in physical abilities over time. For others, coping with the impact of Parkinson's on work, hobbies, family and relationships is most important.

It is key to understand that *you*, as a person with YOPD, can affect how you change and feel with Parkinson's over the years. It is absolutely critical to take control, tend to your health and proactively take the steps needed to do your best with Parkinson's. Using this manual to help you navigate Parkinson's and take the actions necessary for your wellness is an important step toward lifelong wellness. Wellness with Parkinson's means tending to physical mobility, nutrition, general health, cognitive and emotional health, spiritual growth, relationships and intimacy. One of the most important first steps is to prioritize what matters most to you and what adds true quality to your life. For some, this might mean a focus on physical health, exercise or nutrition. Perhaps your priority is to reconnect with loved ones or family. Discuss these priorities and the actions needed to achieve them with your friends and family. Include them in your plan if you feel comfortable doing so. Remember: even small changes can make big differences in how you feel.

" *Especially when you have young onset Parkinson's, you realize so clearly that life is short. Because of Parkinson's, I say now: let's take that trip. Let's do that move. Let's retire way before we ever thought we would. The value of living fully right now is something that we as a family have really emphasized."*

— JILL

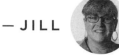

As a person with YOPD, you are in a unique position to take charge of your healthcare. You and your wellness team will be working together to keep you healthy over many years. Keep records during and between office visits to help you in the years to come. Remember, you know yourself best and are in a better position than your doctor or other healthcare professional to understand what has and has not worked for you. Your treatment may change from visit to visit, year to year. By keeping an organized list of these changes, such as medications you take or side effects that occur, you are better able to steer your care in the right direction.

Tools such as the **Goal Summary for Doctor Visits** in the **Worksheets and Resources** section can help you with this and additionally serve as a blueprint for long-term care that fits your needs.

Many questions arise as to the effect of Parkinson's on work, home, relationships and family life. The following sections address some of the unique concerns that face people with YOPD and more detailed information can be found in the **Parkinson's and the Family** section.

EMPLOYMENT

It is unknown precisely how many people diagnosed with Parkinson's are still in the workforce. Some continue full- or part-time work for many years. While the diagnosis of Parkinson's doesn't necessarily call for early retirement, it does require that you look at how you can best do your job and minimize work-related stress.

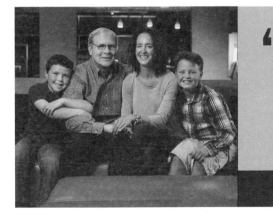

For those of us with young onset, we're still in our prime income-earning years. It's important for our retirement that we're earning and for our marriage that we're contributing. I had a high-stress job that I quit too early, in hindsight."

— LIZ

In looking at how you do your job, it may be helpful to make an outline of your overall responsibilities and then break each area down into specific tasks. Next, consider whether or not your symptoms will interfere with your ability to carry out each task. Look for other ways of doing things. Try to create a schedule that enables you to address difficult or challenging tasks during your peak performance periods and set aside specific hours for time-consuming efforts like writing reports.

The issue of when and what to tell your employer is very much a personal decision depending upon your condition and personality as well as your employment situation. For more on this important topic, refer to "Workplace Issues" in the "Family, Relationships and Work" chapter earlier in this section.

FAMILY

A diagnosis of Parkinson's affects everyone in the family: older parents, children, teenagers and, of course, your spouse or partner. Your loved one, now designated as your care partner, may be wearing multiple hats as sole or co-breadwinner as well as parent. Patience, understanding, stamina and creativity will be required from everyone.

Older parents are often shocked to learn that their middle-aged (or younger) child is diagnosed with a disease that is usually associated with the elderly. Their concern may build if this is someone on whom they're also dependent for emotional or financial support.

> " *I have six brothers and my dad is still living, so there are a lot of assumptions, but also a lot of support in the family. I try to keep them informed, but wonder how much information is too much. I've learned to address the big things, not the little things. I haven't gotten really personal, talking about the daily challenges or depression, because we are so far apart geographically.*"
>
> — BRIAN

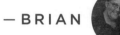

The care partner of a young or middle-aged person with Parkinson's faces particular challenges. The frustration of dealing with incorrect or delayed diagnosis can take its toll; some couples are actually relieved to get the diagnosis of Parkinson's because it is less terrifying than some of the alternatives they may have been considering. Hear Dave, Liz's husband, discuss living with YOPD while raising young kids: ◼◀ **dpf.org/dave**.

It is important for couples to keep an open dialogue about the feelings and experiences of living with a person with Parkinson's. Eventually the care partner may need to assume some of the tasks and roles in the family that the person with Parkinson's had previously managed. This should be an ongoing negotiation and requires constant dialogue around when to hold back help and when to rescue. Listen to Lily talk about what she's learned about when to intervene as a care partner: ◼◀ **dpf.org/lily**.

Couples who manage best in the face of a chronic illness begin talking together from day one about how Parkinson's affects daily operations in the family and what can be done to make things easier. Care partners who manage best are those who learn early to be flexible, state their own changing needs clearly and protect regular blocks of private time to meet those needs over the years. This is not selfish; it is crucial to the well-being of the person with Parkinson's and the family that the primary care partner does whatever it takes to maintain his or her own physical and mental health (see the "Care Partner Health" discussion in the **Parkinson's and the Family** section). Hear how Brian and Lily work together to partner in Brian's Parkinson's care: ◼◀ **dpf.org/brian**.

CHILDREN AND TEENAGERS

Young families have to deal with the unique issues of communicating the diagnosis and sharing the daily ups and downs of living with Parkinson's with young children and teenagers.

Children will absorb the reality of Parkinson's in the family by osmosis and by processing what they are told directly. They seem to intuitively sense a parent's frustration with tremors or difficulty walking and are capable of both empathetic and sympathetic offers of help. Attempting to hide a diagnosis from children is usually not the best approach. They know instinctively when something is not quite right in a family. It is often better to direct energy used to keep Parkinson's a secret into coping with the demands of maintaining a marriage, making a living and raising a family.

" *We've never hidden Parkinson's from the kids; it's always been something they knew. My boys have kept me very active, which has been a blessing. I've always thought: I don't want my kids to grow up thinking of me as sick. I want my boys to think of me as a normal mom, and I think that's been their experience."*

— LIZ

Young children may need reassurance that their mommy or daddy is going to be okay. They may need to hear that both parents will be there for them, that Parkinson's is not an aggressive disease like some cancers, and that it is not contagious like chicken pox. Matter-of-fact answers to specific questions on a need-to-know basis can help children cope with a parent who has special needs.

What about teenagers? Parents in general can be embarrassing to them without reason, so you can imagine how they may feel when their parent is visibly struggling with movement issues.

" *My kids are so aware of other people's needs because of my Parkinson's. They are both very empathetic and socially conscious – they'll automatically help older people with groceries, doors, etc. Part of it is that they're boys with good manners, but a larger part of it is that they grew up having to help their own mom with those things."*

— JILL

It is important to maintain your role as parent, model or mentor and avoid overburdening your teenage child. Older teens may need reassurance that their lives will go on as planned and that mom or dad does not expect them to be a surrogate care partner. On the other hand, a mature teenager can get great satisfaction from helping with chores or chauffeuring tasks that may have once been the responsibility of the parent with Parkinson's. Sometimes adolescents can benefit from professional counseling to help ease the struggle of having a parent who has physical challenges. Hear Brian explain how he talks with his adult children about Parkinson's, and learn more from parents and children living with Parkinson's in the **Parkinson's and the Family** section: ■◀ **dpf.org/brian**.

PREGNANCY

Deciding to have a child is a big decision, particularly for a woman with a progressive condition. Special issues are raised for the small percentage of women who develop Parkinson's under the age of 40. Many have questions about the effect of the medications on the fetus as well as the impact of the pregnancy on the progress and course of the disease.

❝ *My hormones have been very influential in my Parkinson's. Parkinson's for me emerged right after I had my youngest son and when I was breastfeeding him, I had virtually no symptoms. When I stopped breastfeeding, my Parkinson's symptoms went crazy.*❞

— LIZ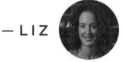

(130)

Young women considering pregnancy should discuss this with both their neurologist and obstetrician. Parkinson's does not affect a woman's chances of becoming pregnant nor does it cause physical or congenital birth defects. Parkinson's symptoms may worsen with the hormonal changes and stress of pregnancy on the body. The safety of medications used to treat the disease has not been studied extensively. However, guidelines do exist based on the experiences of women treated for Parkinson's and other conditions, such as restless legs syndrome. Many Parkinson's medications are not recommended for use during pregnancy. Amantadine has been associated with birth defects and miscarriage. Animal studies also caution against the use of selegeline during pregnancy. Levodopa appears to be safe and should be used at the lowest effective dose to control motor symptoms. Other treatments, like antidepressants and dopamine agonists, should be reviewed carefully with your doctor. It is also helpful to seek the advice of an obstetrician who specializes in high-risk pregnancies. Some medications are excreted in breast milk, so remember to review your medications with your doctor if you plan to breastfeed.

If you are considering having a child, discuss pregnancy and any concerns you may have about your Parkinson's medications with your family doctor, your obstetrician and your neurologist.

LIVING WELL WITH PARKINSON'S

THERE <u>ARE</u> THINGS YOU CAN DO TO LIVE WELL <u>TODAY</u>

In this section, we will discuss what it means to live well with Parkinson's. Living well means much more than simply managing symptoms. Certainly, medication and other therapies play a role, but there are many other ways you can improve your quality of life with Parkinson's through exercise, proper nutrition, connection with family, friends and other people with Parkinson's and more. Hear Steve explain his what living well with Parkinson's means to him: ◼ **dpf.org/steve**.

You deserve the best possible health and your physical health, personal care with Parkinson's, mental and emotional health and spirituality are key to your well-being. A holistic, integrated approach to living well will create a strong mind, body and spirit to improve how you feel, manage and adapt to changes. Living well might require some lifestyle changes. Create your own prescription for better living after you read this section by completing the wellness and lifestyle assessments, symptom checklists and medical snapshots in the **Worksheets and Resources** section of this manual. Share these with your family and wellness team to help them give you the support and resources you need.

By Davis Phinney

When I was first diagnosed with Parkinson's, my foundation for living well was exercise. As a professional athlete, that's what I knew and it was my bedrock. More than 17 years into this journey with Parkinson's, though, the role exercise plays in my view of living well has changed. Now, it's an important part of my day, rather than the focus of it. I do it for the physical benefits, as well as what it facilitates — better sleep, more energy, appetite and positive mood.

The one thing that has remained constant for me in my approach to Parkinson's is my philosophy: celebrate the little victories. I say this with conviction — not only to you, but often, to myself — because this disease so frequently can dampen your enthusiasm for life. It's vital to be able to acknowledge when you've experienced something good. You've got to stop to really see it, to "chalk it up." I don't mark those occasions by raising my arms up in victory like I did when I was a cyclist, but I do make a point of pausing long enough to recognize it. I try to be conscious of those moments — even something as simple as taking joy in reading a funny essay, or feeling the warmth in a hug from my wife, or watching one of my kids compete in a sporting event — and celebrate them.

131

Before Parkinson's, I spent a good amount of my day thinking about the past or things yet to come, obscuring the present moment. Today, I'm much better at bringing myself back to the moment at hand and letting worries or fears pass by. When I do, I'm able to appreciate and celebrate my moments of victory as they unfold.

I make a conscious point of not dwelling in negative thoughts. For me, anxiety is best managed by being present in my thoughts and actions as much as I possibly can, throughout the day. Instead of lamenting what I can't do or how things have changed, this approach frees me to see and savor the joy that occurs in so many ways throughout the day. Put my socks on while standing up? That's a victory. Rode my bike for coffee with friends? Another victory. Got in a few ski runs on fresh powder? Definitely a victory. The occasions may not be momentous themselves, but living with Parkinson's, I firmly believe that *every victory counts!*

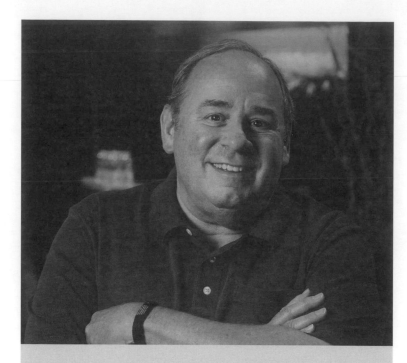

" *I see Parkinson's as both a blessing and a calling. I found it to be a blessing mainly because of the incredible people I've met through it. The people in the 'Parkiesphere' I've met are literally worldwide friends I can call on and get encouragement from daily. As far as a calling, I've found that one of the things I'm good at is gathering information and sharing it with people. It's something I enjoy, and it's an opportunity to share information that's accurate and timely to help people have a better quality of life.*"

— JOHN

PARKINSON'S SELF-CARE

Parkinson's is a chronic illness. As you are learning in this manual, treatment includes medication, lifestyle changes, non-medical therapies and wellness-based treatments for the mind, body and spirit. Treatment can be complex and will change over time. Although you depend on your wellness team to recommend and administer treatments, only you know what is best for

132

you. You are also in the best position to keep track of what has worked and what has not, and you can apply that knowledge to make the best treatment choices over the years. Who better to look out for you than you and your family?

BE ACTIVE: *Take charge, and be a participating member of your wellness team.*

The following steps will help you take an active role in your care:

1. **Be Informed.** Understand your symptoms, medications and their side effects. Ask your provider what you should watch out for when starting new treatment and when to seek additional treatment. Learn what rehabilitation and other therapies can do for you, when they can help and where you can get them. More information on rehabilitation therapy, including exercise, is included throughout this section.

2. **Be Engaged.** Be prepared for your medical visits. This is by far one of the most important and least performed self-care tasks. This manual will help you keep track of your medications, side effects and treatments. Prior to your office visits, be clear about what you want and what can be achieved. Set realistic goals during your appointments, and learn how you can play a role in achieving these goals. Consider involving your care partner, both in helping you to record changes you experience and in helping you to remember and implement the recommendations your doctor makes. Your care partner can be the unbiased voice, almost like a coach. He or she might see you every day, but they also see you with more objectivity than you can likely see yourself. This is a helpful perspective to have, especially when visiting your doctor. The wellness and lifestyle self-assessments, symptom checklists and medical information snapshots in the **Worksheets and Resources** section will help you organize, prepare for and get the most out of your healthcare appointments.

133

BE ENGAGED: *Care partners can attend doctor appointments and, with the doctor's permission, may want to make an audio recording of the discussion to help both of you remember and share an understanding of what was said.*

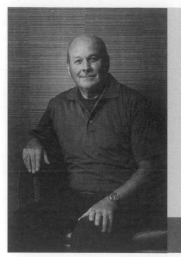

> *I've only missed one appointment in my wife's six years with Parkinson's. I find it very beneficial to be there and fully involved in the discussion. Our neurologist will ask Edie a question and I'll chime in with my opinion so he gets both sides."*
>
> — SCOTT

3. **Listen and Assess.** Listen to your body, and report any uncomfortable changes you feel. Listen to family and others who can be a source of information and support. Listen to your doctor's recommendations. With your new knowledge, you can ask for help and gain the tools you need to customize your treatment to your needs.

4. **Think Holistically.** Holistic health means that you look at the whole body and the whole picture. Step back and look beyond the Parkinson's to see yourself more accurately. Medical treatments, vitamins or supplements focus on only one part of healing. Healing requires an integrated approach to care, which has proven over and over again to result in the best outcomes. A holistic approach treats the whole person, not simply symptoms of the disease, and aids the healing process for any condition, at any stage. Holistic therapy is not easy, since it is not something that your doctor can prescribe in a simple step, like taking a pill or supplement. It is something in which you must both believe and participate if you want to see results. This means a focus on lifestyle, including diet, exercise, stress management, relationships and personal and spiritual growth.

5. **Establish Your Parkinson's Wellness Team.** Each person is unique and has different needs. Therefore, each person will have different members on their Parkinson's wellness team. Your team can include your medical providers, rehabilitation therapists, support group members or other people with Parkinson's, spiritual advisors, counselors, exercise trainers, mind-body specialists, family and friends. Your team can share helpful knowledge and tips, help you through the hard times and celebrate the good times. As you learn more about your Parkinson's and available therapies, your team will likely become bigger. Just knowing you have support and a safety net can be comforting and healing. Your personal support team should also know and celebrate the fact that while you may have down days or periods of time, you will also have good days, too.

" I try to be aware of developing problems and take action before they become acute. My doctors and I work together to stay on top of things and make sure I have things on hand if I need them."

— EDIE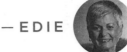

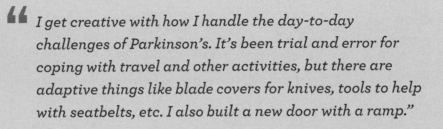

" I get creative with how I handle the day-to-day challenges of Parkinson's. It's been trial and error for coping with travel and other activities, but there are adaptive things like blade covers for knives, tools to help with seatbelts, etc. I also built a new door with a ramp."

— RYAN

GENERAL HEALTH

The first step in living well is to separate your Parkinson's symptoms from any other issues related to your health.

Your primary care physician (PCP) or family doctor will play an important role in problems unrelated to Parkinson's, monitor your general health and make sure you get preventive medical screening tests. This physician also provides general health education and will work with you to diagnose and treat your general medical problems, as well as ensure that you receive routine dental and vision care. **Managing your healthcare without a PCP is like an orchestra playing without a conductor.** Your PCP may help identify potential medication interactions and assist you in finding additional specialists if needed. If you do not have a PCP, now is the time to get one. Ask friends, family or other people with Parkinson's for recommendations. Choose a PCP who listens, respects your input and with whom you feel comfortable. It is sometimes helpful to schedule an interview or "get to know you" visit with a new doctor to be sure there is a good fit before selecting him or her as your doctor. A physician's assistant or nurse practitioner can also serve as your general healthcare practitioner. Learn tips for how to best communicate with your doctor: ◼ dpf.org/communicate-doctor.

135

> *During the year and a half it took me to get diagnosed with Parkinson's, I went to my primary care doctor and told him I thought I had Parkinson's. He said, 'No, you don't. You only have a tremor on one side.' It shows me he didn't know much about Parkinson's. Since I've been diagnosed, I have been teaching him about Parkinson's so he can help other patients."*

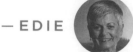

— EDIE

Questions you might want to cover during this "get to know you" visit include:

- Do you currently have any other patients who have Parkinson's? How many?

- What is your experience in treating people with Parkinson's, and for how many years have you been doing it?

- Do you work with movement disorder specialists?

- What is the role of rehabilitation for people with Parkinson's?

- Where do your patients with Parkinson's receive their rehabilitation therapy?

- Since Parkinson's research is rapidly progressing, can I share new information, research or updates about my Parkinson's or treatment with you?

- What is your philosophy regarding the prescribing of various treatments, including medication, occupational or physical therapy, counseling, diet and exercise for Parkinson's symptoms?

Avoid waiting until you have a problem or are sick before you see your PCP. Schedule a yearly examination to focus on your current medical problems, detect new problems and/or prevent future problems. Keep your PCP updated on any changes in your Parkinson's symptoms and treatment as this may influence how other problems are treated and will help avoid medication interactions. Many of the tools in the **Worksheets and Resources** section of this manual will help you do this.

Listed below are just a few of the medical problems or preventative measures that are of special importance to people with Parkinson's. (This list is not complete, but serves to reinforce the important role your PCP has in your general health.)

PREVENTATIVE SCREENING

Screening tests or examinations for skin, breast, colon and prostate cancer, osteoporosis, high cholesterol, high blood pressure, heart disease and diabetes are just a few of the illnesses that can be detected early and treated. Frequent skin examinations are especially important, since people with Parkinson's have a three to five times increased risk of developing melanoma, an invasive form of skin cancer.

> **BE INFORMED:** *It's important to wear sunscreen. People with Parkinson's have been shown to have a melanoma rate three to five times the average. Be sure to have a skin exam each year.*

ACUTE CHANGE IN PARKINSON'S MOTOR OR COGNITIVE SYMPTOMS

Parkinson's is a slowly changing condition. It is important to consult with your PCP if you are experiencing an abrupt change or worsening in movement, new or significant declines in thinking and processing, confusion, hallucination or psychosis. This is because a medical illness, not Parkinson's itself, is often the cause when symptoms change quickly. The most common medical conditions that can worsen your Parkinson's symptoms are infections such as bladder infections, pneumonia, heart problems, dehydration or a blood clot. Side effects of new medication or medication interactions can also be the cause of an abrupt change in symptoms.

BONE HEALTH

Bone health becomes more important as we age and are less physically active. With aging, bones can become thinner and weaker, increasing the risk of fractures from falls. Other changes associated with aging and Parkinson's are flexed posture, spine and joint arthritis and pain. Osteoporosis (bone loss) and osteopenia (bone thinning) are both treatable bone conditions that can have a negative impact on the health of bones, especially the spine. Vitamin D is needed to help your body absorb calcium for strong bones. Ask your doctor about a bone density scan for early detection of osteoporosis or decreased bone density. This is important for both men and women.

If you don't spend much time outside or use sunscreen, both resulting in less sun exposure, your levels of vitamin D could be reduced. Parkinson's itself can be associated with lower vitamin D levels and since vitamin D helps your body absorb calcium needed for strong bones, it is important to monitor your vitamin D levels. A blood test can determine your vitamin D level and whether your current treatment is appropriate.

HEART HEALTH

Your heart supplies blood to vital organs including your brain. Blood pressure control, diabetes care, screening for control of high cholesterol, dietary changes, weight management and exercise are all important tasks that you and your PCP may work on together to maintain a healthy heart and brain. In general, what is good for your heart is also good for your brain.

137

By Jane Busch, DDS (retired), person living with Parkinson's

Regular visits to the dentist are, of course, important for all of us. As a dentist, I encouraged my patients to brush, floss and see me regularly. For a person who has Parkinson's, good dental care is even more critical. That's because the disease can impact the mouth and jaw and make dental care more challenging. I am a retired dentist, but I am also a person living with Parkinson's.

HOW DOES PARKINSON'S AFFECT DENTAL HEALTH?

Parkinson's does not directly increase the risk of periodontal disease (tooth or gum decay). Decay occurs when oral hygiene is poor, either due to inadequate oral hygiene related to loss of dexterity, or from conditions like dry mouth.

Then, there are the general effects of Parkinson's. Fatigue, apathy and depression may make it difficult to even make or keep a dental appointment. A care partner might need to motivate the person with Parkinson's to seek dental care.

There are also the facial symptoms of Parkinson's. A person with Parkinson's has slowness of movement that can make chewing and biting down correctly difficult. Our speech is also slowed, and our voice softened, hurried or hesitant. These symptoms, plus facial masking, can affect how well we communicate. As a dentist, I often looked for non-verbal facial expression cues to monitor the comfort level of the patient, so I know that the lack of these cues can have an impact on communication.

Rigidity, tremor and dyskinesia can occur not only generally, but orally and facially. This can lead to jaw discomfort, cracked teeth, tooth wear and denture instability. In addition, rigidity and tremor of the hands causes a loss of dexterity leading to oral hygiene issues. Dyskinesia may cause tooth grinding. It is more challenging for a dentist to work on a patient whose jaw is constantly moving or is so rigid that it can't open wide enough. Something as simple as timing of medications can make your dentist's job easier and make you more comfortable.

What about the oral effects of Parkinson's? Difficulty in swallowing, or dysphagia, is a big concern. This problem often causes decreased cough reflux, which increases the risk of aspiration. Discuss swallowing challenges with your dentist, as there are precautions he or she can take, such as using barrier protection or more diligent suctioning to keep water and debris from reaching the back of your throat.

Let's talk saliva. Saliva not only assists in chewing and swallowing, it lubricates oral tissues, provides immunity to infection and neutralizes acid, preventing tooth demineralization. What if there's too much saliva? You might think this is the cause of drooling, but it's more likely the result of swallowing issues. Drooling can lead to irritation or infection at the corners of the mouth, so if you have swallowing problems, you should consult a speech-language pathologist about appropriate swallowing therapy.

Lack of saliva or dry mouth (xerostomia) is more common and troublesome. It increases the risk of both dental decay and gum disease. Dry mouth can be caused by drug therapy, Parkinson's itself or even by aging. To treat this problem, your dentist may suggest artificial saliva substitutes. Sugar-free hard candy (especially citrus) can help to stimulate the salivary glands. Try to avoid irritating products, such as alcohol, tobacco, spicy and acidic foods.

PREPARING FOR YOUR DENTAL APPOINTMENT

Your dentist specializes in treating your mouth, but it is tied in with the rest of your body's systems. Thus, the dentist must have a complete picture of your medical status. The information you provide on the medical history form is important. The more your dentist knows about you, the better care they can provide. Tell your dentist about your overall health, the degree to which Parkinson's affects you and list all medications (both prescription and non-prescription). Your dentist might consider consulting with your neurologist to inquire about disease stage, cognitive impairment, drug interactions and treatment modifications. Consider using the **Dental Worksheet** as you prepare for your appointment and bringing the **Medical Summary for Dentists** to help educate your dentist about Parkinson's, both of which can be found in the **Worksheets and Resources** section.

For example, people with Parkinson's taking MAO-B inhibitors such as rasagiline or selegiline need to limit the amount of epinephrine received via local anesthetics, because it can raise blood pressure. A consult with your neurologist is most likely warranted, especially for elective general surgery, as it may be recommended to stop this medication prior to surgery.

Your dentist will evaluate potential for drug interactions and avoid prescribing pain medications that are contraindicated.

HOW OFTEN SHOULD YOU SEE YOUR DENTIST?

I recommend more frequent check-ups for people with Parkinson's and a tooth cleaning at least every six months (every three months, if there is gum disease). Even if you wear dentures, routine visits are necessary to screen for oral cancer and evaluate the fit of your dentures. Restoration of oral health is best completed in the early stages of Parkinson's. If possible, replace old fillings, crowns and bridges and ill-fitting dentures before your symptoms progress. Consider dental implants, especially for overdentures. Dental implants are metal substructures embedded in the upper or lower jaw bone to which an overdenture can be attached. These stabilize the denture from the dislodging forces caused by chewing and swallowing, which helps the denture to last longer.

Ask to keep the dental chair more upright to assist in swallowing. Plan shorter, morning appointments that are about 45 minutes in length. Schedule the start of the appointment about 60-90 minutes after taking your Parkinson's medication. After dental treatment, rise from the chair gradually to prevent dizziness caused by orthostatic hypotension (OH). All instructions given to you should be written, as well as provided verbally.

DENTAL HOME CARE

Oral hygiene in the home starts with your toothbrush. Your toothbrush should have a large handle to grip and soft bristles. A small brush head reaches the corners better. An electric toothbrush is good, some even have timers. Ideally, brush after every meal for two minutes, and be sure to brush your tongue. Try a "one-handed" strategy, using the stronger side of your body. If you can't brush after a meal, rinse your mouth with water. Replace your brush every three months or when the bristles show wear. Floss once daily, preferably at bedtime. Floss aids ("floss swords") can be helpful, and care partner assistance might be needed.

An over-the-counter fluoride rinse is helpful in preventing decay, but you must be able to swish and spit. Your dentist may prescribe fluoride gels applied with a toothbrush or sponge applicator for serious decay issues. Periodontal disease may be treated with a prescription, anti-microbial rinse containing chlorhexidine. If you wear dentures, clean them daily. You may brush them or use a soaking cleanser. You should leave your dentures out at night.

As a dentist, I treated patients with Parkinson's. Now I, too, am living with Parkinson's. My teeth are important to me, as is my overall health. I encourage you to be committed to your dental health and to consider it an essential part of your overall wellness.

Hear more about the important role your dentist plays in your quality of life with Parkinson's: ◼ dpf.org/dentist.

By Daniel Gold, DO

Research has shown that visual symptoms are extraordinarily common in people living with Parkinson's. Visual symptoms may occur as a result of dysfunction of the eyes themselves or due to dysfunction involving the dopamine-enabled visual pathways that course throughout the brain.

HOW VISION WORKS

Vision plays such a critical function in daily life that a very large portion of our brain is made up of pathways connecting the eyes to the visual areas of the brain, in addition to the areas that help to process this visual information (e.g., color, shape, size, motion, etc.). The main purpose of the front part of the eyes (the cornea, lens, etc.) is to produce the clearest possible image, which is then transmitted to the back part of the eye, called the retina. The retina is made up of nerve cells, which communicate with each other via visual pathways using the neurotransmitter dopamine.

Parkinson's causes a lack of dopamine in the visual system, which likely contributes to common visual complaints. Replacing dopamine may lead to some improvement in both color vision and clarity of vision.

HOW PARKINSON'S IMPACTS VISION

Symptoms can be specific: eyes can feel dry, gritty/sandy, may burn or have redness, crusting on the lashes, lids that stick together in the morning, sensitivity to light; or, symptoms can be non-specific: vision just isn't what it used to be, difficulty seeing on a rainy night or in dim lighting, difficulty with reading, etc.

Vision problems can bring many practical challenges. For example, difficulty with color vision and loss of contrast sensitivity (the ability to discriminate an object from its background) can make reading signs or walking down patterned stairs difficult. Problems with motion perception and clarity of vision can affect driving.

Many of the visual symptoms experienced by people living with Parkinson's are mild, and overall visual function is quite good with routine examinations in your eye care professional's office. However, it's likely that multiple, small abnormalities in combination will become problematic and cause more significant symptoms.

COMMON VISION PROBLEMS

General Vision Difficulties

Blurry vision and difficulty with color vision

- This may be related to dopamine depletion in the back of the eye and within the visual connections through the brain. Partially corrected with dopaminergic medications.

Visual processing difficulty: orientation of lines and edges, depth perception

- This can take different forms, including:
  - Troubles with peripheral vision: distracted by objects and targets in the peripheral vision
  - Difficulties perceiving overlapping objects
  - Difficulty copying and recalling figures
  - Difficulties detecting whether motion is occurring and in which direction
  - Difficulties recognizing faces, facial expressions and emotions

Dry Eye

A consequence of decreased blinking and poor production of tears. This can be worsened by certain medications sometimes prescribed for Parkinson's, such as trihexyphenidyl or Artane.

Dry eye improves with liberal use of artificial tears and good eye/eyelid hygiene.

Double Vision Due to Convergence Insufficiency

Convergence insufficiency is a common problem that can interfere significantly with a person's ability to focus on an object as it moves closer to them. This can be diagnosed during a routine examination by your eye care professional and often presents as seeing side-by-side or "double" images when reading. Other symptoms often come while reading or doing close work, including: headaches, eye strain, blurry vision, short attention span, constant adjusting of the distance of a book and loss of place on the page.

When double vision is experienced, the person living with Parkinson's should cover each eye individually. If double vision resolves when covering either eye, this is probably a convergence problem. If there is still double vision in one eye when the other is covered, this is often due to dry eye or an optical/refractive disturbance.

To help with convergence problems, consider:

- Occasionally, eye exercises like "pencil push-ups" can help with convergence problems. Pencil push-ups involve slowly bringing a small object, like the tip of a pencil, from arm's length in towards the nose, repeating 20 or so times a few times a day for a few weeks. There's no clear protocol or prescription for this, and it is usually much more effective in younger people recovering from head trauma, such as concussions.

- Get prisms in your *reading glasses only*. Prisms bend light to compensate for a misalignment of the eyes. Since the eyes can't work together because of convergence, prisms can bend the light to compensate so one clear image can be seen, as opposed to two separate images.

- If nothing else helps, you could try an old trick of covering one eye or putting Scotch tape over one lens of your reading glasses to ensure only one eye is being used at a time.

Hallucinations

Hallucinations can result from Parkinson's itself or be related to medications used to treat Parkinson's. Amantadine and dopamine agonist medications (pramipexole, rotigotine, ropinirole) tend to the be the biggest offenders, although levodopa/carbidopa, entacapone, rasagiline and selegeline can also cause hallucinations.

Common types of hallucinations are:

- **Simple:** Seeing insects or small animals (which are not there) located in the peripheral vision.

- **Complex:** Usually seeing animate objects (e.g., a small, black cat which is not there), often in the center of vision in dim lighting and associated with poorer vision.

- **Illusion:** Mistaking a small pile of clothes in the corner of the room (which is there) for a small cat (which is not there).

Treatments

If hallucinations are mild, ensure the person living with Parkinson's is not particularly bothered by them. If they are moderate to severe or particularly bothersome, discuss with your neurologist and consider possible removal of certain medications. Doctors may consider starting another medication to decrease hallucinations, including pimavanserin (Nuplazid), which is the first FDA-approved drug to treat hallucinations and delusions in Parkinson's. While it never hurts to inform your eye care professional about hallucinations you are experiencing, these should be discussed in detail with your neurologist.

141

Other ocular conditions may affect people living with Parkinson's, but are more common in atypical parkinsonian syndromes, such as progressive supranuclear palsy (PSP).

Uncommon problems include:

- Blepharospasm
  - Involuntary, forceful eyelid closure
- Apraxia of eyelid opening
  - Difficulty voluntarily opening the eyes in the absence of spasms that force the eyes closed
- Vertical eye movement limitations
  - Most common with PSP – e.g., people living with this disorder may be messy eaters or have significant difficulty walking down stairs due to eye limitations in looking down.

TAKE ACTION TO LIVE WELL

While there are no proven ways to prevent most ocular conditions from developing, routine visits with an eye care professional can lead to early recognition and treatment of eye issues before they can have a negative impact on quality of life. Between you, your neurologist and an ophthalmologist, the vast majority of visual complaints can be handled. However, when symptoms remain unchanged and unexplained, consultation with a neuro-ophthalmologist is probably warranted.

A neuro-ophthalmologist is either a neurologist or an ophthalmologist with fellowship training in neuro-ophthalmology. Neuro-ophthalmologists have a unique appreciation for the intersection of the eyes and the brain and perform comprehensive testing in the office to figure out where a visual or eye movement problem could be coming from. Once the location of the disturbance is identified, diagnostic testing (when appropriate), treatments and therapies can be customized depending on the individual and his or her complaint(s).

While your eye care professional may not specifically be aware of common ocular symptoms that people living with Parkinson's experience, explaining the kinds of situations and triggers that bring on eye symptoms is usually enough for your doctor to know where to look during the examination (e.g., front part of the eye, back part of the eye, movements of the eyes). Keeping a journal or diary of symptoms can also be helpful for both you and your doctor.

FATIGUE

Fatigue is a common symptom of Parkinson's, but can also be caused by other problems, which you should consider as part of the big picture. Heart problems, diabetes, thyroid disease, depression, cancer, lung disease, anemia, sleep apnea and medication side effects are just a few medical problems that can also cause fatigue.

Eating smaller meals more frequently, having a bit of caffeine midday and exercising can diminish fatigue. Pay attention to how you feel, and give yourself time to revive with "down time."

SLEEP

Disrupted sleep is very common in Parkinson's and may begin years prior to your actual diagnosis. Poor sleep can cause daytime sleepiness, fatigue, low energy, irritability, poor concentration and attention and feeling tired when first waking. Many people feel better and have fewer issues with symptoms when sleep quality and quantity improves. Treating sleep issues requires a multidisciplinary approach, because sleep problems can be the result of other medical conditions, as well as a symptom of Parkinson's.

Lifestyle choices, such as watching television or using a computer or tablet before bedtime, can also compound sleep problems. The brain's circadian rhythm is typically set to fall asleep in the evening, but blue light from screens can stimulate and confuse it. Limit exposure to electronic devices before bedtime, and try to sleep in a room free from these distractions. Find more resources and ideas for getting a better night's sleep at: **dpf.org/more-sleep**.

Good sleep habits are important. This includes going to bed and getting up at the same time each day, avoiding caffeine at least four to six hours before bedtime and skipping alcohol and heavy, late-night snacks. Gentle stretching can also help sleep when done before bed. Changing your nighttime habits can be challenging, but making healthy adjustments to your routine can often solve many sleep problems.

MOOD CHANGES AND COGNITIVE PROBLEMS

Depression and anxiety are common symptoms of Parkinson's associated with changes in the neurotransmitters inside the brain. Mood changes can occur before any physical signs of Parkinson's or as a reaction to the diagnosis and progression of symptoms. Apathy can result from changes in the brain associated with Parkinson's or may coincide with cognitive declines. Apathy is commonly mistaken for depression due to the changes in motivation or decreased interest in activities or socializing. For more about depression, anxiety and apathy, read the "Emotional Health" chapter in this section.

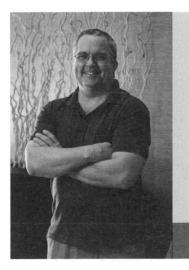

I've found specialists like a psychiatrist or a neuropsychologist to be necessary tools for coping and growing. I'm not afraid to reach out for help. People take their cars in for routine maintenance, and I believe we have to do that with our minds as well. Often we think we can fix something ourselves, but our mind is far more intricate than a car."

— BRIAN

Cognitive or thinking skills can decline as a result of neurotransmitter changes or aging and may begin before diagnosis. Cognitive changes are highly variable in Parkinson's, ranging from mild declines in performance of planning and executing tasks to dementia. Vitamin deficiencies, such as low B12 levels, electrolyte abnormalities, thyroid problems, sleep apnea and cardiovascular disease are examples of medical issues that can cause depression, anxiety or thinking problems. However, the medication cycles and fatigue associated with Parkinson's will also affect your mood and cognition.

GASTROINTESTINAL, BOWEL AND BLADDER CHANGES

Gastric reflux, constipation, urinary frequency and urinary urgency are common in people with Parkinson's because of how the nervous system controls both bladder and digestive functions. In Parkinson's, the bladder muscle can become overactive and the digestive system can become underactive from changes in the nervous system. Review any changes in bladder or bowel function with your doctor to be sure the symptoms are caused by Parkinson's. These problems are all treatable.

Most often, people with Parkinson's experience problems with frequent or urgent urination that can worsen to the point of incontinence. When bladder symptoms progress, urinary tract infections may be more common.

CONSTIPATION

Constipation is frequently reported by many people with Parkinson's and can actually appear years before an official Parkinson's diagnosis. Part of the effect of Parkinson's on the autonomic nervous system seems to be the slowing down the movement of food through the gastrointestinal tract. Like bladder control, constipation can be the result of Parkinson's or it can come as a side effect of medication. Severe constipation can impact medication absorption and is a medical emergency if the colon becomes impacted. If you do not have a bowel movement every three days or experience fullness, discomfort or pain in the abdomen, talk with your doctor.

Certain medications such as pain relievers and antacids, cold medications, antidepressants, high blood pressure medications, high cholesterol medications and cardiovascular disease medications can make constipation worse. If you take any of these medications and experience difficulty with constipation, discuss medication options with your doctor.

Diet also can play a role in constipation. Eating more foods rich in fiber, staying physically active as well as drinking more water can help with constipation. Coffee and some teas are also reported to improve constipation, although too much caffeine may end up making it harder to fall and stay asleep. Some supplements such as aloe vera and magnesium can be helpful in relieving constipation. Your doctor may also recommend an over-the-counter laxative medication that can be used to ease bowel movements.

A daily routine of 30 minutes of some form of exercise is an important part to keeping your gastrointestinal tract healthy and moving and, thus, improving constipation. Consult the **Constipation Worksheet** in the **Worksheets and Resources** section for more ways to improve constipation. Learn more about causes of constipation and how to combat it: ◼️ dpf.org/constipation.

COGNITIVE CHANGES RELATED TO PARKINSON'S

By Mark Mapstone, PhD

Have you ever considered what a remarkable and delicate piece of biology our brains are? They are truly amazing. Everything from moving our bodies, to making complex decisions, communicating thoughts, remembering past events, feeling sad or happy or even just paying attention to things going on around us is orchestrated by this three-pound organ. Each of these complex abilities is the product of many different brain regions working together in large networks and in synchronized harmony. However, when one or more brain regions are not working the way they should, whole networks may be affected and problems can result. Parkinson's causes a specific brain region to slowly stop working and as a result, people with Parkinson's may experience thinking, or cognitive changes due to a decline in specific brain networks.

Most of the cognitive problems that people with Parkinson's experience are linked to bradyphrenia (*brady* means "slowed" and *phrenia* means "thinking"). This is the consequence of slowed signals moving through these brain networks, so some information is delayed or even lost as it moves through the brain. In many ways, bradyphrenia is the cognitive equivalent of the slowness that also affects physical movement in Parkinson's. These slowed signals can affect many cognitive abilities that rely on the speedy transfer of information. These can include executive function (mental skills that help you accomplish tasks, such as time management, future planning and paying attention), language, memory and visuoperception (understanding where things are around you). Some of these cognitive changes may be significant, but it's important to realize that these are typically limited to specific cognitive abilities. While your ability to process information might be different than in the past, that doesn't mean you have a global decline in intellect.

Some of the most common cognitive changes associated with Parkinson's involve executive function. These include difficulty with abilities like making complex decisions, keeping multiple things straight in your mind, organizing actions or ideas or doing tasks in a specific sequence. Executive tasks, like calculating a tip at a restaurant or holding a conversation on a cell phone while grocery shopping may become next to impossible for the person living with Parkinson's because of these brain network changes. Furthermore, these executive problems can be particularly frustrating because we rely on these very abilities to navigate our complex and fast-paced world.

Another cognitive change that people living with Parkinson's may experience involves memory. The most common memory problems affect short-term recall, especially the ability to come up with information from things you have just seen or heard, or to recall information on the spot. Long-term memory of things that have happened in the past is less likely to be affected. One particularly vexing problem involving both memory and language is difficulty finding words. Most of us have experienced a "tip of the tongue" moment where we are searching for a word or perhaps a name that just won't come to us. Eventually, it pops up in a moment of distraction or when our minds have given up the search. It's almost like the harder we search, the more elusive the word becomes. Word finding problems are common for people living with Parkinson's and can be very frustrating and embarrassing.

Any change in thinking can be concerning. Understandably, most people living with Parkinson's, especially those recently diagnosed, want to know if they will experience significant cognitive changes. This is an important question that affects not only the person living with Parkinson's, but those around him or her, including care partners, family members and communities at large. It is difficult to make predictions for any single person and currently we don't have reliable ways to predict cognitive changes for an individual, or to tell them which cognitive symptoms they will develop or how severe any cognitive symptoms may be. That said, most people with Parkinson's will experience some cognitive changes like those described above over the course of their Parkinson's, but not all will have the same combination or severity of symptoms. Some individuals will have subtle cognitive changes while others may develop more severe cognitive problems that impact how they live their daily lives.

A major cognitive concern for many people living with Parkinson's is dementia. Most recent figures suggest that up to one-third of people living with Parkinson's will develop dementia. Dementia is the development of significant cognitive changes that significantly affect how you live your daily life and even your ability to live independently. In addition, Parkinson's dementia may also include the appearance of new symptoms, such as hallucinations and long-term memory loss. Dementia may be difficult to detect, because many of the cognitive symptoms can be related to other problems of Parkinson's, such as depression, low energy or low motivation, or like hallucinations or memory loss, may be side effects of some medications used to treat Parkinson's. For these reasons, it is important to talk openly to your Parkinson's doctor about all of your cognitive symptoms and concerns.

Let's turn now to how to face these cognitive challenges head on.

Many people living with Parkinson's wonder what they can do to stay mentally healthy in the face of all this. First, it's important to realize that you are an active agent in your own health and you can have a very real impact on your cognitive abilities. However, it is important to have realistic expectations. Many of the cognitive symptoms of Parkinson's are the result of structural changes in the brain and there are limits to how much they can be modified. But in most cases, cognitive abilities can be maintained and even improved to some degree. For most people living with Parkinson's, this starts with maintaining physical health. Your brain receives all its nutrients and oxygen from the blood supply, so things that are good for cardiovascular health are good for brain health. Maintaining an active lifestyle with good nutrition and sleep can be a challenge for people with Parkinson's, but these things are vitally important to your physical and brain health. Another key element to maintain brain health is to engage in mental stimulation. Keep mentally active! Have conversations with people around you. Read new books. Teach someone to fly fish. Learn Italian. By encouraging your brain to actively engage and do something it's not used to, you strengthen connections in different brain networks which may help them work more efficiently and ultimately improve the behavior they produce. Watching television is not mental activity and doesn't count.

Finally, make things easier on yourself if you are experiencing cognitive symptoms. Carry a small notepad with you. You can take notes to help remember items at the store or write out the steps for that new recipe so you don't lose your place. Store commonly used objects like car keys, your purse or cell phone in the same place every time so you will know where they will be when you need them. Take a picture of where your car is parked with your cell phone if you have trouble remembering where it is in a parking lot.

For care partners, patience and understanding are key. Cognitive changes may be difficult to comprehend or accept, and as a result, people living with Parkinson's may minimize or deny cognitive changes. In some cases, they may not be able to recognize that these changes are happening. In this situation, repeatedly pointing out and trying to convince your loved one of their cognitive lapses is rarely fruitful. The goal is to be supportive and understanding, and help with tasks to decrease frustration and if necessary, to ensure safety. Have frank discussions about any cognitive changes with your loved one's Parkinson's doctor. For specific cognitive tasks, patience and understanding can go a long way. It may be tempting to finish sentences for someone struggling with word finding, but be patient. Allow a few seconds before jumping in. That mental search strengthens brain networks and it may make it easier to come up with the word next time.

It's important to be aware that cognitive changes can be confusing, frustrating and just as disruptive as motor changes. We all need to understand that people with Parkinson's are giving their best with what they have, and what they have is different now.

OVERACTIVE BLADDER AND INCONTINENCE

People with Parkinson's may also experience incontinence, which is accidental or involuntary loss of control of urine or bowel movements. This can range from occasional minor leakage to complete loss of control of urine or bowel movements.

There are different types of incontinence that people with Parkinson's may experience, such as:

- **Urge incontinence:** a frequent and urgent need to use the toilet.
- **Stress incontinence:** usually occurs in the presence of some kind of physical stressor such as coughing.
- **Nocturia:** the need to get up multiple times in the night to use the toilet.

Turn to the **Bladder Worksheet** in the **Worksheets and Resources** section to learn about changes you can make to your diet and lifestyle to help manage an overactive bladder, as well as treatments to discuss with your doctor and other healthcare professionals. Many incontinence issues can be addressed by therapy with an incontinence specialist, practicing exercises such as Kegels on a daily basis and by taking certain medications.

EXCESSIVE SWEATING

Parkinson's affects the autonomic nervous system (the parts of your body that you do not consciously direct or think about). This includes everything from body temperature, breathing, digestion and your heartbeat. Occasionally, some people with Parkinson's experience excessive sweating that occurs regardless of level of physical activity or room temperature. This can occur at night and impact sleep or can happen during the day.

Some tips to help with excessive sweating include:

- Staying hydrated
- Wearing lightweight, loose fitting clothing made from cotton or other natural fibers
- Choosing clothing that doesn't show sweat
- Identifying and reducing consumption of foods that may trigger sweating (spicy foods, caffeine or alcohol)
- Identifying and reducing stressors that cause sweating (public speaking, crowded rooms, etc.)

If you are experiencing excessive sweating, have a conversation with your doctor to explore how to specifically address this.

While less frequently reported, some people with Parkinson's may experience too little sweating or hypohidrosis, which could be a side effect of an anticholinergic Parkinson's medication. Too little sweating can have a negative impact on your ability to control your body's temperature and thus put you at risk for overheating.

147

If your excessive sweating or lack of sweating begins to negatively impact your daily life, talk with your doctor about adjusting your medication or other treatments, such as botulism toxin (Botox) injections that may help manage excessive sweating.

WEIGHT MANAGEMENT

Some people with Parkinson's gain weight due to diet changes, sweet cravings and/or decrease in exercise. This can lead to many problems including joint disease, pain, fatigue, diabetes, heart disease, sleep apnea, reduced stamina and walking problems. It is easy to see how these conditions could also affect your mobility.

Conversely, some people with Parkinson's have trouble gaining weight due to loss of sense of smell, altered taste, decreased desire to eat, apathy, depression, swallowing problems, stomach bloating, constipation, change in the body's metabolic rate and increased energy expenditure due to tremor or dyskinesia. Unexplained weight changes can also be a signal for other problems such as thyroid disease, gastrointestinal problems and cancer.

Pay attention to your weight, and discuss sudden changes with your doctor.

SMOKING CESSATION

Smoking is directly associated with heart disease, lung problems and cancer. It also can reduce your stamina, making exercise and your everyday movements more difficult. Smoking has a negative impact on your brain health as well. Medication, nicotine supplements and behavioral therapies are available to help you kick the habit.

ALCOHOL USE

You may have heard that one glass of red wine a day can reduce your risk of heart disease. For some individuals with Parkinson's, even this small amount is not recommended. Review your use of alcohol with your PCP and neurologist, since alcohol can exacerbate low blood pressure, affect balance, impair mood, impair thinking functions, worsen apathy and interact with many of your medications. This may not mean you must avoid alcohol altogether, but you should be aware of how it interacts with your medications and assess whether the benefits outweigh the risk.

■ EXERCISE

In all people, exercise can improve heart health and endurance, increase strength, reduce fatigue and make a positive impact on mood, weight management and self-esteem. Hear how John has made exercise and being active a priority after being diagnosed with Parkinson's: ◼ dpf.org/john.

However, exercise takes on an even greater importance in Parkinson's, given the physical changes associated with the disease. Your muscles may feel tighter, weaker or heavier. You may lack the coordination or fluidity of movement that you are used to, and these changes require more energy to complete your daily activities. Despite these barriers, there are many reasons to exercise. Whether you are already in good shape and are trying to maintain what you have, or have lost fitness and need to build a better you – it's never too late to start. Exercise will almost always help you.

❝ *I recently had surgery and wasn't able to exercise as vigorously as I normally do. I didn't realize what a difference exercise was making in my life with Parkinson's. I know they say to 'move it or lose it,' but I really believe it's never too late to start being more active.*❞

— LIZ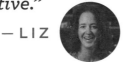

A STRONGER BODY LEADS TO BETTER MOVEMENT

Exercise can help your Parkinson's in the following ways:

- **Improve your physical body.** Exercise will improve your physical strength, agility, flexibility, posture and balance. Your ability to move will improve with practice, just like an Olympic athlete that improves his or her performance with training.

- **Improve your endurance.** An exercise program focused on endurance will help with daytime tiredness, fatigue, heart health, breathing muscles and stamina.

- **Improve your general well-being.** Research confirms that exercise can reduce your risk of heart disease, hypertension and diabetes. It can help reduce pain, improve constipation, manage weight gain and improve depression, cognition, sleep and self-confidence. This is more than any one pill can do, and exercise can be fun!

- **Delay or reduce problems of Parkinson's.** Certain muscle groups stiffen and lose flexibility with Parkinson's. Movements get smaller, arm swing is reduced, posture and balance change. Targeting these areas before they give you trouble can help delay or reduce these problems. This is especially true for balance, posture and flexibility.

EXERCISE IS MEDICINE FOR THE BRAIN

By Jay L. Alberts, PhD

While many great scientific discoveries are rooted in dimly lit laboratory or clinical environments, some are not. In 2003, I pedaled a tandem bike with my companion (a person with Parkinson's disease) on a multiday group bike tour through the corn and bean fields of Iowa. Little did I realize at the beginning of this trek that an important discovery about the effects of exercise on Parkinson's motor function was about to be made.

A few days into the ride, my Parkinson's companion noticed a dramatic improvement in her handwriting as she wrote out a birthday card – effortlessly and legibly. Initially, I thought that maybe our diet of pie and homemade ice cream was responsible for these improvements in motor function. Who wouldn't feel better after indulging in such treats?

Turns out it was neither the pie nor ice cream; it was riding the tandem that was making the difference. What is special about tandem cycling? Couples without Parkinson's jokingly call it a test of marriage, because of the coordination and communication that is required on a bicycle built for two. For us, the tandem enabled us to engage in a type of exercise called "forced-exercise." Forced-exercise essentially means assisting a person in exercising at a rate that is greater than their preferred, voluntary, exercise rate. In this case, the person with Parkinson's could pedal at a rate of approximately 50 revolutions per minute (RPM) when she was exercising by herself. When she rode tandem with me, our pedaling rate or cadence was 80–90 RPM. Thus, I was "forcing" her to pedal faster than she could by herself.

We have published an article in which we compared the effects of eight weeks of voluntary exercise to eight weeks of forced-exercise on Parkinson's motor function, and most recently a review on aerobic exercise and Parkinson's. Our results indicated that participants in the forced group exhibited substantial improvements in their overall motor functioning compared to those in the voluntary group, and the effects of the improvements lasted even after exercise was completed. This data, along with data from the animal studies, suggests that exercise rate or effort may be an important variable in improving motor function in people with Parkinson's disease.

We are currently working to develop a paradigm that does not require the use of a tandem bike (I don't want to be responsible for breaking up any marriages), and also learning more about how home exercises can help improve the lives of those with Parkinson's disease. The Davis Phinney Foundation has greatly helped in funding this research with cycling and home therapy.

Our most recent study allows us to give stationary bicycles to people living with Parkinson's where we can monitor their exercise with the use of telemedicine. In the meantime, you can ask your doctor or physical therapist how to safely integrate some of our methods into your own exercise. As with any exercise program, consistency and compliance are critical if the program is going to be effective. Hopefully, you will, through your own experience, be able to proclaim that exercise really is medicine for Parkinson's.

RESEARCH SUMMARY: THE POSITIVE EFFECTS OF PHYSICAL ACTIVITY ON PARKINSON'S DISEASE

By Lee Dibble, PT, PhD, ATC

As life expectancy increases worldwide, the number of people over age 50 with Parkinson's disease in the world's 10 most populous countries is expected to double, from approximately 4.5 million in 2005 to 9 million by 2030. These numbers highlight the importance of seeking simple, low-cost interventions such as exercise, to minimize disability and improve mobility and quality of life in people with Parkinson's disease.

Over the last decade, evidence has emerged to reveal significant and clinically meaningful benefits of exercise for persons with Parkinson's. Distinct lines of evidence are converging to strengthen the theory that physical activity and exercise can result in tangible benefits. These lines of evidence are: 1) Longitudinal (epidemiologic) studies, 2) Physical activity interventions for diseases associated with sedentary behavior and aging, 3) Exercise studies in animal models of Parkinson's, and 4) Synthesis of human studies of exercise and Parkinson's.

1. Evidence from multiple longitudinal observational studies suggests that persons who regularly engaged in moderate to vigorous exercise had a decreased risk of developing Parkinson's. The apparent risk reduction was substantial and present even if the regular exercise was performed in the third or fourth decades of life.

2. The positive effects of physical activity and exercise are present regardless of age or type of illness. There is strong evidence that regular participation in physical activity and exercise decreases the occurrence and adverse consequences of disorders, such as heart disease, diabetes and obesity. In addition, exercise studies consistently improve cognitive abilities even in the presence of dementia. Through the prevention of other potentially concurrent diseases, physical activity and exercise indirectly improve movement abilities and quality of life in persons with Parkinson's.

3. Multiple exercise studies in animal models of Parkinson's disease demonstrate improvements in mobility, nerve cell function and the potential of increased survival of nerve cells within the affected area of the brain. In contrast, animal studies that impose inactivity demonstrate increased degeneration of nerve cells and loss of mobility. Proposed mechanisms for the observed positive effects include increased production of nerve cell growth factors and the growth of new blood vessels that supply oxygen and nutrients to at-risk areas of the brain. At the very least, these findings suggest that exercise has a positive impact on the brain, as well as on the rest of the body.

4. Research reports that synthesize the combined results of high-quality studies of persons with Parkinson's consistently demonstrate that those who participated in exercise programs, regardless of the type of exercise, enjoyed a better quality of life, walking ability, balance, strength, flexibility and cardiovascular fitness compared to those who did not exercise. Recent specific positive effects of exercise are highlighted below:

    a. Several different research groups around the world (Hong Kong, Sydney, Melbourne and a European/Israeli Consortium) have demonstrated the benefits of exercises targeted at improving balance in the reduction of falls in people with Parkinson's. Despite differences in methods and interventions, these studies found that exercise improved functional mobility and reduced the incidence of falls in the future in people with Parkinson's. This study reinforced the power of exercise and specific balance task practice to improve balance and reduce fall risk.

b. Researchers at the University of Colorado reported that the inclusion of spinal and extremity flexibility exercises significantly improved mobility and performance of daily activities in people with early and mid-stage Parkinson's disease after 16 weeks of exercise. Participants in this study that performed aerobic exercise improved their walking ability and efficiency of walking.

c. Researchers at Northwestern University reported that regular resistance exercises over a 24-month period resulted in significantly improved muscle strength, reduced disease severity and improved mobility in people with early and mid-stage Parkinson's disease. With consistent participation in exercise after the initial exercise period, improvements were sustained for two years.

d. The positive effects of "forced exercise" on a tandem bicycle were reported by researchers at the Cleveland Clinic. Participants in this study rode as the passenger on a tandem bicycle that was mounted on a trainer in the clinic. By keeping pace with the person without Parkinson's who pedaled with them, people with Parkinson's experienced fitness improvements and overall reductions in their motor symptoms.

e. Researchers at Boston University reported that people with Parkinson's disease who were at risk of moving from home to nursing home care benefited from a focused inpatient exercise program conducted by physical, occupational and speech therapists. Participants improved in mobility measures, and many were able to avoid nursing home placement.

f. Improvement of the size of handwriting was reported by researchers in Belgium. Participants in this study practiced handwriting tasks five days a week for six weeks on an electronic tablet. In addition to improvements in the size of the handwriting, participants improved their ability to maintain writing size in the presence of distraction and improved in writing tasks that were not practiced.

152

Exercise helps your body and brain find new ways to move. This can occur in two ways: neuroplasticity or alternative brain pathways. The brain can utilize a process called neuroplasticity to improve function. If there is damage to a particular area of the brain, new nerve cell connections can be made or strengthened, or new pathways or brain areas can be recruited and used for activity. Think of this as boosting current brain circuits, re-wiring your brain circuitry; disconnecting the old wires and redirecting to new wires and different pathways. This is the theory behind "forced use" therapy. It requires repetitive motor training under the supervision of a professional, such as a physical therapist, to avoid injury. Ongoing research suggests that aerobic exercise has a strong potential to slow the progression of Parkinson's symptoms in some individuals.

" *You can lose balance, but you can get it back. Balance is a learned process.*"

— EDIE

Listen to Edie explain how exercise has helped her regain function lost because of Parkinson's: ◼ **dpf.org/edie**. Alternative brain pathways enable you to perform and gain strength in a task you otherwise have trouble performing by using other, stronger brain circuits typically used for similar functions. For instance, people with speech problems might be able to sing, or those with walking problems might be able to dance or march to music, because these tasks also engage different areas of the brain.

MOVE IT! EXERCISE AND PHYSICAL ACTIVITY ARE KEY TO LIVING WELL WITH PARKINSON'S

By Gammon M. Earhart, PT, PhD

When someone asks me what they can do to live well with Parkinson's, my number one recommendation is to keep moving. That may seem like a strange recommendation, since Parkinson's can make it challenging to move, but the evidence supporting the importance of physical activity and exercise is hard to deny. A study of over 2,000 people living with Parkinson's showed that those who were exercising for 150 minutes or more per week had better mobility, physical function and cognitive performance compared to those who were not exercising. The people who were exercising regularly also experienced less disease progression over the course of a year.

Exercise can convey a wide array of benefits, not the least of which is improved quality of life. Studies suggest that exercise can be helpful whether you have been living with Parkinson's for a day or for decades. It is never too early or too late to start, and there are lots of options in terms of types of exercises and activities that are beneficial.

- **Strengthening exercises** can improve the structure and function of muscles, making movement more effective.

- **Aerobic exercise** such as walking or biking, anything that gets your heart pumping harder and faster, can improve cardiovascular health and make movement more efficient.

- **Balance exercises** such as those in yoga or tai chi can help to improve postural stability and may even lead to a reduction in fall risk and number of falls.

- **Stretching and flexibility exercises** such as those in yoga or tai chi can help reduce stiffness.

- **Complex activities** that require learning of new skills, such as dancing, may help with physical function as well as cognitive function.

Since there is no overwhelming evidence to suggest that one form of exercise is better than others, I recommend that people incorporate a variety of different types of exercises into their routines. After all, variety is the spice of life and can help to keep exercise interesting and enjoyable rather than doing the same thing day after day.

Speaking of day after day, we often underestimate the importance of our daily levels of physical activity. It is not just planned or structured exercise that matters; activity level throughout the course of daily life is also important. Being active and spending less time sitting is associated with fewer movement difficulties, along with a host of other health benefits. Ideally, we would all exercise for 150 minutes per week of exercise and get 10,000 steps per day. In reality, any amount of activity is better than being inactive. Do what you can to be active and set goals for yourself to keep moving. To help you do this, here are eight evidence-based recommendations for integrating exercise into your daily life.

- **Believe in yourself.** People who are more confident in their ability to exercise are more likely to engage in exercise. You can increase your confidence by having a plan for how you will exercise in the face of challenges such as bad weather or fatigue.

- **Expect exercise to be beneficial.** The evidence is undeniable – exercise helps! And people who believe in the power of exercise seem to benefit more than people who do not expect exercise to be helpful.

- **Seek professional input to get started.** Before starting any exercise, it is advisable to consult with a medical professional. Consider asking your physician to refer you to a physical therapist who can assess your needs and help you design a program to meet your goals.

153

- **Put exercise on your calendar and set reminders.** Having a specific plan of when you are going to exercise and setting reminders for yourself can increase the probability that you will follow through and get moving. Even people who are already exercisers end up exercising more often when they have reminders to do so.

- **Break your exercise into chunks.** Research shows that as little as 10 minutes of exercise at a time can be effective. Squeeze in 10 minutes here and there, and before you know it, you will be getting the recommended 150 minutes a week!

- **Exercise with a partner or a group.** Having a friend, family member or group helps you to be accountable. People who exercise with others are more likely to stick with it.

- **Use technology to your advantage.** There are many options when it comes to pedometers, activity trackers and smartphone apps that can help you to keep track of your activity. These same devices can also help you to set activity goals, monitor your progress and connect and compete with friends.

- **Have fun!** Whatever you do, make sure you choose activities you like. One of the biggest predictors of whether or not people exercise is how much they enjoy the exercise. And, exercise can be made even more enjoyable by adding music.

Exercise is one of the most powerful tools at your disposal and will help you to live well with Parkinson's. So, keep moving and remember that *every victory counts*!

> " *I can be paralyzed by dystonia and then get on the treadmill and walk. I also roll on a foam roller and roller balls to help work out tight muscles.*"
>
> — LINDA

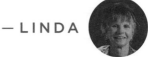

154

Exercise may be neuroprotective. Research is exploring the possibility that exercise helps protect nerve cells that are at risk for damage, degeneration or cell death. In other words, exercise helps cells that are most vulnerable strengthen their line of defense before they sustain damage. The idea that exercise can protect nerve cells is not unique to Parkinson's. Exercise also has been shown to treat depression, limit memory problems associated with normal aging and reduce the risk of developing Alzheimer's disease. It is not known what type of exercise has the greatest potential for neuroprotection, but intensive, high-energy aerobic exercise is actively under study in people with Parkinson's.

COMMON QUESTIONS BEFORE STARTING AN EXERCISE ROUTINE

WHAT SHOULD I DO?

The good news is that exercise can help at any time during the progression of Parkinson's. However, the earlier you start the better. The key to exercise is to make it a part of your life and a long-term commitment. Hear about Brian's experience exercising in Parkinson's-specific group classes: ▪◄ **dpf.org/brian**.

> *"When I was first diagnosed, I stopped running and cycling because I was depressed, and I lost a year of well-being. Don't stop what you've been doing, don't let stuff go. If you sit on the couch, you'll feel worse, and it's going to get harder. Find something you love to do and do it."*
>
> — TIM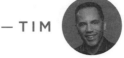

Start an exercise program now to help slow progression of Parkinson's symptoms and of aging. There are many resources available to help you get started or renew your commitment to exercise both in your community and online. Watch "Parkinson's Exercise Essentials" for a comprehensive guide to starting your own exercise routine: 🎥 **dpf.org/how-to-exercise**.

A comprehensive exercise program should include:

- **Aerobic or cardiovascular activity.** This includes exercises that increase your heart and breathing rate such as walking, hiking, rowing, swimming or cycling. You can also try a variety of cardiovascular machines at your local fitness center or community center. See a tour of common cardio machines and how they can help you stay active: 🎥 **dpf.org/aerobic-tour**.

- **Posture and stretching.** The primary muscles that flex your arms, shoulders, hips, knees and ankles can feel tight and stiff with Parkinson's and can be alleviated with dance, yoga and tai chi, to name a few. Regularly stretching these muscles (hamstrings, calf muscles) can reduce the impact of stiffness that affects your body's movement, such as postural changes.

- **Strength.** Stronger muscles lead to less energy expenditure with everyday movement, less fatigue throughout the day and greater stamina. Greater leg strength is also associated with balance control and fewer falls.

- **Balance and fine movement control.** It is important to include exercises that challenge your balance and hand coordination, such as yoga and tai chi.

- **Complex exercises** such as dancing, yoga and circuit training bring together the benefits of aerobic, strength and endurance while engaging the mind and balance system and are typically performed in a social setting.

- **Weight-bearing exercises.** Walking, running or jumping can improve bone strength.

- **Intensity.** Continue to challenge yourself by increasing the intensity of your exercise. Relative intensity can be measured by doing a "talk test" while you exercise. If you are engaged in moderate-intensity exercise, you should be able to talk, but not sing. If you are engaged in vigorous-intensity exercise, it will be difficult to say more than a few words without pausing for a breath.

155

THREE WAYS TO GET MAXIMUM BENEFIT FROM YOUR EXERCISE ROUTINE

By Matthew P. Ford, PT, PhD

By now, you've probably heard that there is no one perfect exercise plan for people living with Parkinson's. There are some fundamental concepts, though, that should apply to whatever your chosen activities may be.

Exercising to live well with Parkinson's means incorporating three things into your daily routine:

- **Physical activity:** any activity you do when not sitting or lying down
- **Exercise:** planned physical activity or movement that is frequent and intense
- **Moving to music:** adding music to stimulate your movement

PHYSICAL ACTIVITY

It's essential to get adequate physical activity each day. Yet, understandably, this is not always easy for people with Parkinson's to do. To get an idea of how physically active you are, measure the amount of time during the day that you are *not* sitting in a chair or lying down. From there, commit to progressively increase that time each day, even if only by a few minutes at a time. If you make that commitment, you will see significant improvements in a week, a month and a year. Just increase your physical activity a little bit each day.

Remember to:

- **Decrease your sit time:** stand up more frequently
- **Use a step counter** (various wrist band types) to measure your physical activity
- **Increase your physical activity** a little bit each day

When you stand upright, you work your leg and posture muscles. From there, you can start to walk around more. There are numerous digital step counters available on the market. A smartphone (such as Android or iPhone) has a counter in it, as well. Keeping track of your daily steps makes it easier to measure process towards your goal of increasing activity each day. It may not seem like a lot, but this simple change in daily habits can significantly add up over time. If you commit to increasing your physical activity at any stage of Parkinson's, you will feel better and see health benefits.

EXERCISE

The next thing to do is add regular exercise to your daily and weekly routine. Exercise could be walking, running, biking, swimming, hiking and/or lifting weights (resistance training). The goal of exercise is to work your heart, lungs and muscles. People living with Parkinson's feel better, get stronger and are more independent when they exercise regularly. While exercise does not cure Parkinson's, it is an essential component of managing symptoms.

You'll be more successful if you:

- **Plan it out** using an exercise calendar or journal
- **Do you something that you enjoy**
- **Exercise with others** to hold yourself accountable
- **Exercise frequently**, two to three times per week
- **Exercise with adequate intensity**, as measured by:
  - Difficult to carry on a conversation *while* exercising
  - Breathing is heavy, but you are *not* out of breath

The most common question I'm asked is, "What is the best exercise for people living Parkinson's?" The answer is that **there is not one type of exercise that is best for Parkinson's**. Pick the exercises you will keep doing! Your exercise routine should include aerobic exercise (walking, biking, swimming, elliptical, treadmill), resistance training (weights) and something for balance and flexibility.

Even as we age, the heart, lungs and muscles still respond very positively to exercise training. People with Parkinson's *do* get healthier when they exercise *regularly*. I recommend that you consult with a licensed physical therapist (PT) in your area in order to establish an exercise program specific for your needs. A consultation with a PT may require one to two initial visits followed by periodic visits throughout the rest of the calendar year. You do *not* need to see a PT three times per week in order to exercise. However, you *should* see a PT to get your "exercise prescription," that is, your proper exercise dosage, considerations related to your form and physical fitness, etc., before you start exercising. Research has shown that the exercise intensity can be the single most important aspect of exercise for relieving Parkinson's symptoms. You will do well if you follow the guidelines above, but a PT can look more objectively at your heart rate (HR) as a measure of intensity. Armed with this information, they can provide you with very specific guidelines and instructions on how to use HR to keep track of your exercise intensity.

MOVING TO MUSIC

Moving, whether just walking around the house or during exercise, can be difficult, even for people with Parkinson's who are active. Listening to music will help you become more physically active and exercise better.

Your brain, even with Parkinson's, is a great internal timer. The connections between parts of your brain, specifically those associated with your muscles, have a rhythm. Your brain can easily process the timing in music (external timer) and facilitate movement by driving your brain's internal timer. We have all experienced this phenomenon. For instance, when you are in the car and hear a favorite song, you start tapping the steering wheel or moving to the beat. It is a natural thing to do. The same thing can happen when you exercise to music. Try it. Play an upbeat song, and see how your walking changes immediately.

To get started including music in your daily routine:

- Purchase a digital, portable music player, or use your smartphone
- Establish a digital music account (iTunes, Pandora, Spotify, etc.) and find your favorite music
- Download your personal playlist to your music player or smartphone

Note: If you're unfamiliar with these technologies, ask a relative or friend to help you. You can learn to use these simple devices, and they will help you exercise better with more enjoyment.

Everyone likes music. There are so many genres, and we have each been influenced by music differently. The first step is to exercise to music that you know and enjoy. Listening to your favorite music will improve your mood, which will in turn, improve your physical activity.

Whatever your preferred style of music — slow, fast, big band, rock and roll — there is one activity everyone can do to their favorite music: **dance!** Start off by dancing at home. Dance by yourself, or find a partner. Use your favorite music to help you move and increase your physical activity. Dancing at home is fine, but I encourage you to find a local dance class and make dancing a part of your weekly routine. Research has shown that regular dancing can help people with Parkinson's improve their balance and overall quality of life. Dancing with a class offers social connection, a more focused routine and a great reason to get out into the community. It also means building in accountability, one of the factors for success I've already mentioned.

The next step is to find songs that facilitate more intensity in your movement. The average adult takes approximately 110 – 120 steps per minute. You can figure out your own walking rate by counting each step you take over the course of 60 seconds, at your comfortable walking rate. To transform comfortable walking into exercise, here's what you can do:

- **Plan a weekly walking schedule**

  - Week 1: Walk 15 – 20 min 2x/week

  - Week 2: Walk 20 – 25 min 3x/week

  - Week 3: Walk 25 – 30 min 3x/week

  - Week 4: Walk 30 min 4x/week (every other day)

- **Progressively increase walking rate**

  - Week 1: 120 – 125 steps/min

  - Week 2: 130 steps/min

  - Week 3: 135 steps/min

  - Week 4: 140 steps/min

(Assumed baseline walking rate of 120 steps/min)

The schedule above is an example of a modest progression of walking. The most important factor is that you stick with the exercise (plan and schedule), and progressively increase the intensity (average number of steps taken in one minute).

You can add music to help increase the intensity of your walking exercise. Login to your digital music platform (explained previously), and follow these steps:

- Search the music platform for music at 120 – 140 beats/minute (bpm)

- Purchase and download playlists:

  - Matching your comfortable walking rate (such as 120 bpm)

  - Greater than your comfortable walking rate (such as 125, 130, 140 bpm, etc.)

- Play the music while you walk, stepping to the rhythm of the music

Some music will be easier to walk to. Take some time to figure out which songs, at which rates, get you walking faster. In addition to playing your music from your playlist, you can also use a metronome to help facilitate your walking. You can use a mechanical or digital metronome, or if you have a smartphone, search "metronome" to find apps. A metronome is the best external timer for facilitating rhythmic movement and increasing the intensity of the movement; however, you won't want to listen to a metronome for extended periods of time. You'll find your own music a lot more enjoyable.

The bottom line is that people living with Parkinson's should be physically active and exercise regularly. Daily physical activity and regular exercise should done safely first, but as you become stronger and more confident, the focus should shift to frequency and intensity. Music will definitely help you move, keep you moving and increase the intensity of your movement. A physical therapist can help you to monitor your program and appropriately adjust your exercise prescription so that you continue to benefit from the work you're putting into your routine.

- **FUN!** You have to pick a program that you enjoy in order to achieve success and continue to do it regularly. Many people find that their interests change over time, so the exercise program you love today might not be the one you choose tomorrow. That's okay; switch things up to keep yourself motivated and active. Use the **Pre-Exercise Self-Assessment** in the **Worksheets and Resources** section to frame a discussion with your doctor before starting or increasing the intensity of your exercise program. The **Worksheets and Resources** section also contains an **Exercise Journal** to help you track your progress.

BE ACTIVE: *Doing something is always better than doing nothing!*

> *Every time I don't feel like going to exercise, my friend drags me out, and when he doesn't feel like going, I do the same thing for him. It's also the social aspect, getting out of the house. We get exercise, we're participating in life and we're counting on each other."*
>
> — COREY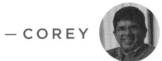

Discover who can help you create a customized exercise plan: **dpf.org/personal-plan**.

HOW MUCH CAN I DO?

This varies from one person to the next and will likely evolve as Parkinson's progresses.

> *When I was diagnosed with Parkinson's, I was training for a marathon. While I don't do nearly the exercise I used to do, I'm still physically active. I'm not running marathons, but I walk on the treadmill. I keep moving, and I tell myself it's okay not to do everything I used to do."*
>
> — LINDA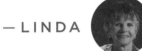

Discuss with your doctor before starting any exercise routine, referencing the "Exercise Guidelines" on the following pages. If you have heart disease, cardiac rehabilitation may be the place to start before starting an exercise program for your Parkinson's. It is better to start slow and develop a habit of exercise rather than try to do too much at once. A physical therapist, especially one who has specific experience with movement disorders, can help you design your exercise program to avoid injury, ensure you are doing the right exercises and help you organize your program to get the most out of your routine.

> *Not only does exercise help Edie with her Parkinson's, it has helped me a lot. We both encourage each other and get to know each other better. It's always encouraging when you see your partner working hard, no matter how far the disease has progressed."*
>
> — SCOTT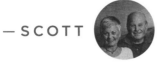

Learn how tracking your exercise can help you measure progress over time:
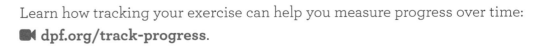 **dpf.org/track-progress**.

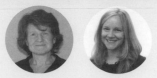

By Terry Ellis, PhD, PT, NCS and Tamara Rork DeAngelis, PT, DPT, GCS

While most people know that it is important to exercise for their health, many have a difficult time staying on track and making exercise a part of their daily routine. It can help to start slowly and do a little more every day to begin to make exercise a daily habit. Use the buddy system and find a partner to exercise with you. Do what you like to do and vary your exercise, if possible, to prevent boredom. Tennis, dance, tai chi and yoga are examples of exercises that can help improve balance, posture, strength, flexibility, engage the mind and can be done with partners or in groups.

Whether it is due to time constraints or simply because you become bored with your exercise routine, the following strategies can help you stay with a program and become a lifelong exerciser.

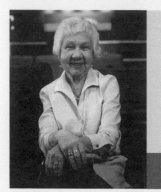

> " *The support of others in my Parkinson's exercise classes keeps me going. Every time I don't feel like going to a class, I force myself to go and always feel better because of the people. Their energy gives me energy.*"
>
> — BRENDA

160

IDENTIFY BARRIERS

Before you begin an exercise program, it is helpful to plan how you will overcome day-to-day challenges that may prevent you from sticking to your routine. Here is a list of some common barriers:

- I have a busy schedule and am not able to fit exercise into my life.

- I have fatigue and I am too tired for exercise.

- I am not confident in my ability to exercise successfully.

- I don't enjoy exercise and therefore find it difficult to motivate myself to participate in a long-term program.

- I don't really know where to begin or which exercises are best for me.

OVERCOME BARRIERS

Once you've identified the barriers that may limit your success with exercise, use the following strategies to help you get started and stay on track:

- **Schedule it.** Just as you would schedule a meeting at work or a visit with a friend, you can schedule exercise. If you put it in your calendar, you are more likely to do it. Schedule a specific time during the day when you feel your best and have more energy.

- **Get Guidance.** If you have difficulty with fatigue or experience sleepiness during the day, speak with your doctor about possible ways to address these issues. Overt time, exercise may increase your energy level and reduce feelings of fatigue.

- **Be Informed.** If you aren't sure what you should be doing for exercise or if you have questions about what exercises are best for you, visit with a physical therapist who can help you get started. Once you've done that, you also can work with a personal trainer or other fitness professional who can help find new ways to make your workout challenging and fun!

- **Make it Fun.** Find activities that you enjoy. There are many different types of exercise and ways to make it more fun. Add music or bring a friend to make your time exercising more pleasurable. Many people also find that participating in a group exercise program adds to both their enjoyment and commitment to exercise.

- **Stay Accountable.** Tell friends, family, coworkers and others that you are going to start an exercise program. When they ask you about it, you can proudly report that you have been reaching your goal to make exercise a part of your life. You can also stay accountable to yourself by keeping an exercise log. Find one online by using the term "exercise log" in your favorite search engine.

- **Be Focused.** For various reasons, you might stop exercising for a short time period. The goal is to get back on track as soon as possible. It is important to keep in mind the reasons for your commitment to exercise and to focus on all of the benefits you experience. There will be bumps in the road to becoming a lifetime exerciser, but as long as you keep going, you can continue to make a difference in your health and well-being.

EXERCISE GUIDELINES

Before beginning any exercise program, you should consult with your doctor to ensure that you are healthy enough to participate in exercise. It is also helpful to see a physical therapist so that you can start off on the right foot and make sure you are choosing the types of exercise that will benefit you most. We all know how difficult it can be to find the time (and sometimes, motivation) to exercise, so it is important to get guidance on making the most of your time while exercising at the gym or at home. By finding the most appropriate exercise at the optimal intensity, you can exercise smartly, safely and effectively.

Several national organizations have published exercise guidelines for the general population (some consider factors, such as age and health status). These national organizations include the World Health Organization (WHO), the American College of Sports Medicine (ACSM) and the National Institutes of Health (NIH). While the specifics of these guidelines differ in some areas, there is general consensus on the recommended amount and type of exercise to include in the optimal program. Based on these guidelines and some considerations specific to those living with Parkinson's, we have outlined the following exercise program recommendations, based on the four main types of exercise recommended for people living with Parkinson disease: Cardiorespiratory, Strength, Flexibility and Balance.

CARDIORESPIRATORY EXERCISE

Cardiorespiratory exercise (also known as "cardio" or aerobic exercise) is exercise that causes the body to consume more oxygen and use large muscle groups. Depending on your fitness level, cardiovascular exercise can include walking at a fast pace, jogging, swimming, biking and hiking to name a few. At this time, we don't know if one form of aerobic exercise is preferable to another for Parkinson's so it is important to find an activity that is safe to engage in at a moderate intensity. While it is very important to remain active throughout your day, it should be noted that regular self-care or household activities such as dressing, meal preparation or housecleaning don't "count" toward your cardiovascular exercise activity. This is because they are not performed at a significant enough intensity to result in positive changes for cardiovascular health.

Monitoring Intensity

The ACSM guidelines define moderate intensity physical activity as "working hard enough to raise your heart rate and break a sweat, yet still being able to carry on a conversation." This is often called the "talk test." If you are exercising and don't have enough breath to get the words out, you might be working too hard and need to decrease the intensity of the exercise. Conversely, if you are able to sing several verses of your favorite song while doing your cardiovascular exercise, you are likely not exercising at a high enough intensity and should be working harder in order to maximize benefits. Another common way that people monitor the intensity of their activity is by checking their heart rate. Your physical therapist will teach you how to safely monitor your heart rate during exercise and will establish your target heart rate, based on your current fitness level.

Cardiorespiratory Exercise Recommendations
(From ACSM Guidelines, 2011)

- Adults should get at least 150 minutes of moderate-intensity exercise per week.

- Exercise recommendations can be met through 30–60 minutes of moderate-intensity exercise (five days per week) or 20–60 minutes of vigorous-intensity exercise (three days per week).

- One continuous session and multiple shorter sessions (of at least 10 minutes) are both acceptable to accumulate desired amount of daily exercise. Therefore, three bouts of exercise for 10-minutes a day is another way to successfully achieve the recommendations.

- Gradual progression of exercise time, frequency and intensity is recommended for best adherence and least injury risk.

- People unable to meet these minimums can still benefit from some activity.

STRENGTH EXERCISE

Strength training is another very important part of any exercise program. The research suggests that there may be some strength loss associated with Parkinson disease. The good news is that people with Parkinson's can increase their strength through an appropriate strength training routine. However, it can be overwhelming when you go to a gym and see all of the strength training equipment including machines, pulleys, free weights, medicine balls, etc. It doesn't need to be fancy to be effective. You could do your strength training at home, if that works best for you.

Your physical therapist can determine specific strengthening exercises that might benefit you most, before starting out on your own. As an example, a therapist might identify during an examination that you have weakness in your postural muscles. He or she can then teach you the best exercises to improve the strength of those muscles and potentially help you stand taller and breathe better.

Here are some general considerations when choosing exercises:

- Some people with Parkinson's may have weakness in their extensor muscles (including large muscles in the back, buttocks and the front of the thighs), so it is important to make sure you address these muscles as part of your program.

- Focus on larger muscles groups, such as those in your legs. For example, doing a squat or a lunge uses several large muscles in your legs as well as requiring you to use your trunk muscles. The leg press machine also uses large muscles in your lower body. For your upper body, rowing or pull-downs use larger muscles groups.

- Remember that more isn't always better. Going through a complete circuit of machines can take a long time. Your time might be better spent with a handful of exercises that combine multiple muscle groups.

If you are otherwise healthy, you should work up to lifting enough weight so that your last few repetitions in the set are difficult. If it's easy for you to continue lifting that weight for another set without resting, then you should slowly increase the weight.

If you have other restrictions or health conditions, such as pain, arthritis, heart disease or any others, you should not begin strength training without first consulting with your doctor or physical therapist. You can still benefit from strength training with these conditions, but always seek advice first.

Strength Training Exercise Recommendations

- Adults should train each major muscle group on two or three non-consecutive days each week using a variety of exercises.

- For each exercise, do two sets of 8–12 repetitions to improve strength.

162

- Focus on larger muscles groups, such as those in your legs. For example, doing a squat or lunge uses several large muscles in your legs plus your trunk muscles.

FLEXIBILITY EXERCISE

Flexibility or stretching exercises are another important component of any exercise routine, but are especially important for people with Parkinson disease. Two of the cardinal signs of Parkinson's, bradykinesia and rigidity, can potentially put you at risk for decreased muscle length or joint range of motion. This is because the stiffness may contribute to smaller movements, like swinging your arms less or taking smaller steps when walking. Many people with Parkinson's also report that stretching helps reduce the discomfort or the feeling of stiffness and makes movement easier.

It is safe (and often advisable) to do some stretching every day. Some people find it helpful to stretch first thing in the morning while others prefer to stretch before bed. There are also some people with Parkinson's that report doing a few stretches in the middle of the night if sleeping is difficult because of stiffness.

It is also important to stretch after you exercise. You will get the most benefit from stretching after your muscles have warmed up.

The following are general guidelines for stretching:

- If you are not able to do all your stretches every day, then do some one day and others the next day.

- Repeat each stretch two to three times and hold for 30 seconds.

- Do not hold your breath while stretching.

- Do not bounce while you stretch; simply hold the position.

- Do not stretch to the point of pain.

BALANCE EXERCISE

There are many ways to improve your balance, such as strengthening and stretching exercises for your legs or exercises to improve your posture. Tai chi and yoga classes can be helpful to improve balance in a group setting. However, if you are experiencing falls or near falls, it is recommended that you consult with a physical therapist to have an individualized balance program designed for you. Listen how Brenda stays active despite balance challenges: ◼ **dpf.org/brenda**.

TOP 10 TIPS FOR EXERCISING WITH PARKINSON DISEASE

1. **Exercise is medicine**, so don't miss a dose. Exercise has been shown to build a healthier heart, lungs and muscles; boost metabolism; prevent diabetes; improve physical function and reduce disability. Some research also suggests that exercise may even be neuroprotective – that is, slowing the progression of Parkinson's – although more research is needed to study this further.

2. **Be realistic.** Something is better than nothing. There is no perfect one-size-fits-all exercise for people with Parkinson's. Don't wait. Start walking around the block. Or dancing. Find a physical therapist that can design an exercise program that is right for you.

3. **Have fun.** Consistency is critical and if you don't enjoy it, you won't stick with it. Do something you like. Dance, yoga, tai chi, cycling and strength exercises have been shown to help reduce physical and/or cognitive symptoms of PD. Try exercising with a group. The research suggests that social support helps people stick with exercise and enjoy it more!

4. **Break a sweat.** Movement only becomes exercise when done at an intensity that is high enough to be physically challenging. Although more research is necessary to determine the optimal intensity of exercise for people with Parkinson's, most studies suggest that at least moderate intensity exercise is important to maximize the benefits.

5. **Do three major types of exercise.** Do aerobic conditioning or cardiovascular exercise for 30 minutes, three times per week; strength or resistance training for 30 minutes, three times per week and stretching or flexibility exercises daily. See a physical therapist for help with balance exercises.

163

6. **Start today, don't wait.** The sooner after diagnosis you begin exercising, the greater your physical reserve and self-motivation are likely to be. Don't wait for the disease to progress further or for problems to emerge. Start strong to stay stronger longer.

7. **Find an exercise buddy.** Exercise with people whose life stage and physical ability are similar to your own. Especially for people with young onset Parkinson's, exercising with peers may be more enjoyable, more motivating and more appropriate than finding a Parkinson's-specific exercise group.

8. **Stick with it.** If you stop exercising, the positive effects you've worked so hard to achieve through exercise will decline and disappear. People with Parkinson's who exercise regularly do better than those who don't.

9. **Exercise for your whole being.** Exercise isn't just good for your body. Other issues related to Parkinson's disease, like depression, sleep, cognition and constipation, could also be positively affected by exercise and activity.

10. **Use exercise to take control of your Parkinson's.** People with Parkinson's can feel a loss of so much control in their lives, but exercise is one thing you can control and in the process, enjoy a better quality of life.

DO I NEED PHYSICAL THERAPY?

Physical therapy can be helpful at all stages of Parkinson's, from recently diagnosed to advanced disease. A physical therapist, especially one who specializes in neurological disorders, can help you get started. This person will evaluate your strengths and areas that need improvement, review your prior exercise experience, analyze your current level of conditioning and review future problems that exercise can prevent. They will also develop an exercise program tailored to you and instruct you in how to perform exercises correctly to avoid injury and safely progress your routine as you become stronger. In early Parkinson's, the focus may be on strengthening and prevention of future problems. Some people find it helpful to work with a personal trainer in the community to continue the exercise program started by a physical therapist. Personal trainers can also offer motivation and encouragement, along with supervision to help you to perform exercises safely and correctly. Since Parkinson's changes over time, it's a good idea to consult your trainer or physical therapist once a year and adjust your program as necessary to accommodate changes to your body and your needs.

Learn how to find a physical therapist experienced with Parkinson's: ◼ **dpf.org/pd-pt**.

▋ DIET AND NUTRITION

A healthy diet will improve your general health, reducing your risk of diabetes, heart disease and stroke. Although there is no specific diet for Parkinson's, general recommendations for healthy eating do apply, and changes in your diet can help some of your symptoms. Avoid the many fad diets that carry promises of health or symptom control.

Eat fresh, wholesome foods when possible, and limit processed food and drinks and fast food. Limit sugar, while focusing on healthy carbohydrates and fiber. Local produce that ripens naturally on the vine contains more nutrients than canned or "fresh" vegetables picked early and shipped from afar. Consider eating organic foods to reduce ingestion of pesticides, herbicides or hormones that may be harmful to your health. The most recent dietary and lifestyle recommendations for people living in the US are published by the American Heart Association and the US Department of Agriculture (☞ cnpp.usda.gov/dietary-guidelines). The USDA nutrition guidelines ("Food Pyramid") have been updated and can be reviewed at ☞ choosemyplate.gov. Health Canada's Food Guide can be found at ☞ hc-sc.gc.ca. Consult similar organizations that exist in your home country for specific guidelines.

Before making any changes to your diet, be aware that the suggestions outlined in the following pages are meant to serve as guidelines only. Review any dietary changes with your doctor and wellness team, especially if you have diabetes, heart or gastrointestinal problems. Ask your doctor about the effects of your dietary choices on your medications.

165

GENERAL NUTRITION

While there is no one-size-fits-all diet for Parkinson's, there are sound guidelines that can serve anyone well. Eating well means getting the appropriate vitamins and nutrients from your diet and not from a pill. Eating well means that your diet will reduce your risk of diseases, such as cardiovascular disease, hypertension, diabetes, obesity, intestinal problems, stroke and cancer.

Food chemistry can be divided into two categories: macronutrients and micronutrients. Macronutrients are the major food categories of carbohydrates, fats and proteins. Micronutrients are vitamins and substances found in food and needed in smaller amounts to promote cell health and catalyze biochemical reactions. We will begin by reviewing each of these major food categories and then provide specific recommendations for your diet.

PROTEIN

Protein is essential for building and maintaining muscle mass needed for energy, stamina, strength, weight control and normal body function. Protein also is needed to build and maintain healthy cells. Inadequate protein can cause muscle (strength) loss, fatigue, poor healing, reduced immunity and skin breakdown in areas such as the elbows, heels and lower back when sitting or lying for prolonged periods. You may need more protein if you are vegetarian, suffering from infection or recovering from an injury.

The building blocks of protein are called amino acids. Essential amino acids can only be obtained from foods. Complete proteins are foods that include all essential amino acids. Meat, dairy and eggs are complete proteins, while many plant-based proteins are not. However, a recent study showed a plant-based diet was noted to be associated with a lower risk of developing Parkinson's, thus many health-conscious people are eating diets that are plant-based. Consider substituting plant-based protein for meat proteins when possible, as you can obtain the necessary essential amino acids in your diet without relying on meat if you eat a combination of plant-based foods. The following foods are examples of plant-based proteins that are easy to add to your diet:

- Nuts
- Beans
- Soy, tempeh and tofu
- Quinoa
- Amaranth
- High-protein vegetables like spinach, kale, Brussels sprouts and broccoli
- Chia and hemp seeds
- Lentils
- Chickpeas and hummus

Although protein can delay the absorption of levodopa, it does not affect medications besides levodopa. _Do not avoid protein for fear that it will interfere with your medications, since protein is a necessary nutrient for health._ Read the "Protein Interference with Medication" section later in this chapter for ways to get the protein you need without interfering with your medication absorption.

CARBOHYDRATES AND SUGARS

Carbohydrates act as our body's main source of energy. Approximately 45–55% of your energy should come from this group. Complex carbohydrates such as starchy vegetables, fruits, grains and milk products are healthy sources of carbohydrates. However, not all carbohydrates are healthy.

Carbohydrates can be divided into simple sugars, complex carbohydrates and starches based on their chemical structure. These differences mean that they are processed differently by the body, so all carbohydrates should not be treated the same way.

Simple sugars are made up of one or two sugar units. Glucose is the most important sugar unit used to fuel cells and the primary energy source for brain cells. Table sugar is an example of a simple sugar that is made up of glucose and fructose. Simple sugars are absorbed quickly, since they require little to no digestion.

Complex carbohydrates are not one to two sugar units, but long and complex chains of sugar molecules. These carbohydrates require more complex digestion and are more slowly absorbed. Complex carbohydrates can be divided into two forms:

- **Starch.** A long chain carbohydrate that is digestible by the body and must be metabolized before absorbed. Starch does not cause glucose to rise as quickly as simple sugars do, meaning your energy stays steadier.

- **Fiber.** A form of carbohydrate that is resistant to metabolic breakdown in the intestinal tract.

Currently, there is a tremendous amount of information warning of the perils of sugar and carbohydrates, as well as often conflicting guidance about which carbohydrates should be eaten or how much to eat. Like everything else, the quality of the carbohydrate you consume is important; there can be a big difference in the carbohydrates consumed in a donut versus that in a vegetable. The glycemic index and glycemic load are two measurements to help assess the quality of a carbohydrate. Glycemic load is a measure of a food's tendency to increase your blood glucose levels after eating it. The glycemic load of food is measured on a scale of 0 to 100. A glycemic load of greater than 20 is considered high and foods with a higher glycemic load lead to a more rapid increase in blood sugar after they are eaten. Determining the actual glycemic load of a food is more complicated, and the following factors impact glycemic load:

- **Food processing.** Puffed, blended, crushed or refined foods have a higher surface to volume ratio, allowing faster digestion and absorption than whole foods. This processing increases glycemic load.

- **Food preparation.** Foods cooked until they are soft have a higher glycemic load since chemical bonds are broken in the cooking processes, making foods easier to digest.

- **Food combinations.** Carbohydrate-rich foods will have a lower glycemic load when eaten with other foods that are high in fiber, fat and protein.

FIBER

Unlike starch, fiber is not digested by the body. There are two types of fiber: soluble and insoluble. Soluble fiber found in fruits, flaxseed, oatmeal and psyllium (Metamucil) in water, can slow digestion and can cause you to feel full. Insoluble fiber found in vegetables, whole grains, raisins and prunes does not absorb water and passes through the gastrointestinal tract to reduce constipation. Fiber is an important treatment for constipation, which is a common problem for people with Parkinson's. The recommended daily intake of fiber is 20-30 grams. You can get this by choosing a diet rich in fresh fruits, vegetables and whole grains.

FATS

Fats provide energy stored in our body for endurance and keep cells healthy. Naturally occurring fats are divided into three types:

- **Saturated Fats.** These fats are solid at room temperature and are found primarily in red meat, tropical oils (like coconut) and dairy. A diet high in saturated fats can increase cholesterol levels, risk of atherosclerosis, stroke and heart disease.

- **Monounsaturated Fats.** These fats are liquid at room temperature, but get cloudy when refrigerated. Examples of monounsaturated fats include olives and olive oil, canola oil, nuts and nut oils and avocado. These oils are a better substitute for saturated fats, can reduce cholesterol levels and improve insulin activity. Olive oil, a staple in the Mediterranean diet, is a versatile and healthy ingredient for cooking, salads and spreads.

- **Polyunsaturated Fats.** These fats are liquid both at room temperature and when refrigerated. Polyunsaturated fats can be divided into two types: omega-6 and omega-3. Omega-6 fats include sunflower oil, safflower oil, corn oil, most seeds and oil from grains. Omega-3 fats are found in walnuts, flaxseed, chia seed, pumpkin seeds, purslane and cold water fish, such as salmon, tuna and sardines. Omega-3 fats are found in highest concentration in the brain and are important to brain cell function. Omega-6 fats will increase inflammation in the body when eaten in excess of omega-3 fatty acids. The American diet is high in omega-6, largely from processed foods. A diet high in omega-3 fats relative to omega-6 can reduce inflammation and your risk of heart disease, certain cancers, depression, stroke, dementia and asthma. Diets high in omega-3 may have more positive brain effects due to reduced inflammation and oxidative stress. However, there is no research that shows omega-3 fats reduce Parkinson's risk or symptoms.

Read food labels before you eat fried foods, processed foods or processed spreads like peanut butter, shortening or margarine, and avoid trans fats and hydrogenated fats. These fats increase shelf life and add a creamy, smooth texture. They should be avoided because they boost blood levels of bad cholesterol (LDL) and decrease good cholesterol (HDL), increasing risk of heart disease and stroke.

Reduce your saturated fat intake by limiting the amount of red meat you eat to twice a week or less. Choose low-fat milk and dairy products. Use olive oil for cooking and salad dressings instead of corn oil and other oils that are high in omega-6 fats. Aim for two servings of cold water fish weekly. Add whole nuts to your diet.

Many pre-packaged snack foods and meals contain large amounts of simple carbohydrates (sugars) and saturated or trans fats, which contribute to low energy, constipation, weight problems, heart disease, diabetes and poor overall health. Packaged foods are usually labeled with information about the types of carbohydrates and fats they contain.

CAN FOOD CAUSE PARKINSON'S?

While there is no food or diet proven to slow the progression of Parkinson's, there are foods that change the risk of developing Parkinson's. The following table[1] lists foods or diets found to influence Parkinson's risk, along with possible reasons why.

INCREASED RISK	DECREASED RISK	PROPOSED REASON(S)
Milk (not cheese or yogurt)		Low urate, pesticides and contaminates
Diet high in meat		Iron in heme (red meat)
	Prudent diet Mediterranean diet	High in antioxidants, low in inflammatory fats and processed sugars
	Beta carotene (carrots)	Antioxidant (beta carotene)
	Peppers	Nicotine
	Berries	Antioxidant, acanthocyanins
	Coffee	Antioxidant, adenosine blockade
	Green tea	Antioxidant

Eating a Mediterranean diet is associated with a lower risk of Parkinson's (studies have shown this can reduce the risk of Parkinson's anywhere from 14% to 48%) and later age of disease onset. Similar studies suggest a lower risk between a diet that is rich in fruit, vegetables and fish, healthy plant-based fats, whole grains and low in meat and processed sugars compared with the typical Western diet. This is strengthened by consistent findings that the Mediterranean diet is proven to reduce the risk of many other diseases, such as stroke, hypertension, heart disease, diabetes, depression, dementia and cancer, proving its global impact on health and disease.

169

---

[1]   Used with permission from *Optimal Health with Parkinson's: A Guide to Integrating Lifestyle, Alternative and Conventional Medicine* (2015) by Monique L. Giroux, MD.

Recommendations based on the Mediterranean or prudent diets include:

- High in fruits and vegetables: 8-10 servings daily
- High in fish: 2-3 times per week
- Low in meat (especially red meat): 1-2 times week
- High in plant protein: nuts, seed, beans

- Olive oil as primary oil
- High in whole grains
- Low in processed, refined sugar
- Foods in their whole state (rather than processed)

SHOULD I ONLY EAT ORGANIC FOOD?

Exposure to pesticides is the strongest link between the environment and Parkinson's. Eating organic foods can reduce ingestion of pesticides, but organic produce, dairy and meat do cost more than conventional products. Be sure to wash all produce in warm water with mild soap, especially if organic foods are not an option. Foods with thick skins or peels often contain lower pesticide levels. The "Dirty Dozen" and "Clean Fifteen"[2] are lists published annually of foods with higher and lower pesticide exposure, respectively, to help you choose which foods to eat organic. Here are the lists from 2017:

DIRTY DOZEN	CLEAN FIFTEEN
• Strawberries	• Sweet corn
• Spinach	• Avocados
• Nectarines	• Pineapples
• Apples	• Cabbage
• Peaches	• Onions
• Pears	• Sweet peas (frozen)
• Cherries	• Papayas
• Grapes	• Asparagus
• Celery	• Mangos
• Tomatoes	• Eggplant
• Sweet bell peppers	• Honeydew melon
• Potatoes	• Kiwi
	• Cantaloupe
	• Cauliflower
	• Grapefruit

2   Learn more about the annual "Dirty Dozen" and "Clean Fifteen" lists from the Environmental Working Group, a non-partisan, nonprofit organization dedicated to protecting human health and the environment at ewg.org.

DIETARY RECOMMENDATIONS FOR SPECIFIC PARKINSON'S SYMPTOMS

CONSTIPATION

- Increase your intake of fruits and vegetables that are high in soluble fiber. Try broccoli, beans, hummus or chickpeas, cauliflower, Brussels sprouts, prunes, figs, apples, berries, pears and citrus.

- Aim for 20-30 grams of fiber daily. In addition to fruits (guava, blackberries, raspberries and pears are especially high in fiber) and vegetables (beans, corn, peas and lentils are high in fiber), add high fiber or bran cereals and breads, foods made from wheat, rye, oat or barley flours instead of refined or white flour breads and cereals.

- Limit low fiber items. Examples include cheese, eggs and meat high in fat.

- Choose complex carbohydrates found in fruits, vegetables and whole grains over simple sugars and processed foods.

- Drink plenty of water. Inadequate fluid intake is a common problem.

- Exercise. Simply walking can help promote movement in your bowels.

LIGHTHEADEDNESS

- Eat smaller, more frequent meals.

- Reduce your consumption of alcohol and caffeine.

- Increase the fluid you drink daily (talk with your doctor if you have heart or kidney disease before you increase fluids or salt).

- Increase salty and high electrolyte fluids. Examples include V8 juice, broths and non-sugary sport drinks (avoid sugary drinks, especially if you have diabetes).

- When moving from sitting to standing, try to engage your muscles by bending your knees a little. This muscular activity will help to keep blood from pooling in your legs. Pause before taking your first step to allow your vascular system time to adjust to the change in posture.

FATIGUE AND ENERGY LOSS

- Increase your fluid intake to prevent dehydration.

- Eat breakfast.

- Pay attention to the amount or ratio of carbohydrates, proteins and fat in your diet. Aim for a balance of each of these food groups. Many people snack on high sugar processed foods for energy, yet this can deplete your energy level.

- Eat a balance of simple and complex carbohydrates. Simple sugars supply faster energy, but can later lead to energy drain. (The boosting effect of sugar lasts only 30 minutes). Healthy simple sugars for energy include fruits and honey. Complex sugars are found in whole wheat and grain products, and starchy vegetables like peas and corn.

- Eat smaller amounts of energy-boosting foods more frequently, rather than eating fewer big, heavy or fatty meals.

- Eat energy-boosting foods, such as fruit, yogurt, almonds, walnuts, lentils and oats.

- Drink caffeine (coffee, hot chocolate, tea) in the morning, but avoid it later in the day.

- Eat chocolate! A small (one ounce) amount can be an energy booster, but avoid overeating as the effect can backfire and cause sleepiness due to its highly processed sugar and fat content.

SLEEP PROBLEMS

- Avoid heavy meals before bed.

- Drink most of your fluids before 5:00 p.m. to reduce your nighttime need to urinate.

- Think tryptophan. Tryptophan is an amino acid that can enhance your feelings of sleepiness. Foods high in tryptophan include chicken, turkey and milk.

- A light snack consisting mainly of complex carbohydrates and a small amount of protein, such as cheese or peanut butter and crackers, is thought to help your brain produce serotonin and increase tryptophan. Carbohydrates cause the pancreas to release more insulin, which in turn helps tryptophan enter the brain.

- Valerian root and chamomile teas are both calming and touted to help sleep. Ask your doctor before taking any supplement or herb. If you use sleep aids, discuss these with your doctor.

- Avoid caffeine, nicotine or excessive alcohol before bed.

NAUSEA AND STOMACH BLOATING

- Ask your doctor to review which medications can be taken with food to reduce nausea. Take Parkinson's medications with food (see "Protein Interference with Medication" below).

- Drink plenty of water. Ask your doctor how much is too much.

- Take vitamins and supplements with dinner or at the end of the day, as these can cause nausea.

- Try grinding (pulverizing) your meds and mixing with fluids if approved by your doctor.

- Use ginger root, candied ginger, crystallized ginger or ginger tea to control nausea.

- Snack on starchy foods without spice, such as crackers, rice, toast, cereal or oatmeal.

172

- Eat smaller, more frequent meals.

- Papaya, pineapple, yogurt and peppermint tea can ease bloating and gastric upset.

- If nausea and bloating persist as a result of medication, your doctor may prescribe supplemental medication to treat these symptoms.

" *A few years ago I started getting really bloated after I ate. I had a bunch of tests done and they found four ulcers. Even though those have gotten better, I still can't eat much. My body doesn't digest all the food I eat, so I end up throwing up a lot. It's no fun because I love to eat.*"

— LINDA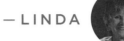

DROOLING AND SWALLOWING

- Take big "swallows" when you feel saliva build up in your mouth. Chewing gum can facilitate swallowing.

- Try papaya or papain extract if you are bothered by thick secretions in your mouth.

WEIGHT LOSS

- See your primary care physician for a general medical check-up and preventative care.

- Add high-calorie nutritional drinks and protein supplements to your diet.

- Eat smaller portions more frequently, rather than three big meals. For some people, a full plate may seem less appealing.

- Focus on flavors and spices that you like.

- Add higher calorie sauces and gravies, especially if you have difficulty swallowing thin liquids or dry solids.

- Don't be afraid to use your hands if managing a fork or spoon is daunting. Think "caveman" with a napkin!

PROTEIN INTERFERENCE WITH MEDICATION

Protein can interfere with absorption of carbidopa/levodopa, but not other Parkinson's medications. This may delay the onset of levodopa effectiveness, causing the benefits to take awhile to kick in or have a reduced effect on your motor symptoms. You may not notice this effect if you do not have "on/off" fluctuations or dyskinesia. Consider spreading out your protein intake, and avoid large amounts of protein at any one time. You can make these adjustments to your diet even before the onset of dyskinesia or wearing "off" problems.

- Try to take carbidopa/levodopa medication at least one hour before or one hour after meals.

- Don't skimp on protein. Protein is needed to build your muscle mass and strength.

Eating smaller amounts more frequently is a strategy that can help offset protein interference.

- If medication absorption is significantly impacted, try to eat most of your protein at less active times of your day, such as in the evening.

- Try concentrated sources of protein (yogurt, nuts, tuna) as a snack between medication doses.

- Try drinking a carbonated beverage, like sparkling water or club soda, to speed delivery of your medication.

NUTRITION FOR A HEALTHY BRAIN

Although researchers have not yet reached a definitive conclusion on the full benefits of certain foods, nutrients and supplements on brain health, the following general guidelines offer sound nutritional advice:

- A general multivitamin offers a good supply of vitamins and minerals to fill in what is missing from your diet. Some vitamins are specially formulated for seniors or have added levels of antioxidants. Do not take mega doses of vitamins except under the supervision of your doctor.

- Vitamin B may have special importance in Parkinson's as well as aging. In one study, vitamin B6 reduced the risk of developing Parkinson's. Lower levels of vitamin B12 can be found in older individuals and may contribute to thinking problems. Vitamin B12 and folate can reduce homocysteine levels elevated as a result of levodopa metabolism (abnormally high levels of homocysteine can increase your risk of heart disease or stroke). Ask your doctor about adding a vitamin B complex or if you should have your vitamin B12 level checked. Some people require injections of this vitamin to obtain normal blood levels.

- Vitamin D is lower in people with Parkinson's and in those who live in areas with less sunshine. Ask your doctor if you should have vitamin D levels checked to guide how much vitamin D you should add to your diet.

- Screening for diabetes, high blood pressure and high cholesterol is recommended. These conditions increase your risk of atherosclerosis, a problem that can damage blood vessels in the heart and the brain. The steps you take to improve your diet and exercise can help these problems. Seek advice from a dietician or nutritionist if you have these and other chronic medical conditions.

- Add heart healthy omega-3 fatty acids to your diet. Foods high in omega-3 fats include salmon, tuna, sardines, crushed flaxseed and walnuts. Aim for two servings of fish per week. Ask your doctor if you should take a fish oil capsule if you do not eat these foods.

- Antioxidants can slow cell damage that can otherwise go unchecked when free radicals are produced during cell oxygen metabolism. Heart disease, macular degeneration (eye disease), brain health, diabetes and cancer are just a few of the health conditions that are associated with these by-products. Foods bright in color, such as berries, pomegranates, cranberries, grapes, yellow and dark green leafy vegetables, have strong antioxidant properties. Chocolate, red wine, green tea, walnuts and flaxseed also make the list.

VITAMINS AND SUPPLEMENTS

There is a great amount of interest and effort that goes into the search for a supplement or herbal pill to offset symptoms of Parkinson's or aging. Although taking a pill is easier, the best defense and best results occur when nutrition, vitamins and minerals come from a healthy diet, not a pill.

Supplements or alternative medication compounds are not regulated by the FDA, meaning there is no external, unified oversight of the quality or consistency of the supplements you may find on the store shelf. Just because something is an "herbal preparation" or "natural compound" does not necessarily mean it is any safer than prescription medication. Search for products that carry USP (United States Pharmacopeia) or similar verification for your home country. This independent laboratory tests the purity, potency and bioavailability of products. In effect, this test ensures that what is on the bottle label is, indeed, what is contained in the pill or supplement. Otherwise, the actual purity and strength of the substance might differ from what the bottle label claims. Consumer Lab (⌖ **consumerlab.com**) tests different brand names and can provide you with similar information.

For your safety, the potential for interactions between supplements and your prescribed medication should be discussed with your pharmacist and doctor. For example, warfarin (Coumadin) is a blood thinner that may be prescribed for blood clots, stroke therapy or heart problems. Garlic, ginseng, ginger and ginkgo supplements can interfere with the intended blood thinning action of warfarin. This highlights the importance of informing your doctor or pharmacist of all supplements or complementary treatments that you are using or considering. The supplements noted below are a reasonable addition if your diet is limited due to your Parkinson's; however, a balanced diet is your safest source for health and wellness.

Vitamins that are important for the aging adult with Parkinson's include:

- **Vitamin B12.** Over time, inadequate B12 can lead to fatigue and weakness from anemia and possibly numbness and tingling from nerve cell degeneration. Constipation, weight loss, appetite loss, confusion, memory problems and tongue soreness can also occur from too little vitamin B12. Medications used to reduce heartburn or acid reflux and Metformin, a medication used for diabetes, can reduce the absorption of vitamin B12. Supplements containing the crystalline form of B12 are recommended for older adults due to better absorption since vitamin B12 absorption normally decreases with aging. Vitamin B12 (and the B vitamin folate) can reduce homocysteine levels thought to play a role in reducing heart attacks and possibly stroke. The recommended dietary allowance for vitamin B12 is 2.4 mcg per day. Ask your doctor about taking a vitamin B complex pill that includes B12, thiamine and folate.

- **Vitamin D3.** The recommended dietary allowance for vitamin D intake is 1000 IU (international units) per day. Three cups of D-fortified milk, one cup of D-fortified orange juice and 600 IU vitamin D supplement would provide the recommended 1000 IU of vitamin D. Vitamin D levels tend to be lower in people living with Parkinson's and those in areas with less sunshine, so ask your doctor to check your level before adding vitamin D as higher doses may be needed.

- **Calcium.** Inadequate calcium intake can lead to bone thinning, abnormal blood clotting, dental problems and can affect heart and nerve function. The Institute of Medicine recommends 1200 mg of calcium intake per day for individuals over the age of 50. Recent research suggests getting calcium from food may be better than taking calcium supplements. In fact, a study evaluating the effects of long-term calcium supplements in women revealed an increase risk of heart disease in those taking higher doses. This is an important reminder that vitamins and supplements do not have the same benefits as nutrients obtained from food.

- **Antioxidants.** Antioxidants are vitamins and chemicals that combat the effects of free radicals and are found in many food sources. In Parkinson's, free radicals can potentially contribute to nerve cell death. Antioxidants include supplements and vitamins such as Coenzyme Q10, vitamin A, E, C and selenium. Other, less common antioxidants include ligans, flavinoids, lycopene and lutein. The medical evidence for supplementation with antioxidants is in the early stages and effective doses are still unknown. Some may even cause harm, such as high dose vitamin E. Food sources of antioxidants provide an abundance of other nutrients important for optimal health. Antioxidants obtained from foods may prove to be better than antioxidants in pill form. A healthy diet, high in antioxidants, includes pigmented or brightly colored vegetables and fruits. See the **Nutrition Self-Assessment** in the **Worksheets and Resources** section for common food sources that contain each of the above types of antioxidants.

By Kathrynne Holden, MS, RD (retired)

Why is food important to people living with Parkinson's? Because, no matter how perfect your medication regime, no matter how often and how hard you exercise, you need nourishing food for good health. While there is little scientific evidence supporting consumption of any specific food or probiotic, with Parkinson's, nutrition takes on a new role: the role of supporting the brain and nervous system. So, let's take a look at food considerations that theoretically can help to fortify the brain and the body.

Thumbs up:

1. **Plant foods:** Whole grains, fresh vegetables and fruits, legumes. These provide complex carbohydrates, vitamins and minerals, antioxidants and fibers.

   Whole grains? Yes! Whole barley, rye and oats have all been found to improve aspects of our health, such as improved colon health, regular bowel movements, control of blood glucose and cholesterol and strengthening the immune system.

   Blueberries may help prevent or slow neurodegeneration and appear to boost memory. Apples and onions contain quercetin, a flavonoid and antioxidant, that may help protect against damage to DNA.

   Legumes, dry beans, split peas, lentils, chickpeas are rich in protein, fibers and the B vitamins so important in Parkinson's.

2. **Animal foods:** Fish and seafood, meat, poultry, eggs and dairy foods all contain vitamin B12, which is not found in plant foods. They also have complete protein, meaning protein that contains all nine essential amino acids.

   Big plus — fatty fish and seafood, and to a lesser extent, eggs, also have omega-3 fatty acids and vitamin D. These are especially important in Parkinson's. The gray matter of the brain is largely made up of omega-3 fats and deficiency is associated with dementia and depression. Omega-3 fats also support heart health.

   Fatty fish and eggs are among the few foods that naturally contain vitamin D. This includes the more powerful form called twenty-five hydroxy-D 25(OH)D, which is not found in supplements. There is widespread deficiency of vitamin D among people with Parkinson's, for reasons not entirely clear. Deficiency can mean loss of muscle mass and bone density, falls, fractures, cancers, irritable bowel syndrome and cognitive decline.

   If you use levodopa, you probably already know that for many people, protein can block levodopa absorption. This is especially true as Parkinson's advances. But it's still important to include enough protein every day.

   You require about **two** grams of protein per pound of body weight per day. It's necessary in order to restore and repair cells, hair, skin and nails, and muscles (including the heart). I would divide this amount about equally among morning, midday, and evening meals, taking levodopa about 30 to 60 minutes before the meals. This will help to time protein and levodopa.

   Then, if you need to take levodopa medication in between meals, wait at least an hour after eating, to allow the stomach to clear and give the levodopa medication quick access to the small intestine and bloodstream.

177

NOTE: Some people are very sensitive to the milk of cows, sheep and goats. These contain an especially high ratio of the amino acids that compete with levodopa for absorption. If milk severely blocks levodopa absorption, choose a milk alternative such as almond, soy or rice milk.

3. **Prebiotic and probiotic foods:** These are especially important for those with Parkinson's, because research is increasingly finding a relationship between the brain, the gut and the microbiome. It appears that the microbiome may influence the onset and progression of Parkinson's. Some speculate that Parkinson's actually begins in the gut, due to poor health of the gut microbiota.[3]

   - Probiotic foods contain living organisms that make up the microbiome.

   - Prebiotic foods contain fibers that are indigestible by humans, but are needed as food by the probiotic organisms.

   Probiotic foods. These are fermented foods that have the living, friendly bacteria and yeasts that make up our microbiome. Examples are yogurt, kefir, fermented pickles and miso.

   NOTE: If you are using Azilect, use caution when eating aged or fermented foods, as they have high levels of tyramine. Such foods can cause hypertensive crisis. One exception is yogurt, which is safe for those using Azilect.

   Yogurt can be a good choice; look on the label to be sure it contains living cultures. The more different strains it has, the better.

   Kefir is a fermented drink that may be made with milk, water or coconut milk. It has more different strains of probiotic bacteria than yogurt. If you are sensitive to milk protein, try water kefir or coconut milk kefir.

   Fermented pickles are made by immersing vegetables in a salt and water brine solution that promotes fermentation. They are not the same as those made with vinegar, which are not fermented and do not have probiotic properties. Fermented pickles must not be canned or otherwise heat-treated; that will destroy the live organisms.

   Sauerkraut is fermented cabbage and is a good source of probiotic bacteria. Kimchi is a Korean version and is spicier. Both must be unpasteurized, as heat will kill the organisms.

   Miso is fermented soybean paste. It must be eaten uncooked, because cooking will destroy the probiotic organisms.

   Prebiotic foods. Whole wheat, oats, onions, leeks, garlic, asparagus, Jerusalem artichokes, lettuce, eggplant, sweet potatoes, bananas, tomatoes, cashews, peanuts and legumes (dried beans, peas, lentils). Each of these foods has different types of indigestible fibers, known as prebiotics. Also, *dark chocolate!* Surprised? Yes, a high-quality dark chocolate is a prebiotic food.

   Prebiotics are used as food by the colony of friendly bacteria in our gut. Each prebiotic food supports different kinds of friendly bacteria, so it's important to eat a variety of these foods. One study found that people eating whole grains had an increase in one kind of the friendly gut bacteria and a decrease in harmful bacteria. An animal study discovered that prebiotic foods improved sleep. Don't skimp on fiber; keep those good microbes well-fed.

Thumbs down:

Refined and highly-processed foods. Some examples: white flour, refined sugar, canned soups, boxed macaroni and cheese, frozen ready-to-eat meals. Refined foods have been stripped of nutrients and prebiotic fibers. Highly-processed foods have refined ingredients and also have potentially harmful additives, such as emulsifiers, synthetic dyes and preservatives.

---

3 Mulak A., Bonaz B. Brain-gut-microbiota axis in Parkinson's disease. (2015 Oct 7). *World J Gastroenterol*, 21(37): 10609–10620.

Food ingredients that have been sprayed with pesticides and herbicides. We've long seen an association between agricultural use of herbicides and increased incidence of Parkinson's among farming communities. Now research is beginning to uncover possible causes. Some degenerative diseases appear to be linked to glyphosate, a weedkiller. Animal studies show that it may interfere with the normal working of the gut, which eventually damages motor neurons.[4]

Plan your meals to promote living well with Parkinson's

By assembling meals that are planned to provide nutrients that promote digestive health and support overall dietary needs, you can do something each day to fortify your mind and body. Let's plan some menus to do just that. Then, we'll assess how well each menu meets our plan to nourish the brain and body and keep our microbiome healthy.

FOR PEOPLE USING LEVODOPA

1.

Breakfast
Take levodopa 30-60 minutes before eating.

- Oatmeal or cooked steel-cut oats
- Milk (if sensitive to milk protein, choose a milk alternative such as almond, soy or rice milk)
- Fruit or fruit juice
- Coffee or tea

Snack (protein-free)
- Water kefir
- Banana

Midday Meal
Take levodopa 30-60 minutes before eating.

- Sandwich of whole-grain bread, sliced turkey and cheese, lettuce, mayonnaise
- Deviled egg
- Deli-style fermented pickle
- Milk or milk alternative, or fruit juice
- Coffee or tea

Snack (low protein - about 7 grams)
- One ounce of raw nuts a mix of almonds, walnuts, filberts, pecans, Brazil nuts

2.

Breakfast
Take levodopa 30-60 minutes before eating.

- Eggs, fried or poached
- Sausage patty
- Whole-wheat toast, butter
- Yogurt with sliced banana
- Fruit juice
- Coffee or tea

Snack (protein-free)
- Smoothie made with fruit and kefir
- Rye or whole-grain cracker with peanut butter

Midday Meal
Take levodopa 30-60 minutes before eating.

- Lentil or split pea soup
- Whole-grain crackers
- Cheese
- Mediterranean olives
- Vegetable juice
- Coffee or tea

Snack (protein-free)
- Popcorn

4 Seneff S., Morley W.A., Hadden M.J., Michener, M.C. Does glyphosate acting as a glycine analogue contribute to ALS? (2017) *J Bioinfo Proteomics* Rev 3(1): 1- 21.

Evening Meal

Take levodopa 30-60 minutes before eating.

- Miso soup
- Stir-fry of shrimp, snow peas, carrot, mushroom and onion
- Kimchi
- Brown rice
- Soy sauce
- Dates or figs

How did we do?

For the body, brain and nervous system:
Oat cereal, milk, fruit and fruit juice, whole-grain bread, turkey, cheese, egg, nuts, shrimp, vegetables, brown rice, dried dates/figs.

For the microbiome:
Prebiotic foods: Oat cereal, banana, lettuce, peanuts/cashews, onion.
Probiotic foods: Water kefir, fermented pickle, miso, kimchi.

Evening Meal

Take levodopa 30-60 minutes before eating.

- Grilled salmon
- Cooked quinoa or baked potato with butter
- Asparagus
- Sliced tomato
- Sauerkraut
- Whole-grain dinner roll
- Cantaloupe half

How did we do?

For the body, brain and nervous system:
Eggs, sausage, whole-grain bread, yogurt, banana, fruit and fruit juice, whole-grain crackers, peanut or almond butter, lentil/split pea soup, cheese, olives, popcorn, salmon, quinoa/baked potato, asparagus, tomato, whole-grain dinner roll, cantaloupe.

For the microbiome:
Prebiotic foods: Whole-wheat toast, banana, peanut butter, lentil/split pea soup, asparagus, tomato.
Probiotic foods: Yogurt, kefir, sauerkraut.

FOR PEOPLE USING AZILECT (RASAGILINE)

Note: Rasagiline is a Parkinson's medication that increases dopamine by blocking an enzyme called MAO-B (monoamine oxidase type B). Earlier MAO inhibitors (such as reserpine) blocked both the type A and type B forms of the MAO enzyme. This caused interactions with certain foods that are high in tyramine, such as aged meats and cheeses. While this interaction with food is less of a concern with MAO-B inhibitors such as rasagiline, caution should be used with certain foods.

All vegetables and fruits eaten should be fresh, not overripe; meat, poultry and fish should be fresh, not aged or smoked, or else canned or frozen and eaten immediately after opening or thawing. Eggs, cooked dried beans, peas and small quantities of nuts and peanut butter are safe. Avoid aged cheeses and meats, foods containing meat extracts such as bouillon or beef broth, fermented soy products such as tofu, soy sauce and miso, other fermented foods except for yogurt, which is safe. Because fermented foods are limited, you may wish to consider a probiotic supplement, such as gelcaps.

1.

Breakfast

- Oatmeal with milk
- Whole-wheat toast, butter
- Orange juice (fresh, or frozen and reconstituted)
- Coffee or tea

2.

Breakfast

- Eggs, cooked as you like
- Fresh sausage
- Whole-wheat toast, butter
- Mixed berry compote (fresh, or thawed from frozen)
- Coffee or tea

Snack

- Whole-wheat blueberry muffin, butter

Midday Meal

- Tuna salad sandwich on whole-wheat bread
- Raw carrot, celery, radishes
- Fresh milk or vegetable juice, coffee or tea

Snack

- Plain yogurt, with sliced banana and honey if desired

Evening Meal

- Beef steak (fresh, not aged)
- Brussels sprouts, lightly steamed with fresh lemon juice
- Baked sweet potato with butter and honey
- Whole grain dinner roll, butter
- Baked apple with maple syrup

How did we do?

For the body, brain and nervous system:
Oatmeal, milk, whole-wheat toast, whole-wheat blueberry muffin, tuna, whole-wheat bread, raw vegetables, milk/vegetable juice, yogurt, banana, beef, Brussels sprouts, sweet potato, whole-grain dinner roll, baked apple.

For the microbiome:
Prebiotic foods: Oatmeal, whole-wheat toast, muffin, whole-wheat bread, banana, sweet potato.
Probiotic foods: Yogurt.

Snack

- Cottage cheese, cantaloupe

Midday Meal

- Vegetable soup (made with fresh ingredients and legumes, no aged meats or meat extracts)
- Whole-grain crackers
- Fresh milk or vegetable juice, coffee or tea

Snack

- Yogurt smoothie with banana, honey

Evening Meal

- Grilled shrimp with whole-grain linguine, extra-virgin olive oil, garlic
- Fresh spinach salad
- Roasted carrots
- Whole-grain garlic bread
- 1 ounce dark chocolate

How did we do?

For the body, brain and nervous system: Eggs, sausage, whole-wheat toast, berry compote, cottage cheese, cantaloupe, vegetable soup, whole-grain crackers, milk/vegetable juice, yogurt, banana, shrimp, whole-grain linguine, spinach, carrots, garlic bread, chocolate.

For the microbiome:
Prebiotic foods: Whole-wheat toast, vegetable soup with legumes, banana, garlic, chocolate.
Probiotic foods: Yogurt.

SUMMARY

To best fight Parkinson's disease, maintain a healthy body and support the brain and nervous system:

- Choose Parkinson-fighting foods, like fatty fish, blueberries, apples, onions and foods rich in vitamin D, such as eggs and salmon.
- Select both prebiotic and probiotic foods to sustain the gut microbiome.
- Avoid anti-nutrients, such as refined grains and sugar, highly-processed foods and foods and ingredients sprayed with toxic pesticides and herbicides.

Eating the highest-quality foods will nourish your brain and nervous system, your microbiome, your heart, muscles and bones. You'll have more energy, feel more alert during the day and sleep better at night. And those millions of friendly microbes in your gut will thank you.

By Davis Phinney

Meditation may sound like something only for monks or mystics, but isn't so different from other training we do for Parkinson's, like physical or speech therapy. In all instances, we're trying to gain control of our thoughts and encourage ourselves to respond in a certain way that we've predetermined. Sometimes that response is to "do nothing" or to watch the thoughts pass through our mind without reacting or judging. Sometimes the response is to calm rising anxiety and slow down our breathing. Gaining control in any sense takes practice, just like it takes practice to walk in new ways or to swing your arms when they no longer want to swing naturally.

182

They say mindfulness – or focusing completely on the "here and now" – is a form of meditation. Living with Parkinson's, I'm forced to be more mindful of the present moment. Things that were once automatic are not automatic anymore. I can't just hop out of my car and run up a flight of stairs to the door without hesitation. I need to see the stairs, focus my concentration on the task at hand and then climb them with purpose. That's mindfulness: I have put my attention in the moment in order to accomplish the task. My dedicated practice is like a form of training for my mind that helps make these moments of practical mindfulness come more

EMOTIONAL HEALTH

Your mind *will* influence how you feel as a person living with Parkinson's. There is growing evidence that behavioral health therapies, such as stress reduction, treatment of depression and anxiety, biofeedback, medication and other therapies can help many chronic conditions, from Parkinson's to heart disease to cancer. Despite these important findings, we often spend very little time or energy on this part of our health.

> **"** *We feel that we need permission from others or ourselves to be a certain way instead of just acknowledging this is who I am, how I am and dealing with the circumstances that are what they are. I've let go of some of those things and acknowledge what life is, what I need and how to be more balanced and healthy."*
>
> — TIM

MIND-BODY CONNECTION

What was once a philosophical discussion is now an emerging area of healthcare called mind-body medicine. Specialists who practice mind-body medicine share the belief that thoughts and emotions can influence healing and well-being. Rather than viewing the brain and body as separate entities, this philosophy views them as linked together to form each person's unique existence. Health and wellness are optimized when equal attention is given to each of these areas. All too often, modern Western medicine focuses on the physical body and puts an emphasis on quick treatments with pills or surgery – ignoring the impact that emotions, mind and spirit have on the healing process.

Many believe the "power of the mind" is one of the biggest strengths when it comes to healing. This is understood all too well by people who experience tremor. An increase in life stress is directly tied to

easily throughout the day and my various activities. Extending that basic concept of mindfulness into other areas of life is a form of meditation.

For me, mindfulness ebbs and flows throughout the day. While I do set aside time at the beginning and end of each day to practice intentional meditation, it's really throughout the day that I can see the benefits of those dedicated practices, not during the practice itself. Meditation can be spiritual, or it can be secular. How you approach it has much to do with your worldview and what you hope to get out of the experience.

Meditative practices and mindfulness in general help me specifically to calm my overloaded Parkinson's mind. Five years ago, if I had ten things to do during the course of my day, I would have become overloaded with distractions and suffered brain freeze. Now, I find that it's become much easier. First, I have an appreciation of how anxious Parkinson's can make me, so I know that I need to counteract that in some way. Second, through practicing mindfulness, I have learned how to quiet my mind down and focus on accomplishing one thing at a time before I turn to something else. This might sound simplistic, but it really works for me. I find that I can get through whatever tasks the day holds with less stress and more ease. I don't know if people that don't have a Parkinson's-affected brain can fully understand the anxiety and feelings of overwhelm that rush in when, as a person with Parkinson's, you're faced with a big menu of choices. It's like your brain freezes, wondering what you're going to decide. It's in situations like this that mindfulness really helps me sort out, prioritize and complete tasks or make choices.

The better I understand anxiety and how it takes root in my mind, the less I'm carried away by the anxious thought process. Going into a social situation if I'm tired after a long day of flexing my brain and my vocal cords, if my voice quality is poor and my thought process is muddy, it's a sure recipe for anxiety. But, if I've planned my day right and managed my schedule so that I show up to a dinner party rested and with a bit of reserve in the tank, I am much better equipped to handle a challenging social situation. Putting the components in place to help me be mindful, organize my thoughts and manage my energy gives me a great foundation to not only handle, but enjoy that dinner party or any other social situation.

Try this: whatever you're doing right now, give yourself a few moments to take ten deep breaths, focusing only on your breath. What did you notice? Did thoughts try to muscle their way into your consciousness? Was it hard to stay focused on just your breathing? If you didn't immediately settle into a zen-like calm, don't be discouraged.

Meditation and mindfulness takes practice, intention and work. Sometimes people tell me, "I don't have time," or, "I can't quiet my brain." But here's the thing: if you practice mindfulness for only five minutes per day, it's like trying to train for a marathon by running only five minutes per day. You won't get very far with that approach. Instead, just start where you are today, and begin training every day. Pretty soon, you'll start seeing the fruit of your labors, and it will get easier. When mindfulness begins to come more naturally, you'll appreciate how many times throughout the day you rely on this simple technique to clear your mind and make it easier to live well today.

an increase in tremor. Relaxation, in turn, can reduce tremor. The "power of the mind" is so important that modern-day scientific studies are designed with this mind-body connection. For instance, medication studies are designed so that a medication's effect is compared to that of a placebo or sugar pill. Simply wishing, expecting or believing that a treatment will work increases the likelihood that it will. In fact, there has been recent attention paid to the influence of the placebo effect on clinical trials specifically related to Parkinson's.

DEPRESSION IN PARKINSON'S

By Melanie M. Brandabur, MD

Over my many years of taking care of people with Parkinson's, I met with hundreds of people living with Parkinson's, even more if you include the ones I have met at support groups and conferences. The vast majority of the people living with Parkinson's I have met are optimistic, intent on living life to the fullest, despite their diagnosis.

During an office visit, when I ask people living with Parkinson's if they are depressed, most of them say, "no." I commonly hear, "I get down once in a while, but I can snap myself out of it." However, studies have found that depression is extremely common in Parkinson's, present in up to 90% of people living with Parkinson's depending on the type of depression scale that is used. What accounts for this apparent discrepancy?

It is my belief that the problem arises in part from the terminology. The word "depression" tends to imply a degree of sadness that is overwhelming, perhaps incapacitating, with overt displays of emotion, tears or even suicidal intentions.

Most people living with Parkinson's do not report having anywhere near this degree of emotional upheaval, though of course there are exceptions. For example, people who have recently been diagnosed with Parkinson's or a related condition such as MSA (Multiple Systems Atrophy) may become quite depressed as they struggle to come to terms with the diagnosis and all of the potential implications on their life, work and loved ones. This is a perfectly natural response, though counseling and/or antidepressants may be helpful during this period. Typically, most people living with Parkinson's get through this time with amazing strength and resolve as they learn to "fight back" against their Parkinson's with exercise, medications and family support.

For the less acutely depressed group, we probably need a better term, something that means "not as happy as usual; a bit down" to describe the mood of people living with Parkinson's.

Family members frequently tell me that the person with Parkinson's does have some degree of depression, even when he or she does not complain of a mood problem. Of course, this must be differentiated from the motor aspects of Parkinson's, which may cause the face to appear less animated, even if the person is not actually depressed. Spouses and adult children may say that their loved one no longer does things that he or she used to enjoy, avoids going out and no longer participates in previous activities (clubs, sports, volunteering).

What is to blame for this lack of momentum? Many people living with Parkinson's blame Parkinson's, but this lack of interest and difficulty in initiating activity often turns out to be depression. Once the depression is treated, many people living with Parkinson's are more interested in re-engaging – and they still have Parkinson's.

Anxiety is a frequent companion to depression in Parkinson's and is sometimes a bigger problem. Treating both of these symptoms is an important step in improving quality of life for many reasons. In addition to effects on important elements of a good quality of life, such as appetite and motivation to exercise, both depression and anxiety can cause insomnia and early morning waking. Sleep, vital to everyone for maintaining good health, is especially important in people with Parkinson's. When people living with Parkinson's who report having "good days and bad days" are questioned closely, they often note a strong relationship between a sleepless night and poor motor function the next day.

So how do we treat depression? In an ideal world, I would refer every patient to a well-rounded program that includes individual and family counseling, meditation, stress management, perhaps even a week at a spa or a yoga retreat in a beautiful setting. The realities of life, insurance, time constraints and often unwillingness on the part of people living with Parkinson's make most of

Examples of techniques that focus on the mind-body connection include:

- Biofeedback
- Cognitive behavioral therapy
- Hypnosis
- Breathing techniques
- Meditation and guided imagery
- Relaxation techniques and stress reduction
- Therapeutic yoga
- Spiritual practice such as prayer or chanting

DEPRESSION

Depression is common in people with Parkinson's. Depression can be a lifelong problem, a reaction to struggles with Parkinson's or a symptom of Parkinson's due to biochemical brain changes. The important thing to remember is that depression can change every aspect of how you feel – much in the same way that dark glasses color the way you see the world. It's also very important to know that just as you did not choose to have Parkinson's, you did not choose to experience depression. You don't have to feel weak or beaten because you are experiencing this, but be aware that it will affect you in many ways and may or may not be a temporary experience for you.

Depression is treatable. There is a tendency to turn to antidepressant medications as the sole treatment of depression based on the findings that it is related to biochemical changes with Parkinson's. Although antidepressants are a very important and often necessary part of treatment, it is equally important to explore other therapies that influence your mind and well-being.

The techniques listed above under "Mind-Body Connection" can be a helpful addition to your medical treatment if you have depression or as a step to reduce the risk of developing depression. This includes cognitive therapy, counseling, exercise and diet.

this holistic approach hard to come by.

Moreover, studies have shown that Parkinson's can cause changes in the levels of some brain chemicals related to mood, such as serotonin and norepinephrine. Therefore, drugs that restore these substances to a more normal balance are often the most effective therapy. People living with Parkinson's are often reluctant to take these drugs because they have heard negative things about them. But when prescribed appropriately, they usually are safe and effective in people with Parkinson's.

Two troubling symptoms that may or may not respond to therapy for depression are fatigue and apathy (loss of motivation). In fact, fatigue is noted by most people living with Parkinson's whether they have depression or not. Apathy may occur as part of a spectrum of depressive symptoms but may remain after depression has resolved. We work hard to treat these troubling symptoms in people living with Parkinson's. We have yet to find a solution that works for everyone.

As someone living with Parkinson's, the best way to approach these issues is to work with people who know you well enough to identify mood issues that could be having a negative effect on your overall quality of life. Then, bring them to the attention of your doctor and prepare to be open-minded about possible solutions. Remember, a positive attitude is one of your most important assets in fighting Parkinson's!

185

By Roseanne D. Dobkin, PhD

Depression and anxiety are very common in Parkinson's and have a major impact on physical and cognitive functioning, quality of life and family relationships. But, despite these detrimental effects, there is good news: you have control over depression and anxiety. You didn't have a choice in your Parkinson's diagnosis; however, you have every choice in how you cope.

COGNITIVE BEHAVIORAL THERAPY

Cognitive behavioral therapy (CBT) is a skills-based, non-pharmacological treatment that teaches practical strategies to help people living with Parkinson's and their family members more effectively navigate the challenges of living with Parkinson's. It is a kind of psychotherapy or "talk therapy" that focuses on examining the connections between thoughts, feelings and behaviors, in order to provide individuals with the skills needed to change thinking patterns (e.g., negative thoughts about self, world and future) and behaviors (e.g., procrastination, social isolation and withdrawal, lack of structure in the day) that may be related to uncomfortable feelings like depression or anxiety. Unlike some other talk therapies, CBT is highly instructive in nature and involves active one-to-one collaboration between the person living with Parkinson's and the therapist. Sessions are usually structured, and specific techniques/coping skills are explained during each session. CBT is tailored to each person's unique goals and people are encouraged to practice their newly acquired coping skills between sessions in order to work toward their goals.

CBT is generally a brief, time-limited treatment (three to six months). However, the number of sessions varies, depending on the needs of each individual. With ongoing practice, you can continue to benefit from your newly acquired coping skills, long after treatment has ended. Learning new information is not enough: true change requires putting different coping skills into action in daily life, ongoing. Relatedly, here is an analogy I think that we can all understand: If you fill your prescription for your Parkinson's medication, but don't actually open the bottles and swallow the pills, your tremor and stiffness will not likely improve. Similarly, if you learn innovative tools to combat depression and anxiety in the face of Parkinson's, but you do not use them on a daily basis, they will not help you. Consistent practice over time is key.

There are several different CBT strategies which can be used to help you cope more effectively with depression and anxiety, as well as with the daily stress of living with Parkinson's (Table 1). Some tools focus on what you are doing or not doing in response to the current challenges that you are experiencing, while others focus on how you are thinking about yourself and your changing life circumstances. Behavioral tools include daily goal setting, increasing involvement in meaningful, pleasurable and/or social activities, and safely increasing daily exercise. All of the people living with Parkinson's that I work with are encouraged to set three realistic, achievable goals per day (one exercise goal, one social goal and one other goal, which might be something productive, like paying a bill or self-soothing, like taking an Epsom salt bath). An example of a realistic social goal could be answering the phone when your sister calls, rather than letting it automatically go to voicemail. Effective behavioral goal setting often involves collaborative problem-solving and thinking outside of the box in order to meet the challenging demands of Parkinson's. This point is nicely illustrated in the case of Howard (Table 2).

Lifestyle Changes

Sleep hygiene, relaxation training and worry control approaches also provide practical insights for mood management. When insomnia is part of the clinical picture, daily exercise, relaxing before bedtime, keeping regular sleep hours (i.e., going to bed and getting up at the same time everyday) and avoiding excess time in bed, daytime naps, caffeine or alcohol in the evening and large evening meals may be helpful. Most importantly, individuals suffering from insomnia are taught to only use their bed for sleep (and sex), not for other activities, such as paying bills, watching TV or trying to solve the problem of the day. A daily practice of yoga, mindfulness meditation, relaxation exercises (e.g., deep breathing, visualization, progressive muscle relaxation), as well as placing strict limits around the time that you allow yourself to worry each day are also useful strategies.

Managing Your Thoughts

Regaining control of your thoughts is another necessary ingredient for improving your mood. In the CBT model, negative feelings like depression and anxiety don't come out of the blue; feelings come in response to your thoughts and interpretations of the situations you are facing. Often, thoughts might come so quickly that you might not even be aware of the fact that you are having them, yet they linger long enough to have a negative impact on how you are feeling and how you act. Importantly, the negative thoughts we observe in depression (and anxiety) are often not as true as they feel and are guided more by emotion than by fact.

To further illustrate this point, let's consider the fictional case examples below. "Mary" and "Joe" are both newly diagnosed with Parkinson's and suffer from similar physical symptoms, with comparable levels of impairment. They both experience tremor when they eat in public and struggle to button their clothes. Mary thinks, "My life is ruined and I have no control." In response to this thought, Mary is likely to feel scared and isolate herself. She may avoid going out to eat in restaurants and decline social invitations from her friends. She is unlikely to be proactive regarding her own self-care. Joe, on the other hand, thinks, "I wish this didn't happen, but I know I can still have a meaningful life even with Parkinson's." While Joe is certainly not happy about his diagnosis, he is likely to feel more hopeful than Mary and remain active and engaged in his life. His likelihood of obtaining all of the Parkinson's multidisciplinary services that are recommended to optimize his health and well-being (physical therapy, occupational therapy, speech language therapy) is very high, and he may even proactively seek referrals from his doctors.

This vignette highlights the fact that different thoughts about the same situation can lead to different feelings and behaviors. A primary goal of cognitive therapy is to "press pause" on negative thoughts, evaluate them to determine if they are as accurate as they feel and to replace them, as appropriate, with more balanced, realistic thoughts. There are several different tools that can be used to facilitate these efforts. Tables 3 and 4 illustrate examples of two common techniques that can be used to test out your thoughts to see if they are indeed as accurate as they feel or if modification is necessary. The goal of "cognitive restructuring" (revising your thoughts after further examination) is not to think more positively; the goal is to turn excessively skewed and negative thoughts that impede successful coping efforts into balanced, realistic thoughts that fuel healthy responses to life stress.

Table 5 presents a sampling of self-assessment questions. If you suspect that you are suffering from depression or anxiety, and/or that there is room for improvement in your mood and coping efforts, there are both external resources and practical strategies available to you that you can implement in your own life to help you manage these symptoms. You have the power, control and inner strength to make the changes necessary to improve your health and quality of life today!

So ask yourself:

- Am I the most proactive member of my treatment team?

- Are my thoughts balanced?

- What would a jury of my peers decide?

Table 1: Practical Strategies

- Increased involvement in meaningful and social activities
  - Bring back the OLD
  - Try something NEW
  - MODIFY an OLD or NEW activity to meet your current needs
- Daily goal-setting
- Exercise
- Problem solving for physical limitations
  - Pacing of activities
  - Realistic daily goals/less rigid demands
  - Plan around "off-time"
  - Follow through with referrals for PT, OT and Speech
- Anxiety management and relaxation
  - Breathing exercises
  - Meditation
  - Progressive muscle relaxation
  - Guided visualization
  - Limit worry time
- Sleep hygiene
  - Using bed for sleep and intimacy only – not TV, paying bills etc.
  - Relaxing before bedtime
  - Keeping regular sleep hours
  - Limiting excess time in bed, daytime naps, caffeine or alcohol in the evening
- Thought monitoring and restructuring
  - Rethink the big picture
    - Catch the negative thought
    - Press pause
    - Rewind
    - Replay in a more balanced way
- Self-help books and community-based resources

Table 2: Behavioral Activation Example

Howard was a volunteer firefighter for over 40 years. He stopped responding to calls when he felt that he was no longer physically able to do so as a result of the worsening of his Parkinson's symptoms. At this point, he became quite depressed and no longer went down to the firehouse to spend time with friends. He also stopped participating in all firehouse related activities, including those that required no physical exertion, like the monthly chili dinner.

Part of Howard's treatment included reconnecting with the local fire department. He began to bring coffee down to the station and visit with old friends one evening per week. He slowly began to explore ways in which he could remain connected to this organization that was near and dear to his heart. Four months later, he was spearheading all fundraising efforts for the local department and his mood greatly improved. Even though Howard was no longer in the physical condition needed to fight fires, he found an alternative way to make a meaningful contribution to the cause.

Table 3: Examining the Evidence

This technique involves examining the "facts" that support and do not support your negative thought. Use the evidence that is gathered to come up with a more balanced thought, as appropriate.

- Situation: Freezing in the bathroom
- Automatic Thought: I'm helpless
- Evidence For: I was alone in the bathroom in the middle of the night and unable to move.
- Evidence Against: This happens quite a bit, so I planned in advance. I had my cell phone in my pocket. I called my wife on the house phone and she helped me back to bed.
- Rational Response: Even though I was physically unable to move my feet, I was able to help myself out of the situation (thus, I am not helpless).

Table 4: Behavioral Experiment

This technique involves engaging in a specific behavior designed to test out a negative prediction and evaluating the outcome.

- Negative Thought or Prediction:
  - It will be impossible to have dinner in a restaurant because of my tremor.
- Experiment:
  - I will go to the Olive Garden with my spouse on Saturday at 6:00 pm.
- Outcome:
  - I was able to eat dinner at the Olive Garden. I ordered food that did not need to be cut and requested a straw and lid for my Diet Coke. I enjoyed getting out of the house. There were no leftovers to bring home.

Experiment results suggest that the negative prediction was not accurate.

Table 5: Self-Assessment Questions

- Is your mood as good as you would like it to be?
- Think about your average day, step by step.
- Which of these activities are you currently engaged in?
  - Socializing with family members and friends?
  - Exercising?
  - Engaging in hobbies?
  - Engaging in other leisure activities?
  - Volunteering?
  - Working?
- Describe activities that you engage in that bring you meaning, joy and pleasure.
- Since your Parkinson's diagnosis, are you as actively involved in things you used to enjoy? Describe.
- Have you decreased the time you spend on any of your activities? Have you stopped any activities altogether? Describe.
- What does the Parkinson's diagnosis mean to you?
- What strategies are you using to cope with the daily challenges that Parkinson's presents?
- Does fear often guide what you do or don't do?
- Do you predict the future negatively?
- Do you often focus on the worst-case scenario?

Newly diagnosed and early Parkinson's
Are you overestimating the extent of your physical disability and functional limitations?

More advanced Parkinson's
Are you underestimating your ability to cope effectively with the challenges Parkinson's presents?

Cognitive behavioral therapy explores how thoughts shape feelings and reactions to events, often without your awareness. Through cognitive behavioral therapy, we can recognize when life events trigger negative thoughts and reshape how we respond to these events or thoughts.

You can improve a depressed mood with laughter, engaging in spiritual interests, social activities or networking by connecting or reconnecting with people who provide support, love and a boost to your self-esteem. See the **Emotional Wellness: Depression** worksheet in the **Worksheets and Resources** section for more helpful hints to improve your mood.

ANXIETY

Anxiety is more common in people with Parkinson's and can occur with or without depression. Anxiety affects your everyday activities in much the same way that depression does and can lead to withdrawal.

❝ *Physical activity always reduces my anxiety."*

— BRENDA

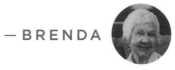

Everyone experiences anxiety and stress, and this is the easiest place to start when trying to understand and work with the mind-body connection. You will find many instances in which you will feel better or worse, based on your levels of stress or anxiety. You may notice that anxiety increases your tremor, muscle stiffness, shoulder tightness or motor freezing. This is an example of the impact of stress on your movements. Equally strong is the power of relaxation – some refer to it as the "vacation effect," in which many people with Parkinson's notice a decrease in tremor when they are relaxed and rested on vacation. Pay attention to this, as the first step to treatment is to simply recognize these changes. You can explore various relaxation techniques to impact these changes once you recognize them.

See the **Emotional Wellness: Anxiety** tool in the **Worksheets and Resources** section for non-medication suggestions to help you manage anxiety. Listen to Liz's experience managing Parkinson's anxiety: 🎥 **dpf.org/liz**.

190

By Joanne Hamilton, PhD, ABPP-CN

Living better with Parkinson's starts with addressing the health of the body and the mind. In the past 10 years, there has been heightened focus by researchers and healthcare providers on the non-motor symptoms of Parkinson's. We are now realizing that depression, anxiety, suspicion, hallucinations and aggression affect a large percentage of the people we serve. Moreover, we now recognize that these symptoms — not tremor, not rigidity and not motor slowness — cause the greatest distress among people living with Parkinson's. They are also a common reason for a move out of the home and into a care community.

Too often, healthcare professionals fail to assess for emotional symptoms of Parkinson's. There are many reasons for this. Some providers do not realize that serious psychological issues, including depression, anxiety and hallucinations, affect roughly 30% of individuals living with Parkinson's. Some providers may not feel comfortable asking questions about intimidating topics like suicide or irrational thoughts. Some providers mistakenly believe that you will spontaneously bring these issues up. Our failure as providers to ask challenging questions perpetuates the stigma that these symptoms of Parkinson's are unusual, or worse, unimportant. Neither is true.

WHEN TO SPEAK UP

We are slowly getting this word out to providers and people living with Parkinson's, but like most aspects of healthcare, being your own advocate is essential. It is important to recognize when emotional symptoms need to be addressed. First, it is natural to feel some sadness, worry and grief related to the challenges of Parkinson's. However, when sadness and loss of pleasure starts to interfere with your day, your desire to get out of bed or your relationships with your family, it is time to speak up. If feelings of worry, fear and dread are continuously rolling in your head, making it hard to sleep or eat and keeping you from relaxing, it is time to speak up. If you are bothered by visions that others cannot see or thoughts that others do not share, it is time to speak up.

If you are spending more time thinking about death and suicide, if you have a plan to end your life or if you are starting to settle your affairs, it is time to speak up.

How? Many of you may be embarrassed to tell someone about your experiences. That is understandable because these are tough topics. Making an appointment with your healthcare provider is an excellent place to start. Telling your provider that you have been bothered by difficult thoughts can start the conversation. Describe in your own words what you are experiencing. Do not be concerned if you do not know the "lingo." Be open about the frequency and severity of the problems. You are not being judged, you are not "crazy" and you are not alone. Remember, 30% or more of the Parkinson's community experience these same problems. Comprehensive evaluation can greatly improve your quality of life.

MANAGING YOUR EMOTIONAL HEALTH

Medication

There are many ways to manage these symptoms and promote good emotional health and wellness. Your healthcare provider may suggest medication, especially if the problems are becoming dangerous. Many people have misconceptions about the way these drugs work, so it is important to have a collaborative relationship with your doctor. Tell your doctor what concerns you about these medications. Are you worried that they are addictive, that they will affect your motor symptoms or that they will change your personality? Ask your doctor what you should expect from the medications. Remember, antidepressants take a month, on average, to reach their full effectiveness. Discuss the benefits and potential risks of the medications. Realize that there are many classes of medications, each with their own pros and cons. There is even a new type of medication to treat hallucinations and unusual thoughts that may not affect your motor symptoms. In some cases, your healthcare provider might not feel that she has enough expertise in these emotional matters to develop an optimal treatment plan so she might ask you to visit with a mental health specialist. I encourage you to request this consultation if you have questions about your treatment plan. This is how you start to develop a solid wellness team.

Talk Therapy

Medication is not the only treatment path for serious emotional issues. There are well-validated methods of talk therapy that can treat depression and anxiety as effectively as medication. Cognitive-Behavioral Therapy, Acceptance and Commitment Therapy and Interpersonal Therapy are each proven to improve emotional functioning. How do you find a therapist? Ask your doctors, ask your spiritual leader or ask your friends. ⏏ WebMD.com publishes an excellent article entitled, "How to Find a Therapist" that explains the difference between all the different mental health providers and gives search strategies. Do not be afraid to interview your therapist. It is essential that you have a collaborative relationship with your therapist.

Physical Activity

Exercise is essential for promoting emotional (and cognitive) health and wellness. The Physical Activity Guidelines Advisory Committee from the Department of Health and Human Services (2008) concluded that exercise can protect against the harmful effects of stress, minimize the risk of developing anxiety and depression and enhance emotional well-being. Physical exercise may be equally effective at treating major depressive disorder as antidepressants and certainly enhances all types of mental health treatment. So, what kind of exercise? Walking, biking, swimming, yoga, tai chi, dancing and non-contact boxing, to name a few, are powerful forms of exercise. You can kill two birds with one stone and enjoy group exercise programs like chair aerobics to increase socialization as well. Silver Sneakers is a benefit of the Medicare program and offers exercise programs in gyms across the US (⏏ Silversneakers.com).

Social Activity

Social involvement can enhance mood, reduce stress and prevent boredom. As isolation increases, so does the risk of major depressive disorder. People may become more isolated because they stopped driving, feel embarrassed about their motor symptoms, have trouble with speech or moved to a new community. Think about joining a group exercise program, spiritual group, book club or senior program if you need help getting out there. Think about a singing group like Tremble Clefs to promote both socialization and communication. Also, consider becoming a volunteer for an animal shelter, children's reading program or local library. Focusing on others can improve mood and reduce stress by giving purpose and moving your attention away from your own struggles, at least for a while.

Stress Management

We all need to think about our emotional well-being and the harmful effects of stress on our bodies and our minds. Not all of us manage stress particularly well. Fortunately, there is greater and greater focus on stress management techniques. Many larger healthcare organizations now include integrative medicine departments that can help you get started. In the community, there are opportunities to practice mindfulness, prayer, meditation, tai chi, yoga and belly breathing. This may sound like nagging, but I can't stress the importance of exercise and staying active enough. Exercise and laughter.

To be clear, Parkinson's is a challenging condition that affects the whole body and the whole family. Taking a proactive and positive approach to all the symptoms of Parkinson's will improve quality of life and emotional well-being. In the same way you would address your tremor if it started to interfere with your eating, why not address your emotional symptoms when they start interfering with your sleep, appetite, relationships, activities and general quality of life?

192

COUNSELING

Counseling can be helpful even before things become overwhelming to you, your care partner and/or family. Combined with mind-body techniques and medications when needed, counseling helps mood, adjustment to stress or symptoms, disease changes, grief, feelings of isolation and loneliness. Just as it is important to address physical health issues early, it is equally important to address the emotional and psychological impact of living with Parkinson's. Trying to manage your symptoms, avoid complications and just living with a chronic disease can drain both you and your family or care partner. Support, knowledge, understanding of available resources and knowing where you can turn for help are some of the best defenses to avoid feeling overwhelmed and burned out.

Counseling can help you, your family and personal relationships. Some of the types of counseling available to you include:

Individual Counseling. Many find it easiest to deal with emotional issues by working with a counselor on an individual basis. In this setting, you can discuss any concerns you have in a private, one-on-one session.

Group Counseling. Group counseling can provide a social outlet for individuals who are experiencing common problems. In this type of counseling, individuals with similar problems form a group with a counselor to discuss their problems together. This type of counseling differs from community support groups in that the counselor helps facilitate the discussion and directs proactive outcomes. It is sometimes easier to gain insights and identify positive coping strategies when learned through the experience of others.

Relationship and Family Counseling. Parkinson's can be difficult for you, your care partner or family. Many times, the spouse becoming the care partner changes the dynamics of a relationship. The goal of relationship counseling is to provide a safe place for communication and honesty. This, in turn, may help to redirect time and energy on the quality of the relationship. You can also read more about how Parkinson's affects other family members in the **Parkinson's and the Family** section of this manual.

> " *I saw a psychologist because of the depression I've experienced with Parkinson's. It took me awhile to find a good one who would really challenge me, but once I did, it's been really encouraging. My wife, Lily, started to drive me there once my driving got worse, and then it became couples therapy, which has helped us tremendously."*
>
> — BRIAN

By Al Condeluci, PhD

Any of us who have experienced or have supported someone who has Parkinson's know that along with the everyday challenges of life, one of the biggest risks is that the condition will lead to social disconnection from friends and families. If this begins to happen, research shows that further compromise to health, safety and overall well-being is accelerated. We know today that if a person becomes socially isolated, this can be as lethal to a person's health and well-being as smoking two packs of cigarettes each day! This article focuses on how people can maintain, and even add social connections in their lives, regardless of Parkinson's or other compromises they might experience. To this end, the first strong recommendation for social well-being is that folks stay as active as possible in their current communities. One of the most important facets of community is that it promotes an opportunity to not only maintain, but to grow social connections for the members who belong. These connections and friendships are often referred to by sociologists as "social capital," and provide an amazing amount of positive benefits.

WHAT IS SOCIAL CAPITAL?

Social capital refers to the connections and relationships that develop around community and the value these relationships hold for people in that community. Like physical capital, the tools used by communities, or human capital, the people power brought to a situation, "social capital" is the value brought on by our relationships. Educator L.J. Hanifan first introduced the idea of social capital in 1916, defining it as: "those tangible substances that count for most in the daily lives of people: namely good will, fellowship, sympathy, and social intercourse among the individuals and families who make up a social unit...The individual is helpless socially, if left to himself...If he comes into contact with his neighbor, and they with other neighbors, there will be an accumulation of social capital, which may immediately satisfy his social needs and which may bear a social potentiality sufficient to the substantial improvement of living conditions in the whole community."

Robert Putnam, the renowned Harvard sociologist, defined social capital as: "referring to connections among individuals-social networks and the norms of reciprocity and trustworthiness that arise from them... [It] is closely related to... civic... virtue... A society of many virtuous but isolated individuals is not necessarily rich in social capital." Other sociologists suggest that social capital is enhanced by social currency. This idea is how social fodder links people together. For example, a popular person who is the life of the party might be regularly included in activities. To this extent, he is strong in social capital. His jokes and storytelling, the items that make him popular in the gathering, are the social currency he exchanges.

All of us, regardless of situation, bring social currency to our relationships. Think about the many communities with which you are involved. People who might be different from you in many ways surround you – your family, your neighbors, your church, your clubs or associations – but the commonality of the community tends to override the differences you have and create a strong norm for connections. The exchange is based in social currency. Further, these relationships become helpful to you for social reasons. Sociologists call this helpfulness "social reciprocity," and this is the core of the value we reap from our relationships.

The fact that social capital keeps us safe, sane and secure cannot be understated. Most of us tend to think that institutions or organizations are key factors to safety. Places like hospitals or systems like law enforcement are thought to keep us safe, but the bold truth is that these systems have never really succeeded in keeping people fully safe or healthy. Rather, it is the opportunity for relationships that community offers us as well as the building of social capital that is at the core of safety or health.

Simply stated, your circles of support and the reciprocity they create are the most important element in your safety. So, what are the things you should consider to maintain or build social capital?

REGULARITY OF EXCHANGE

Cultures and communities have many features, but one key ingredient is regularity. That is, for a community to be viable it must have some regular points of contact and connection. For a family community, this might be annual reunions or the celebration of holidays together. For a religious community, this would be weekly services and holy days for celebration. For organizations, this would be regular staff meetings or stakeholder gatherings. For clubs, groups or associations, regular meetings or gatherings formalize the group as a community. The more people come together, the more they find other ways that they are linked. That is, when a person first comes to a community they are drawn by the common interest of the community. As they attend again and again, they will find other similarities with people in the community and create a deeper sense of bonding.

SIMILARITIES/COMMONALITIES

Other features of community include the notions of consent, creativity and cooperation. Years ago, the sociologist Robert Nisbit suggested that community thrives on self-help and equal consent. He felt that people do not come together merely to be together, but to do something together that cannot be done in isolation. Others identified community for its sense of interdependence. The community builder John McKnight described community as a collective association driven toward a common goal. Indeed, if we think about communities that we know, they all work toward some identified goal that the members agree upon. From teaching people new skills, to saving souls, to addressing a common problem, to launching a government, all of these ventures capture the power of community, and then, through their behavior, create a culture. The most vibrant and successful of these communities are the ones that have built more social capital.

A diagnosis of Parkinson's is life-changing. When my dad was diagnosed, we were all taken aback and wondered what the future would hold. Still, having Parkinson's (or any other type of disability) does not mean that one must now drop out of community, or only can be friends with other people with Parkinson's. We know that community engagement nurtures social capital, and the value reaped by these relationships provide amazing opportunities for all of us to be healthier, happier and have a stronger sense of self. Relationships are waiting for you – all you have to do is seize them!

195

CONNECTING WITH YOUR COMMUNITY

" *It gives me a lot of emotional strength to be in a group of people with Parkinson's. It's nice to hear others talk about their experiences with Parkinson's because then you don't feel so alone.*"

— BRENDA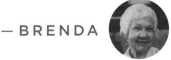

It is so very important to connect with people you love, people that share your common interests or have similar medical conditions such as Parkinson's. It helps to talk about what you are going through and share both good and bad experiences.

HELP OTHERS, HELP YOURSELF: THE IMPORTANCE OF GETTING INVOLVED IN YOUR COMMUNITY

By Karen Jaffe, MD, person living with Parkinson's

You would think that being a physician would have given me a leg up in knowing what to do after I was diagnosed with Parkinson's. The truth is...it didn't.

I was 48 years old and knew no one else with this diagnosis. In fact, it was a full year before I met anyone else walking in these Parkinson's shoes.

I now know that I was not the only one being told early on to think twice about attending a support group. The notion that seeing people more symptomatic than me could be unsettling was a warning I took seriously. In hindsight, this was a missed opportunity for community.

Going at it alone only added to the stigma attached to Parkinson's that keeps many of us silent. With the constant worry about getting worse and thus, being found out, it wasn't long before I had, in my head, become the person with Parkinson's who happened to be a physician, instead of the physician who happened to be a person with Parkinson's.

With the support of my family, in time, I let go of my Parkinson's secret and began to engage with others in the Parkinson's community. One of my greatest strengths as a physician was

> **"** *I have a lot of support from my family and community. It works because I know it's there, but I'm not smothered by it. As people with Parkinson's, we need space to swim and still do things independently!"*
>
> — EDIE

Support groups are a great place to start connecting in your community and a place in which you feel that you are "not the only one." You may also find sharing your experience and wisdom about living with Parkinson's could be very helpful to someone else needing help coping with the disease.

Some support groups focus on special interests such as care partners, young onset Parkinson's, working people with Parkinson's, athletes, women, children of people living with Parkinson's and deep brain stimulation groups. Support groups also offer many educational opportunities to learn more about Parkinson's, community resources and events and are a wonderful opportunity to ask questions and get help when needed. Try different support groups to find one that fits your needs and interests. Consider starting your own if your area does not have a support group. Listen to Jill describe the process of starting her own support group: ◼ **dpf.org/jill**.

> **"** *All the years I've dealt with Parkinson's, I am learning new things as my wife and I co-lead a support group. It's a huge reward for us to help people get information they need that they didn't know how to access. Our support group has become like a family."*
>
> — BRIAN

Your community will likely include others living with Parkinson's, in your immediate area and beyond. However, just as there is more to you than the fact that you are living with Parkinson's, try to

my ability to listen and offer guidance. As I began to do this for other newly diagnosed people with Parkinson's, I discovered my inbox was suddenly full of people whose stories were identical to mine: scared and alone, often keeping their diagnosis secret and knowing no one else who was with living with Parkinson's. Many were not sure what to ask their physician. Almost everyone wanted to know what I was doing to stay well. Looking back, I see now that these conversations were the spark for my dream of opening a center to help people to live well with Parkinson's.

Propelled by the easing of symptoms that exercise gave me, my recommendation for others was for robust activity whenever possible. But for most people, especially those who were not avid exercisers, the lack of organized exercise programs specifically designed for people with Parkinson's proved to be a barrier. I had a hunch that what people were looking for did not exist: a place where there was no stigma; a place that defined community.

In 2013, I joined forces with four other like-minded people in my hometown of Cleveland: my founding partners, Allan Goldberg, Lee Handel, Dr. David Riley and Ben Rossi, to begin the design and implementation of InMotion, a wellness center for people with Parkinson's (beinmotion.org).

InMotion provides our local community of people with Parkinson's and other movement disorders a place to turn for physical, emotional and spiritual support where the stigma of Parkinson's is left at the door, and everyone is encouraged to take charge of their well-being. The center offers a variety of exercise classes such as dance, cycling and boxing, to name just a few of the activities that help clients strengthen their bodies. InMotion also has art and music therapy, as well as a drumming circle to soothe the mind and spirit. A peer program and separate support groups for people living with Parkinson's and their care partners complement the classes. InMotion also hosts expert presentations to help bring the latest movement disorder research and news to light.

The wellness center provides a common ground along with fresh energy and hope, which reinvigorates entire families. Every day, many newly diagnosed people that have not even thought about exercising in years enter our circle of support, creating new friendships and building community.

We face this disease together, with grit and determination. We sweat, we sing, we laugh, and occasionally, we even have to help each other up off the floor. What makes this group so special is that we know that it is working. The impact is evident in our improved outlooks, better health and more knowledgeable and invigorated Parkinson's community.

Perhaps hearing my story has you thinking how you, too, might become a Parkinson's advocate, or as Davis Phinney likes to say, "doing it for the Tribe."

In my experience, the Parkinson's community is one that knows how to roll up their sleeves to get things done. There are many things within your reach if you feel inspired to try. I have friends who started support groups where none previously existed. Groups bring many voices to the table and from there, ideas become reality. There are a growing number of specialized Parkinson's exercise programs to choose from, some of the more widely known including: PWR4Life, Dance for PD, Rock Steady Boxing, Pedaling for Parkinson's and Delay the Disease. Consider bringing an existing program in your area, and expand offerings as interest grows. I know many people who have been given space for their Parkinson's classes at the local Y, in boxing gyms and in community centers simply because they asked. It turns out that folks can be quite generous.

My best advice for how to begin making a difference in your community is this: **share your story**. Almost everyone knows someone who is living with Parkinson's, many of whom are looking for someone to talk to. Be the one who starts the dialogue in *your* community, and that might lead to something bigger than yourself.

not lose sight of other community endeavors with friends and connections outside of your Parkinson's community.

> *Even though I am very active in my local Parkinson's community, I've made it a priority to keep up with my groups and friends who are outside of Parkinson's."*
>
> — BRENDA

This could include old or new hobbies as well as involvement in personal and professional associations. Hear how volunteering helps Jill stay engaged and live well: 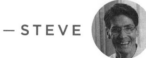 **dpf.org/jill**.

> *About five years into my journey with Parkinson's, I realized that I was getting really run down and it was hard to keep up. I was still working full-time and that meant long days, evening networking events, etc. It was starting to really affect how I felt. I loved doing all that stuff, but it was just killing me. I made the difficult decision to sell my business and went from being ultra-busy to just nothing. I quickly found out that wasn't good either. Depression was 'something that happens to other people,' but suddenly I realized that I was feeling really lonely. I got involved with volunteering and mentoring, and now life feels balanced."*
>
> — STEVE

Listen to Steve explain the importance of building a personal support network: ▪ **dpf.org/steve**.

CREATIVITY

People are creative beings. Bring creativity to your life through art, dance, poetry, photography and play. Dig in your garden, plant bulbs and enjoy their bloom. If you don't have a green thumb, start a cactus garden. Dust off your old hobbies or work with your therapist (counselor, recreational therapist, occupational therapist) to find new ones. Draw, paint, sing, act or simply play.

> *I used to be a technology teacher, but I've lost a lot of my ability to multitask and do math because of Parkinson's. However, recently I've taken up building and it's fired me up in a way I haven't been since I retired from teaching. I'm outside creating something and even though it takes me a lot, lot longer to do things, it's new and challenges my brain. I don't care how long it takes me to finish; I care that I did it."*
>
> — BRIAN

ART THERAPY FOR PEOPLE LIVING WITH PARKINSON'S

By Sophie Canadé, ATR, LPC

Regardless of what motivates you to investigate art therapy, the benefits that can be found are far reaching. There is speculation that dopaminergic medications can result in a surge of creativity in people living with Parkinson's.1 I mention this research as a factor that might encourage someone to try art therapy, even if it is something completely new. As much as that idea has its appeal, it would be an oversimplification of a complex condition and the myriad of reasons that making art could be compelling as you learn to manage the changes that come with a Parkinson's diagnosis. So, let's take a moment to consider some of the reasons art-making can benefit you and help you make this transition:

- **Finding Pleasure.** Art-making is enjoyable. There is no such thing as a "wrong" mark. Every expression is valid.

- **Experiencing Control.** Parkinson's robs you of control. Art making is an activity in which the artist — you — can experience choice (through color, medium, line, subject matter, etc.) and control over your environment.

- **Valuing Individuality.** Free creation can encourage spontaneity which can, in turn, improve confidence in your own ideas and in yourself, overall.

- **Expressing Yourself.** Art is another language for communication that can be done at an artist's own pace. The pressure to communicate quickly, accurately or without hesitation does not exist.

- **Relaxation.** Art-making has been proven to lower blood pressure, reduce repetitive, uncontrollable (anxious) thoughts and lift depression.

- **Finding Flow in Mind-Body Connection.** In a relaxed state with focus on the expression rather than on the physical movement itself, motion can become more fluid.

- **Strengthening Concentration, Memory & Executive Functions.** Art-making increases the bilateral activity in the brain. When drawing or painting, you are using both the right and the left hemispheres of the brain. This is wonderful way to take greater advantage of mental resources.

ART THERAPY AND PARKINSON'S SYMPTOMS

In addition to the intangible and ethereal ways that life can be enhanced through creativity and expression, art-making can be used therapeutically to address some specific symptoms of Parkinson's.

- **Tremors.** Approximately 70% of people living with Parkinson's are affected by tremors, and these can be exacerbated by stress. Relaxation is key. In an art studio or other safe space where acceptance is nurtured and focus is on the process rather than on the product, art-making can lower blood pressure, slow down breathing and calm the central nervous system. Acceptance of a tremor can actually soothe the tremor.

- **Freezing**. When the body is on autopilot, often during repetitive movement, and is interrupted, neuromuscular freezing can result. When you are deeply immersed in art-making, the focus shifts to creating with deliberate, novel motions and you are less likely to freeze.

- **Impaired speech.** The physical and cognitive symptoms of Parkinson's can result in impaired speech. Self-expression and communication with others is essential to well-being. Art-making opens a door for non-verbal communication. The act of creating benefits you, the artist, and the act of sharing what you've created strengthens your relationships with others.

- **Isolation and Depression.** The social and emotional connections you form by sharing a safe, creative space are invaluable for combating isolation and depression. An art therapy support group

199

can be beneficial for those living with Parkinson's as well as for care partners and caregivers. I have witnessed firsthand the emotional support, information and inspiration that members of these groups provide to one another in a way that only someone who has experienced living with Parkinson's could do.

WHAT KIND OF ART MAKES GOOD THERAPY?

In my years working with people who have Parkinson's, preferences for art materials have varied as much as personalities. The choices of medium are influenced by each person's progression of symptoms, as well as by the sort of relationship a person is ready to have with those symptoms. I have found that wet-on-wet watercolor painting can be satisfying for many people, as this method of painting easily creates a satisfying mark with minimal pressure. This approach to painting can be soothing, and we already know how much relaxation plays a part in reducing tremors. However, a few members of my current art therapy support group have really appreciated the use of water color pencils, because they add precision to the medium. These artists choose to focus intently on making deliberate, unique marks, knowing that it is a balance between gaining control through attention to movement (reducing the likelihood of freezing) and putting too much pressure on themselves to make precisely the mark they expect, which brings stress.

While there is no perfect medium for every art therapy participant, I have a few approaches that I have found increase the therapeutic benefits and ease of engagement for most people.

- **Work large.** If you are able, find large paper or canvas and try to fill it. This will invite greater extension of your limbs and greater awareness of your physical space.

- **Work with both hands.** Working bilaterally with the body stimulates greater synaptic activity in both hemispheres of the brain. Using your non-dominant hand will enable you to make the most of your mental resources.

- **Start with a circle.** Starting by marking your surface (such as paper or a canvas) with a large circle drawn can sometimes be the jump start you need to begin an artistic motion. The circle on the page can be a visual signal indicating where the mark is to be made. The very presence of the circle creates something for you to respond to, the way a laser cane can unfreeze a step.

- **Turn on some music.** Rhythm and melody can act as external cues that can keep a paintbrush gliding, and art-making can become a dance. This is consistent with the positive effects music has on any movement, whether exercise, dance class or routine, everyday movement.

FINDING YOUR CREATIVE VOICE

There are so many forms of expressive art that I have not even touched upon which might appeal to you. Participation in creative therapy can improve mobility and increase independence, including greater participation in leisure activities. Visual art-making and music have been shown to stimulate the production of dopamine and serotonin. As I have not trained in music therapy, dance movement therapy or drama therapy, I can't write authoritatively about the wonders of engaging in these modalities. Just know that there are many imaginative ways for you to incorporate creative therapy into your wellness routine. My advice is to be brave enough to try something new, and to be kind enough to love yourself no matter what the "result" looks like. Creative therapies offer an opportunity to not only live with Parkinson's, but also to "meet yourself" again, without judgment. Celebrate free expression, for when you are creating art, there are no wrong answers!

You may be able to find an art therapy group in your area by talking to the clinic where you receive Parkinson's care. Senior Living Centers and Older Adult Day services also sometimes offer Parkinson's-specific art therapy groups. If there are no groups in your area, consider starting one! To locate an art therapist in your area, you can visit the American Art Therapy Association's website at **arttherapy.org**.

SPIRITUAL CARE AS A PATH TO LIVING WELL WITH PARKINSON'S

By Rabbi Rena Arshinoff, BCC

Body, mind and spirit are human components that are intertwined. The concept of spirituality is complex and sometimes used interchangeably with religion, yet religion refers to an institutionalized set of dogma, practices and rituals of a particular faith. Spirituality does not; rather, it is about well-being, one's sense of wholeness, connection to others and the search for one's place in the universe. For some people, spirituality includes religion, but not for all. Everyone has a personal spirituality, but people living with a chronic illness can overlook their sense of wholeness and connection, albeit understandably, to focus on physical symptoms and medications. Spiritual care, therefore, must be given special attention.

Illness challenges our notions about how the world works. A basic Judeo-Christian spiritual belief is that we are created in God's image. The Bible says: "For in His image did God make man" (Genesis 9:6). Often we think of the image of God in physical terms, because this is what is familiar to us, but the Divine image encompasses other attributes, such as speech, will, reason, spirituality, kindness and moral sense. We carry God within us, regardless of how our physical body functions. The Hebrew word "shalom" means peace. Another word from the same root is "shalem," which means wholeness. Wholeness is experienced by the many gifts life offers, such as love, friendship, morality, contributions and shared ideas. Together, *shalom* (peace) and *shalem* (wholeness) bring contentment to our lives. Easier said than done with Parkinson's.

The Webster-Merriam dictionary defines "body image" as "a subjective picture of one's own physical appearance established both by self-observation and by noting the reactions of others." How we look affects our sense of self; how we feel about ourselves influences our identity and quality of life. Body image in Parkinson's has a powerful influence on one's sense of dignity and wholeness. People may struggle with their identity wondering, "Who am I now?" and questioning their personal value as physical symptoms change and/or appear. In his book *Facing Illness, Finding God*, Joseph Meszler wrote: "Even this new person in the mirror we do not want to accept has meaning and value to God." People living with Parkinson's may wonder if they are being "punished" by God or may express anger at God and sometimes feel guilty about having such thoughts. **It is acceptable to be angry at God.**

Spirituality for some people does not include God. For some, spirituality may come from nature or a world cause. Whatever it means for you, spirituality is important in living with Parkinson's, a condition which entails losses on many levels that need to be grieved. Loss is accompanied by suffering, and suffering can be accepted, if not completely explained, through spirituality. In his book about his time spent in concentration camps during World War II, *Man's Search for Meaning*, Viktor Frankl wrote about the meaning of suffering:

> *We must never forget that we may also find meaning in life even when confronted with a hopeless situation, when facing a fate that cannot be changed. For what then matters is to bear witness to the uniquely human potential at its best, which is to transform a personal tragedy into a triumph, to turn one's predicament into a human achievement."*

Can one turn the predicament of living with Parkinson's into a human achievement? Without a known cure for Parkinson's, you may feel disconnected and lost at times. Talk and think often about important roles you have had and still have. Grieve your losses, and feel your sadness, anger, worry or jealousy. A Jewish concept teaches, "Do not separate yourself from the community," — remain involved with your community and in your personal world. Go to day programs, exercise programs and activities that involve being with others. Isolation is a first step to social withdrawal, so it is important to not let it happen. Friendship is an important spiritual experience that brings wholeness to all parties involved;

maintain friendships because they are so very fulfilling. For some, attending religious services brings joy and contact with others. It may be challenging to get to a service or, once there, hard to stay for an entire service. If so, have members of the religious community come visit you at home. Asking for a session with clergy or a counselor can bring profound insight as you speak about topics difficult to share with family.

Some people with Parkinson's worry about being a burden to their family, which can cause great spiritual angst. Meszler asks this question: would we consider God to be a burden? As you are an image of God, you are not a burden. He writes "You are a creation of God, capable of inspiring others. You have a unique perspective on life that is worth sharing." Others living with Parkinson's benefit from sharing with you, just as you benefit from them. Support groups and other gatherings are worth attending.

Another spiritual concept is caring for your body. Sometimes help is needed to do so. Seeking and accepting help is not a weakness, but a strength, and is a way of caring your body and yourself. Reframe thinking from what you cannot do to what you can do. This is a reminder of who you are now and always have been and contributes to your sense of personal value, despite having Parkinson's.

Remember that spirituality is an important element of living well with Parkinson's. Your personal sense of spirituality can be expressed and honored in many ways, but it almost certainly always involves love and gratitude for the people in your life. Express to loved ones your appreciation for their help and love, or express your frustrations. Martin Buber spoke of the space in relationships where trust and sharing take place: this space is where we find the Divine. Sharing both your love and your sorrow, your joys and your concerns with those important to you will help bring them and you *shalem* (wholeness) at the same time.

Remember that your stories are important; they reflect who you are spiritually and what matters to you. Do what brings you joy to experience *shalom* (peace) and *shalem* (wholeness). Even better, do it with the people who are special to you. In living with Parkinson's, remember that you matter. You are not your Parkinson's; you are an image of the Divine. Your dignity and identity are important to yourself, your loved ones and your community, all of whom make up the person that you are.

SPIRITUALITY AND PERSONAL BELIEFS

Your culture, upbringing, values and religious beliefs directly affect your health and well-being. For some, spiritual solace can be the biggest source of guidance and support. Many people with Parkinson's say that their religion or spiritual connections help keep them grounded and hopeful. Studies have proven the healing effect of prayer and the importance of religious and spiritual connections in surviving with conditions such as cancer and AIDS. Since each person is an individual, your spiritual path, commitment or needs will differ from anyone else's.

Some turn to their religious community as a source of support and guidance. Others may find spiritual connection at a different level, such as with nature, meditation, social activism or at some other level.

> *"For us, our faith is important. It gives me another aspect of community that I wouldn't have otherwise, and it's where we get our strength. You're not in control of most things that happen in life, Parkinson's being one of them. This is what we've been given. We move forward with God to lean on, and it gets us through the tough times."*
>
> — NANCY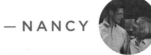

Your personal and cultural beliefs surrounding healing are also an important part of your well-being. Entire systems of care exist – some with a history steeped in cultural traditions, such as Native American medicine, ayurvedic medicine and Chinese medicine. For instance, acupuncture is used in combination with traditional medicine to treat mood disorders, tremor, pain and gastrointestinal problems. These ancient healing systems of care can complement standard Western medical treatments.

Listen as Edie explains how faith motivates her to live well: ◼ **dpf.org/edie**.

HOPE

Hope deserves special mention, because it is so very important to be hopeful in your quest for wellness. For many, religious beliefs give a sense of hope. For others, hope is alive in a desire to experience new things, reach new goals or deal with new struggles. Hear tips for cultivating a sense of hope and resiliency from veteran Parkinson's nurse, Susan Imke: ◼ **dpf.org/resiliency**.

> *"As life goes on, there are all kinds of interruptions and things that are much more difficult than Parkinson's. We still have each other, we still enjoy life and we are grateful."*
>
> — NANCY

CHOOSING TO MAKE A DIFFERENCE

By Evan Siddall, person living with Parkinson's

Albus Dumbledore told Harry Potter in the *Harry Potter* books: "It is our choices... that show what we truly are." Facing a diagnosis of Parkinson's in early 2015, I faced an important choice myself. It was a choice that would set the course for the rest of my life.

Shaken by the news, my life's plan forever changed, and facing the uncertain future of this mysterious degenerative illness, I still had to choose. Not choosing, or surrendering to my potential decay, was itself a choice.

Thankfully, I opted for a different path.

I suppose it was comparatively easy for me. After all, I am white, male, Canadian and financially secure. That's an awfully strong hand of cards to play in life. Much more than any of that, I am supported by the most amazing friends anyone could have. These people have been my salvation.

My closest friends had seen my symptoms when I was riding my bike. What I now understand to be dystonia would slow me down on long climbs; the loss of power in my left leg was noticeable. Much more obvious were the uncontrollable tremors that would follow a high-intensity sprint.

My first choice was to be honest with them: to openly share the reasons behind my symptoms.

"I have Parkinson's and I'm trying to deal with it; I'm trying to figure out what it means for the rest of my life." Their unhesitating, unconditional support was exactly what I needed.

They weren't going to let Parkinson's take over my life. Together, we decided that we would take charge. **That was my second important choice. I would live with Parkinson's. It would not overtake me.**

That attitude led in a matter of weeks to an 11-hour "Sufferfest," literally, that raised $36,500 for the Davis Phinney Foundation. We used our quest for Sufferlandrian "knighthood," involving riding to a series of ten cycling videos non-stop, to raise the money. The people behind "The Sufferfest" (yup, that's what it's called) had long supported the Davis Phinney Foundation. Amazed at the support we felt in just a few weeks, we conceived of the Growling Beaver Brevet (GBB), an annual ride to benefit the Davis Phinney Foundation.

We deliberately designed the GBB to be different. It is hard, *stupid* hard. The feature "brevet" ride is 200 kilometers, largely on hilly dirt roads. It takes a full day for mere humans to finish. Even the shorter 100 kilometer route is grueling.

We say the event is "for cyclists, by cyclists." Our organizing committee consists of experienced cyclists, including two former pros, and all of us have participated in local and international events. We believe that the value of a participant is not the money she contributes through registration fees, it is the network she brings as an enthusiast, as a devoted supporter and fundraiser. In two years, we have raised $500,000. We have uncovered something magical, something that took us by surprise.

The ride is much more to us than a fundraiser. It is a celebration of cycling, friendship, health, community and generosity. Taking place late in our cycling season, it attracts friends connected by cycling and charity. Unlike almost every other organized cycling event, we don't time the ride: people ride together, not against a clock, and take long breaks at local checkpoints.

The Growling Beaver Brevet was born of friendship. I am no Davis Phinney, but I am still a dedicated cyclist. Cycling is typically a group activity. An old African proverb that is popular among cyclists says that, "If you want to go fast, go alone. If you want to go far, go together."

We raise money for Parkinson's through our ride but these messages of "going far together" and "living well today" are universal. They inspire healthy people in their own lives.

I have felt the love of my friends, the devotion of my family and the affection of near-strangers. **My diagnosis has been a gift: I have deeper friendships and more people with whom I enjoy every day more fully.**

Through the Growling Beaver, I made a third crucial choice: to invite people into my diagnosis, into the challenges I face. They never let me down. The innocent passage of each day is lost; I trust it less. In its place is something more precious: the embrace of my family and friends. This "social therapy" is medication to me.

We should all feel the privilege of seeing our reflection in someone else's eyes. After all, it is all that matters. I believe that the only thing we leave behind after we are gone is the impact we had on others.

And the opportunity to transform my illness into an inspiration for people has made all the difference.

Live Well Today.

■ MEDICATION

MEDICATION OVERVIEW

Medication is an important part of your overall care. Professionals trained to help you with medications include neurologists, primary care providers, pharmacists, physician assistants and advanced practice nurses.

Initially, Parkinson's symptoms may be mild and not interfere with daily routines. Choosing when to start medication for Parkinson's varies from person to person. A general rule of thumb is to start medication when the Parkinson's symptoms become restricting or disruptive in some way. In addition, if you are starting to make accommodations or are giving up activities you've previously enjoyed, it is time to consider medication.

> " *I was taking 28 pills a day and had really bad reactions to a couple of the drugs. I started seeing the world in a very manic way. When I stopped sleeping and my previous doctor's solution was to add a sleeping pill to the mix, I found a new doctor. Medication helps, but I wanted a more integrated approach to managing the disease, not just adding more and more pills."*
>
> — JILL

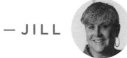

Most Parkinson's medications used to treat movement symptoms are designed to increase or enhance the neurotransmitter that declines with nerve cell loss: dopamine. Fortunately, there are many different classes of medications that offer options for people with mild to advanced symptoms. In addition, treatment discoveries are progressing at a rapid pace and new medications continue to be added to this growing list.

Currently, medication treatment can be divided into motor and non-motor symptom categories.

MEDICATION FOR MOTOR CONTROL

DOPAMINERGIC MEDICATION

Dopaminergic medications replace or enhance depleted dopamine. Dopaminergic medications can be used to treat tremor, stiffness, slowness and walking problems. They can sometimes have a beneficial impact on sleep, mood and cognition as well. Dopaminergic medications make up the majority of medications used to treat Parkinson's, and they can sometimes be used in combination due to the different ways they act in the body. The following are dopaminergic medications, including cautions and common side effects:

Levodopa

Levodopa is one of the oldest medications used for Parkinson's and is still the most effective, even at low doses. Levodopa is absorbed in the intestine and transported to the brain. Dopamine nerve cells absorb the levodopa and convert it to dopamine. Levodopa is now always combined with carbidopa. This blocks conversion of levodopa to dopamine in the gut, reducing the possible side effect of nausea. It also allows more of the levodopa to get to the nerve cells in the brain, where the dopamine is needed. Carbidopa/levodopa/entacapone is described separately under "COMT Inhibitors." The addition of entacapone extends the length of time that a dose of medication is effective.

There are multiple forms and strengths of carbidopa/levodopa. The following chart outlines these different types. Be sure you know which formulation you are taking.

GENERIC NAME	TRADE NAME	WHAT YOU SHOULD KNOW
Carbidopa/Levodopa immediate release	Sinemet	Immediate release, sometimes referred to as "fast acting."
Carbidopa/Levodopa extended release (ER)	Sinemet CR	Controlled release or extended release, which is available in generic preparation. However, this form does not always give a predictable or quick response.
Carbidopa/Levodopa dissolvable	Parcopa	Dissolvable form for people with swallowing problems.
Carbidopa/Levodopa extended-release capsules	Rytary	Extended release, designed to offer longer-lasting effects than immediate release.
Carbidopa/Levodopa gel formulation enteral suspension	Duopa (US) Duodopa (Canada, Europe, elsewhere)	Intestinal gel form of the medication constantly infused via a tube in the intestine. More information about this therapy can be found in the "Surgical Therapies" chapter later in this section.

Levodopa Paradox

Levodopa is the most effective medication for motor symptoms, and it has fewer short-term side effects than many other medications. Initially, levodopa treats motor symptoms smoothly throughout the day. As Parkinson's progresses, motor complications such as "on/off" fluctuations and dyskinesias can arise. Although these motor complications can occur with any medication, they are somewhat more likely to occur over time with levodopa. Other medications, such as dopamine agonists, have a lower risk of motor complications over time, so occasionally these medicines are used early in the disease rather than levodopa. However, dopamine agonists are generally not quite as effective as levodopa in treating motor symptoms, and they have a higher risk of other side effects, such as sleepiness, leg swelling, impulsivity control and confusion. Other medications, such as rasagiline, also have a lower risk of motor complications over time, but are not as effective at reducing motor symptoms as either levodopa or dopamine agonists. Herein lies the levodopa paradox: levodopa tends to have fewer short-term side effects, but has a higher risk of the long-term side effect of motor complications. Thus, the decision of which medications to start depends on each individual, based on factors including the severity of your symptoms and your age. Talk with your doctor and wellness team about the which medications may be best to help you manage your symptoms.

Amantadine Hydrochloride (Symmetrel)

Amantadine is a medication originally used to treat the common flu, but later found to improve the symptoms of Parkinson's. Amantadine can be used alone or in combination with other Parkinson's medications, and it is also sometimes added specifically for the treatment of dyskinesia. It can also improve freezing of gait and has a stimulant effect, which can help with fatigue.

GENERIC NAME	TRADE NAME	WHAT YOU SHOULD KNOW
Amantadine Hydrochloride	Symmetrel	Amantadine is metabolized through the kidneys, and people with kidney disease may require lower doses.

Amantadine Cautions

Amantadine can cause a brown rash, most often seen on the legs with long-term use. Other side effects can include dry eyes, dry mouth, constipation and tissue swelling, especially in the legs. Amantadine should also be used with caution in people experiencing thinking problems or hallucinations.

> " *When I get stressed, my medications don't work right. I've found the rescue drug, Apokyn, to really help when my medications are wearing off. I average about one shot of Apokyn a day."*
>
> — LINDA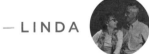

Dopamine Agonists

Dopamine agonists are a group of medications that mimic the effects of dopamine. These medications have a longer-lasting effect and can help control symptoms over a longer period of the day. The following table lists dopamine agonists commonly used in the US.

GENERIC NAME	TRADE NAME	WHAT YOU SHOULD KNOW
Apomorphine	Apokyn	Apomorphine is injected under the skin to provide quick action, typically within 20 minutes, and is used as needed as a "bridge" or "rescue" treatment when wearing "off" is abrupt or unpredictable. Anti-nausea medication such as trimethobenzamide (Tigan) should be used in conjunction with this medication when it is first started.
Ropinirole immediate release	Requip	
Ropinirole extended release (XL)	Requip XL	
Rotigotine	Neupro Patch	
Pramipexole	Mirapex	
Pramipexole extended release (ER)	Mirapex ER	

Dopamine Agonist Cautions

Dopamine agonists, ropinirole (Requip), rotigotine (Neupro) and pramipexole (Mirapex), can be associated with sedation and what are called "sleep attacks." Sleep attacks include falling asleep during activities, such as eating, talking or driving. Some people feel a sense of excessive sleepiness while on these medications, and this serves as a warning sign of risk for sleep attacks.

> *When my doctor put me on a dopamine agonist, I knew there could be compulsive side effects, but I was thinking in terms of the extremes: gambling, hypersexuality, etc. For me, the compulsivity came in the form of rearranging closets at night or chopping every vegetable we had in our fridge and taking hours to make dinner. I didn't think this had anything to even do with Parkinson's, but the minute I told my doctor about these behaviors, she took me off the dopamine agonist. Even if you think something isn't related to your medication, you should always communicate a change in behavior to your doctor."*

— LIZ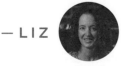

Dopamine agonists can increase your risk of impulse control problems, such as pathological gambling, excessive spending, hypersexuality and excessive eating. Although impulsivity control problems and sedation are more common with dopamine agonists, these problems can occur with any dopaminergic therapy. This medication group may also have higher risk of cognitive changes, hallucinations, leg swelling and dizziness, when compared with carbidopa/levodopa.

Hear Brian talk about his experience learning to manage compulsive behavior: ■◀ dpf.org/brian.

COMT Inhibitors

Catechol-o-methyltransferase (COMT) inhibitors help slow the breakdown of levodopa in the body. This group of medications is used to increase the duration of effectiveness for a levodopa dose. COMT inhibitors increase "on" time and reduce "off" time, especially end-of-dose wearing "off." The following table lists COMT inhibitors commonly used in the US.

GENERIC NAME	TRADE NAME	WHAT YOU SHOULD KNOW
Entacapone	Comtan	Entacapone must be given at the same time as your carbidopa/levodopa dose. Entacapone has no benefit when taken without carbidopa/levodopa.
Tolcapone	Tasmar	A combination pill, Tolcapone is used less frequently, due to potential liver toxicity and requires blood testing of liver function.
Carbidopal/Levodopa/Entacapone	Stalevo	Stalevo combines carbidopa/levodopa and entacapone into one convenient pill, which is also available in generic form.

COMT Inhibitor Cautions

Entacapone can cause dark-colored urine and permanent stains on clothes. Entacapone, tolcapone and carbidopa/levodopa/entacapone can all cause diarrhea. If diarrhea occurs, the medication should be stopped to avoid dehydration and electrolyte abnormalities.

MAO-B Inhibitors

Monoamine Oxidase Type B (MAO-B) inhibitors also slow the breakdown of dopamine in the body and brain. These inhibitors are often used as early treatment, when symptoms are mild, and can also be added when problems with wearing "off" occur and symptoms return between medication doses.

GENERIC NAME	TRADE NAME	WHAT YOU SHOULD KNOW
Rasagiline	Azilect	
Selegiline	Zelapar, Eldepryl	Selegiline is metabolized to an amphetamine, so must be used with caution in people with anxiety, insomnia, cognitive decline or hallucinations.
Safinamide	Xadago	Safinamide was recently approved for the treatment of "on/off" fluctuations and dyskinesia. It has additional actions, such as blocking the neurotransmitter, glutamate, that must be balanced for optimal movement control.

MAO-B Inhibitor Cautions

Talk with your doctor if you are taking an antidepressant, as some medications may interact with selegiline (Eldepryl, Zelapar) or rasagiline (Azilect). Do not take these medications with the pain medications meperidine (Demerol), methadone (Dolophin) or tramadol (Ultram) or propoxyphene (Darvocet), due to a potentially life-threatening drug interaction. Other medications that cannot be used with MAO-B inhibitors include: any over-the-counter cough medication containing dextromethorphan, St. John's Wort or cyclobenzaprine (Flexeril). Antidepressants should be used with caution and only under the close supervision of your doctor.

Note: This list is not complete, so talk to your doctor or pharmacist about these and other medications that you should not take with MAO-B inhibitors.

Overall Dopaminergic Medication Side Effects

General side effects of dopaminergic medication can include:

- Nausea and vomiting
- Heartburn
- Lightheadedness, dizziness, low blood pressure
- Sedation, daytime sleepiness, sudden sleep attacks (especially with dopamine agonists)
- Impulsive or compulsive behaviors such as gambling, overeating, hypersexuality, excessive spending problems (especially with dopamine agonists)
- Confusion, hallucinations or memory problems
- Leg swelling

Overall Dopaminergic Medication Cautions

Alcohol can intensify or increase the risk of sedation, confusion, low blood pressure and falls when taking dopaminergic medications. Speak with your doctor and dentist if your medication causes dry mouth (xerostemia), as this can cause increase risk of gum disease, tooth decay or bad breath. Complete the **Dental Worksheet** in the **Worksheets and Resources** section and bring the **Medical Summary for Dentists** tool to help with your dental care.

Remember that dopaminergic medications are sometimes used in combination, which can increase the risk of side effects and potential interaction with your other medications. New side effects are often experienced when a new medication is added. If you experience a side effect from a new medication, it could be related to that medication or to the combined effect of other Parkinson's medications you are taking. It is important to tell your doctor right away about any side effects you experience.

BE ENGAGED: *Keep a current list of all medications you take for Parkinson's as well as medications that you take for other problems, such as depression, anxiety, sleep, confusion, hallucinations, bladder function, constipation, muscle spasms or blood pressure control. Include prescription and non-prescription medications and update this list regularly. The* **Daily Medication Log** *in the* **Worksheets and Resources** *section is a helpful tool to do this.*

In addition to keeping a list of your current medications, consider creating a long-term record of medications with the **Overall Medication Log** in the **Worksheets and Resources** section. List all the medications you've tried for Parkinson's, and any benefits (such as reduced stiffness) and side effects (such as nausea, sleepiness or changes in behavior). Medications will change as your symptoms evolve over time, so this information will help you and your doctor review what has already been tried and what did or did not work in the past to optimize your current medications.

211

ANTICHOLINERGIC MEDICATION

Anticholinergic medications block a neurochemical called acetylcholine. Anticholinergic medications help to reduce rest tremor and dystonia *only*, so they are *not* used for other motor symptoms of rigidity, slowness or walking problems. These medications are not for everyone and should be used cautiously, as they can cause the side effects listed below. The following anticholinergic medications are commonly used for Parkinson's.

GENERIC NAME	TRADE NAME	WHAT YOU SHOULD KNOW
Trihexyphenidyl	Artane	It is recommended that anyone taking this medication have a gonioscope evaluation, which occurs during an eye exam to check the internal drainage system of the eye. Monitoring eye pressure while taking this medication is also recommended.
Benztropine	Cogentin	
Biperiden	Akineton	
Ethopropazine	Parsitan	

Anticholinergic Cautions

Anticholinergics can cause various side effects, such as dry mouth, blurred vision, dry eyes, drowsiness, constipation, nightmares, difficulty with urination, lightheadedness, unsteadiness and falls, hallucinations, memory loss and confusion. These side effects are more common in older people, people with existing cognitive problems and those with many other medical conditions taking different medications. Long-term anticholinergic medications also have been linked to increased risk of dementia. Any of the anticholinergic medications can cause or worsen glaucoma.

WHICH MEDICATION OR COMBINATION OF MEDICATIONS IS BEST FOR ME?

As you have learned, there are multiple medications used to treat motor symptoms. Which medication is best for you depends on many factors, including your age and side effect risk. Any of the available medications can be used early in the progression of Parkinson's, depending on these factors.

In later stages, motor symptoms can become more unpredictable, with what are known as motor complications. There are two types of motor complications. One is known as motor fluctuations: medications wear "off" before the next dose is due, may wear "off" suddenly or may not "kick in" at all (this is called dose failure). If these symptoms occur, adjustments may be made to reduce these "off" periods. These adjustments may include taking medication doses closer together, using more longer-acting medications, such as dopamine agonists, or using levodopa boosters, such as MAO-B inhibitors or COMT inhibitors. The other motor complication that can occur are dyskinesias, which are irregular, jerky or wiggling movements. Dyskinesias can become a problem as medication dosages are increased. To treat dyskinesias, medication dosages may be reduced, or sometimes amantadine can be added specifically to help reduce dyskinesia.

HOW SHOULD I FEEL WITH MEDICATION?

As is the case with any medication, different people tolerate the same Parkinson's medications very differently. Some people respond well to low dosages of medication, others may require a higher dosage. Some people can experience medication side effects severe enough to warrant a change of course. If you experience side effects with your medication, especially if side effects begin interfering with your ability to go about your normal activities, it is important to discuss this right away with your doctor. Your dosage might need to be adjusted, or your doctor might choose a different medication or combination of drugs.

Parkinson's symptoms may be mild for several years, requiring small doses of medication. During the first few years of treatment, controlling motor symptoms is also generally smooth. Missing a dose or two of medication may not even be noticeable. However, as the number of years with Parkinson's increases, fluctuations in the benefits of medication may emerge, and symptoms may begin to break through before the next dose is due. "On" time is when the medicine is working well to control motor symptoms, and "off" time is when the medicine effect has worn off and motor symptoms return. During "off" time, problems with gait freezing, anxiety, speech, imbalance, tremor, stiffness, slowness and posture can be very pronounced. You may start to feel like you are on a roller coaster: feeling good at times, and worse at others.

As mentioned above, there are strategies to help prolong the effects of the medication. Treatment is focused on achieving the most "on" time and limiting "off" time as much as possible. However, as medications are increased, dyskinesias can become troublesome. If either wearing "off" or dyskinesias are very troublesome, other treatment options such as deep brain stimulation or a levodopa enteral suspension infusion pump can be considered, both of which are discussed more in detail in the "Surgical Therapies" chapter of this section.

Your doctor can work with you to adjust your medications to maximize benefits and minimize side effects. It is critical for you to discuss changes you are experiencing during your appointments. Keep a diary of your symptoms and share it with your doctor if you experience these problems. The **My Symptoms** worksheet and the **Current Symptoms Summary** in the **Worksheets and Resources** section are good starting points. Throughout the day, record your "on" times, "off" times, dyskinesia and when you take your medication in the **Daily Medication Log** in the **Worksheets and Resources** section.

MEDICATION FOR NON-MOTOR CONTROL

Parkinson's-Related Neurogenic Orthostatic Hypotension (nOH)

Neurogenic orthostatic hypotension (nOH) is defined as a drop in blood pressure when moving from lying to sitting, or from sitting to standing. In this condition, the neurologic control of blood pressure is slow, and blood pressure drops with pooling of blood due to the effects of gravity when standing. The primary symptom is dizziness when standing, but other, less obvious problems could include headache, nausea, fatigue, increased fall risk and cognitive change. Non-medication strategies for lightheadedness, dizziness and nOH are covered under "Non-Motor Symptoms" in the **What You Need to Know About Parkinson's** section. Three prescription medications are commonly used to treat this problem when non-medication strategies fail:

Droxidopa (Northera) is metabolized into the hormone norepinephrine, which raises resting blood pressure and reduces the changes that occur upon standing. A doctor may need to adjust your medications if you are taking droxidopa in conjunction with medications that raise blood pressure. Complete the **Low Blood Pressure and Dizziness** worksheet in the **Worksheets and Resources** section to track your symptoms and start a discussion with your doctor.

GENERIC NAME	TRADE NAME	WHAT YOU SHOULD KNOW
Droxidopa	Northera	Because droxidopa may cause high blood pressure when lying down, it is suggested the last dose should be taken three or more hours before bedtime.
Midodrine	ProAmatine	Similar side effects as droxidopa.
Fludrocortisone	Florinef	Similar side effects as droxidopa. Fludrocortisone can cause leg swelling, is not for people with congestive heart failure and requires testing for blood potassium levels.

Parkinson's-Related Dementia

Brain levels of acetylcholine, often referred to as the memory neurotransmitter, are reduced in Parkinson's-related dementia. Acetylcholinesterase inhibitors block the breakdown of this neurotransmitter. There are two commonly used medications for treating Parkinson's-related dementia: rivastigmine and donepezil. Rivastigmine has been studied and proven to be helpful. Although donepezil has not been studied for Parkinson's, it is a commonly used cognitive-enhancing medication. Neither of these medications should not be taken if you have history of bleeding ulcer or heart conduction block, which can be diagnosed with an electrocardiogram (ECG). Refer to the **Cognitive Wellness** worksheet in the **Worksheets and Resources** section to learn what you can do if you or your loved one with Parkinson's may be suffering from dementia.

GENERIC NAME	TRADE NAME	WHAT YOU SHOULD KNOW
Rivastigmine	Exelon pill Exelon patch	Side effects can include nausea, vomiting, loss of appetite, diarrhea, dizziness, drowsiness, tremor and skin irritation at the application site if using the patch.
Donepezil	Aricept pill Aricept dissolvable pill	Side effects can include nausea, vomiting, loss of appetite, diarrhea, dizziness, drowsiness and tremor.

Parkinson's-Related Depression

Up to 50% of people with Parkinson's experience mild or moderate depression. Depression is a symptom of Parkinson's that can appear even before motor symptoms become obvious and should be discussed with your doctor. If symptoms of depression interfere with your daily life, consult with your doctor about treatment options, which may include medication, counseling, exercise and cognitive-based therapy. Complete the **Emotional Wellness: Anxiety** and **Emotional Wellness: Depression** worksheets in the **Worksheets and Resources** section to track your symptoms and triggers and learn helpful hints for improving mood. The table below lists medications that may be considered for treating depression in Parkinson's.

Many factors will influence which medication is best for you. For example, selective serotonin reuptake inhibitors (SSRIs) can help anxiety, so are often chosen when anxiety coexists with depression. Another antidepressant medication, mirtazapine, causes sedation, so it is sometimes combined with SSRIs to help insomnia. Buproprion (Wellbutrin), is also sometimes combined with SSRIs and has the least effect on erectile dysfunction and restless legs syndrome. This medication can also be used for smoking cessation. Finally, serotonin-norepinephrine reuptake inhibitors (SNRIs) can help both depression and chronic pain.

Selective Serotonin Reuptake Inhibitors (SSRIs)

Selective serotonin reuptake inhibitors (SSRIs) increase the presence of the neurotransmitter, serotonin, in the brain.

GENERIC NAME	TRADE NAME	WHAT YOU SHOULD KNOW
Fluoxetine	Prozac	Side effects can include nausea, fatigue, insomnia, headache, dry mouth and sexual dysfunction.
Citalopram	Celexa	Side effects can include nausea, fatigue, insomnia, headache, dry mouth and sexual dysfunction.
Paroxetine	Paxil	Side effects can include nausea, fatigue, insomnia, headache, dry mouth and sexual dysfunction.
Sertraline	Zoloft	Side effects can include nausea, fatigue, insomnia, headache, dry mouth and sexual dysfunction.

215

GENERIC NAME	TRADE NAME	WHAT YOU SHOULD KNOW
Escitalopram	Lexapro	Side effects can include nausea, fatigue, insomnia, headache, dry mouth and sexual dysfunction.
Fluvoxamine	Luvox	Side effects can include nausea, fatigue, insomnia, headache, dry mouth and sexual dysfunction.
Vilazodone	Viibryd	Side effects can include nausea, fatigue, insomnia, headache, dry mouth and sexual dysfunction.

Serotonin-Norepinephrine Reuptake Inhibitors (SNRIs)

Serotonin-norepinephrine reuptake inhibitors are medications that increase the presence of two neurotransmitters: serotonin and norepinephrine.

GENERIC NAME	TRADE NAME	WHAT YOU SHOULD KNOW
Duloxetine	Cymbalta	Side effects can include nausea, fatigue, headache, dry mouth, sexual dysfunction, dizziness, weakness and sweating.
Venlafaxine	Effexor, Effexor XR	Side effects can include nausea, fatigue, headache, dry mouth, sexual dysfunction, dizziness, weakness and sweating.
Desvenlafaxine	Pristiq	Side effects can include nausea, fatigue, headache, dry mouth, sexual dysfunction, dizziness, weakness and sweating.

Tricyclic Antidepressants (TCAs)

Like SNRIs, tricyclic antidepressants increase the presence of the neurotransmitters, serotonin and norepinephrine. These medications are not as frequently used to treat depression due to the higher potential for side effects. They are used for other problems, such as the treatment of pain or insomnia.

GENERIC NAME	TRADE NAME	WHAT YOU SHOULD KNOW
Amitriptyline	Elavil	Side effects can include dry mouth, blurred vision, constipation and urinary retention, drowsiness, increased appetite, sweating, a drop in blood pressure between sitting and standing, confusion and memory loss.
Nortriptyline	Sensoval, Aventyl, Pamelor	Side effects can include dry mouth, blurred vision, constipation and urinary retention, drowsiness, increased appetite, sweating, a drop in blood pressure between sitting and standing, confusion and memory loss.
Imipramine	Tofranil	Side effects can include dry mouth, blurred vision, constipation and urinary retention, drowsiness, increased appetite, sweating, a drop in blood pressure between sitting and standing, confusion and memory loss.

Other Antidepressants

Bupropion (Wellbutrin XL) increases the presence of the neurotransmitters, norepinephrine and dopamine. Mirtazapine (Remeron) and trazodone (Desyrel, Oleptro, Trialodine) can cause sedation and are often given at night to help depression as well as insomnia.

GENERIC NAME	TRADE NAME	WHAT YOU SHOULD KNOW
Bupropion	Wellbutrin, Wellbutrin XL	Side effects can include dry mouth, nausea, stomach pain, headache, dizziness, ear ringing, sore throat, muscle pain, mild itching, mild rash, sweating, increased urination and changes in appetite.
Mirtazapine	Remeron	May cause sedation and therefore can also be used to help with insomnia.
Trazodone	Desyrel, Oleptro, Trialodine	May cause sedation and therefore can also be used to help with insomnia.

Overactive Bladder

Parkinson's can change how the nervous system controls the bladder, resulting in challenges such as urinary frequency and sense of urgency. A urologist can help determine if urine control problems are related to changes in nerve control or other problems, such as prostate disease in men, infection or incontinence due to weakening of bladder and pelvic floor tissue from surgery or childbirth in women.

The most commonly treated bladder problem in Parkinson's is overactive bladder (OAB). Overactive bladder is described as a sense of urgency and needing to urinate quickly, even if the bladder is not full. There are two major categories of medications to treat OAB:

- **Antimuscarinic agents.** These medications block the neurotransmitter, acetylcholine, to relax the bladder muscle. Toviaz, Enablex, Vesicare, oxybutynin and tolterodine are examples of antimuscarinic medications. Although these medications work mostly at the level of the bladder, some medication does move into the brain. Remember acetylcholine is an important neurotransmitter for cognitive function, so these groups of medication must be used with caution in older people or those with cognitive problems.

- **Mirabegron.** Available as Myrbetriq, mirabegron treats OAB without worsening memory or cognition. This medication can increase blood pressure and should not be used if you have kidney disease.

Hallucinations

Hallucinations in Parkinson's are more often visual and less often tactile or auditory. Risk of experiencing hallucination increases with age, high-dose dopaminergic medications and in people with cognitive problems, such as dementia. The dopamine agonists selegiline and amantadine have higher risk of hallucinations in vulnerable individuals compared with levodopa and rasagiline. Hallucinations should be treated when they interrupt your daily activities or are frightening. Begin by having a conversation about what you are experiencing with your wellness team, as reducing dopaminergic medications and/or stopping any new medication that may have triggered the hallucinations is often the first step.

> " *I had to take a lot of medication for a while, before I had DBS. I had visual, auditory and olfactory hallucinations. I smelled things that weren't there. I was aware that what I was seeing and experiencing was not real, but it's still disturbing to be sitting alone at 3 o'clock in the morning, seeing animals scurrying around on the floor and hearing whispering in the shadows. I felt like I was living in my own private version of* The Shining."

— COREY

Hear more about Corey's experience with hallucinations: 🎥 **dpf.org/corey**.

There are several options when medication is needed:

- Rivastigmine can help mild hallucinations and is a good option when dementia is present.

- Pimavanserin (Nuplazid) is the only anti-hallucination medication approved specifically for people with Parkinson's.

- Quetiapine (Seroquel) and clozapine (Cloazril) are older antipsychotics that can help. Side effects include sedation and low blood pressure. Clozaril requires strict monitoring of your white blood cell count.

- Other antipsychotics should be avoided, since they can aggravate movement symptoms by reducing dopamine activity in the brain.

Consult the **Parkinson's Psychosis Self-Assessment** in the **Worksheets and Resources** section for more information if you or your loved one are experiencing hallucinations.

Warning: The medications listed above have a Black Box Warning (high-level caution use by the FDA) to prescribers that their use can increase risk of death when used to treat older people with dementia-related psychosis. The balance between benefits and risks of these medications should be discussed with your wellness team.

OTHER NON-MOTOR SYMPTOMS

Non-motor symptoms can impact quality of life as much as the motor symptoms of Parkinson's. Most non-motor symptoms can be improved with medication, rehabilitation and non-medical therapies. Work with your doctor and pharmacist to optimize medication interactions and to learn about new medications that are available to treat these symptoms. Symptom checklists and worksheets in the **Worksheets and Resources** section that can help prepare you for discussions include **Constipation**, **Overactive Bladder**, **Emotional Wellness: Anxiety**, **Emotional Wellness: Depression**, **Fatigue** and **Insomnia and Sleep**.

Medication Strategies

Medications are tailored to the individual and will vary from person to person. The following section reviews common strategies used as Parkinson's changes over time, primarily focused on the medication strategies to manage motor symptoms.

> " *It's almost 10 years since my diagnosis. I'm not as strong as I was before. I love to hike and mountain climb, but it's a lot more difficult to do a really hard day of climbing or to get on my bike and do a long ride. I need to practice what I preach: eat well, exercise, rest. I'm much more realistic about where I am now than I was in the beginning.*"

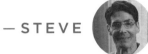

— STEVE

Mild Symptoms

Mild symptoms in Parkinson's may not need to be treated. A tremor that does not interfere with activities may be more tolerable than the potential side effects of medications. Some physicians advise a watch-and-wait approach during the early years of disease. However, because rigidity and slowness can cause subtle changes you may not be aware of, medication treatment may be recommended early on. While medication strategies may vary from person to person, frequent exercise, overall good health habits and reducing stressors should be the main goals early in disease.

Moderate Symptoms

For younger people with mild to moderate symptoms or in the early stages of Parkinson's, a levodopa sparing strategy may be recommended. For instance, you may start off taking dopamine agonists, amantadine or MAO-B inhibitors, and adding levodopa when your symptoms worsen or cause a loss of function. This strategy is not for everyone. A person's age and presence of other problems, such as confusion, hallucinations or balance problems may determine which medications should be used. For example, older people who are at high risk for sedation, hallucinations or thinking and memory problems may do better when levodopa is chosen as initial treatment. In this case, low doses are usually effective when compared to dopamine agonists, which may require higher doses to obtain similar improvement in symptoms at the risk of more side effects.

As noted in the prior section, it's important to remember that levodopa is an effective, safe treatment in all stages of Parkinson's, including the early stages. For this reason, levodopa is sometimes used as the first medication, even in younger people with Parkinson's. This might be considered if tremor is significant, or if motor symptoms are interfering with work or other daily functions. Work with your doctor to decide which initial treatment is right.

Over time, multiple medications are used if symptoms become more challenging to control. Wearing "off" and dyskinesia typically cause a roller coaster experience: symptoms improve, yet dyskinesia occurs as the medication peaks and then symptoms return when the medication wears "off" before it's time to take your next dose. Dopamine agonists, COMT and MAO-B inhibitors can help extend the length of time that levodopa is effective in controlling symptoms, allowing you to reduce the amount of levodopa you are taking to help limit dyskinesia. Amantadine is the only medication available that may help both movement and reduce dyskinesia. Wearing "off" and dyskinesia can be improved by taking smaller doses of levodopa more frequently during the day and sometimes at night. Deep brain stimulation can help reduce "off" times, reduce dyskinesia and possibly reduce the amount of medication that is needed to control symptoms. Deep brain stimulation is explained in detail in the "Surgical Therapies" chapter later in this **Living Well Now** section.

Advancing Symptoms

As Parkinson's changes over time, speech, posture, balance and slowness can worsen. The brief inability to move, called freezing, can be a very serious problem. These symptoms may not respond well to additional medication. The importance of integrative care, rehabilitation therapies such as speech therapy, swallowing therapy, physical therapy, occupational therapy, music therapy, targeted exercise and mind-body therapy may be especially important to enhance safety and quality of life in advanced stages. These therapies are discussed more in the "Complementary Therapies" chapter later in this **Living Well Now** section and you can find strategies to help improve walking and balance in the **Gait, Balance and Freezing** tool in the **Worksheets and Resources** section.

■ SURGICAL THERAPIES

ENTERAL SUSPENSION MEDICATION DELIVERY: THE LEVODOPA PUMP

Levodopa in pill form has the potential to wear "off" before your next scheduled dose. Many people taking levodopa are concerned about the potential for "on/off" fluctuations and dyskinesia that can come as a side effect of the levodopa medication when Parkinson's progresses and the total daily dose of levodopa increases. When "off" times and dyskinesia are significant, there are fewer medication options that deliver a predictable medication response.

Carbidopa/levodopa enteral suspension (called Duopa in the US, known as Duodopa outside of the US) is a Parkinson's medication delivery system for people experiencing persistent "on/off" fluctuations, especially for those with advanced Parkinson's. A carbidopa/levodopa gel suspension is delivered directly into the small intestine through a surgically-implanted tube, where the medication is absorbed. This delivery of medication directly into the small intestine has the added benefit of bypassing the stomach, the emptying of which can become unpredictable or delayed for people with Parkinson's. The small pump, which you carry or wear, allows infusion of a constant medication dose over a 16-hour period each day with ability for your doctor to prescribe additional doses at certain times.

Research shows that Duopa reduces "off" time and increases "on" time by almost two hours a day, when compared to carbidopa/levodopa pills. This effect was especially noted after four weeks of therapy and persisted over 12 weeks in a study of 71 people with Parkinson's.

Duopa can improve motor fluctuations by delivering continuous dosages of levodopa. Dyskinesia can still

DUOPA: HELP FOR MOTOR FLUCTUATIONS IN ADVANCED PARKINSON'S

By Martin J. McKeown, BEng, MD, FRCP(C)

Effective therapy in Parkinson's requires learning about all the potential alternatives, weighing the potential risks and benefits of each, and then choosing the best one for the individual. Early on in the disease, response to medications, such as carbidopa/levodopa pills, is robust and can be dramatic. However, as Parkinson's progresses, the "therapeutic window" (the difference between medication levels in the brain that are too little or too much) diminishes, making it challenging to maintain the correct dose. Normal dopamine levels in the brain are usually fairly constant without large fluctuations, so taking dopaminergic medication intermittently involves a balance between ensuring the medication you take keeps dopamine levels in the brain fairly constant versus the inconvenience of taking pills many times a day.

THERAPEUTIC OPTIONS FOR MOTOR FLUCTUATIONS

Some people with Parkinson's oscillate between being "off" (i.e, slow and stiff), and "on" with dyskinesia (writhing involuntary movements), when the ideal is to be "on" without troublesome dyskinesia all the time. This is called motor fluctuations. For people experiencing severe motor fluctuations, there are a few options. Continuous Subcutaneous Infusion of Apomorphine (CAI), an ongoing stream of apomorphine coming into your bloodstream through a needle in the skin, is a possibility for some people, but runs the risk of nodules under the skin and increasing the risk of psychosis. This treatment is currently not yet available in the US, but in advanced clinical trials. Deep brain stimulation (DBS) is a proven therapy, with significant improvements in rigidity, tremor, "off" times and reduction in dyskinesia. However, DBS is an invasive surgical therapy with some inherent risks. Around the time of the operation, there can be a small, but still significant, chance of bleeding in the head, and postoperative complications such as confusion, infection, etc. must be carefully watched for. Some people are just not good candidates for DBS, including those with dementia, a history of psychosis unrelated to dopaminergic drugs or severe mood problems.

DUOPA: ANOTHER THERAPEUTIC OPTION

What other options are available if you experience fluctuations with medications, but you're not a candidate for CAI or DBS? Enterally administered levodopa/carbidopa gel (Duopa) is an excellent alternative in some circumstances. Duopa (referred to as Duodopa outside of the US) is a gel formulation of standard levodopa medication normally given in pill form, but is administered with a pump

occur, although it may be reduced in many cases as delivery of medication levels out. The total daily dose of levodopa needed using Duopa may be less than that for pills. This treatment can also be an alternative for individuals who are not candidates for or who do not wish to consider deep brain stimulation (DBS) as a means of controlling motor fluctuations and dyskinesia.

ENTERAL SUSPENSION SIDE EFFECTS

The most significant side effects of this surgical therapy include complications related to insertion of the intestinal tube. The tube is surgically placed through the skin over the left upper abdominal region and then advanced through the stomach and into the intestine. A gastroenterologist or interventional radiologist usually performs the procedure in an outpatient setting. Other complications of surgery include bleeding, inflammation and infection related to surgery, perforation of the stomach or intestine with insertion. People with abdominal adhesions, gastrointestinal cancer or inflammatory bowel disease may be at greater risk for Duopa complications. Individuals using Duopa must also be monitored for peripheral neuropathy, which is damage to nerves in the feet that can cause decreased sensation, pain and balance problems.

DEEP BRAIN STIMULATION: THE BRAIN PACEMAKER

If you have Parkinson's, sooner or later you will hear about deep brain stimulation (DBS). If you are a good candidate for this procedure, DBS has been demonstrated to be an effective treatment for many Parkinson's symptoms.

DBS involves the placement of tiny wires into regions of the brain that are affected by Parkinson's. The wires emit continuous electrical impulses (referred to as stimulation) from a device, similar to a heart pacemaker. When placed in the brain, the device is

via a tube that passes through the abdominal wall into the gut. The medication itself is contained in a reservoir bag inside a hard, plastic cassette that fits into a portable, battery-powered pump worn around the waist. Each cassette contains 100 mL of Duopa, with each mL containing 20 mg levodopa and 5 mg carbidopa, as well as carmellose sodium and purified water. The cassettes must be stored in a refrigerator (2-8°C or 36-46°F), protected from light, used one time only and should not be used for more than 16 hours.

Meta-analyses have suggested Duopa results in both significantly improved motor scores, but more importantly, improvements in quality of life measures in people with Parkinson's. An article in the prestigious journal, *Lancet Neurology*, in 2014 demonstrated the clinical improvements that can be seen with Duopa and has led to even more widespread acceptance of this therapy.

POTENTIAL RISKS OF DUOPA

Like all therapies, there are potential downsides to Duopa. The majority of these are seen within the first two weeks of the surgical procedure to insert the tube through the abdominal wall. The tube may become clogged or "kinked," and there may be infection around the insertion site. Once the tube is in place and the insertion site is suitably healed (typically after a couple of weeks), a careful titration process takes place to ensure that the medication levels are just right for you. This procedure varies across jurisdictions, but relies on frequent (at least hourly) observations by trained personnel to ensure that the rate of medication infusion is optimal. This sometimes requires staying overnight in the hospital or nearby for a couple of days.

After the tube has been inserted and there are no complications, and the appropriate dispensing of medication has been achieved, many potential side effects are familiar to people who are already taking the pill form of levodopa: upset stomach, dyskinesia or feeling dizzy when standing up. However, a couple of issues appear more commonly with Duopa: a decrease in weight and a possible increased risk of peripheral neuropathy. The reasons for the weight loss are unclear. Often people with severe, disabling dyskinesia can lose weight because of their continual movements. Once the dyskinesia is reduced with Duopa, they may be able to regain some of their weight back. However, some people still continue to lose weight, for unknown reasons. The peripheral neuropathy, often also seen with the pill form of levodopa, may result from vitamin deficiencies, which can be prevented with oral supplementation.

WHO SHOULDN'T BE CONSIDERED FOR DUOPA THERAPY?

People with mild Parkinson's symptoms who are responding well to oral medication would not need to proceed with Duopa. Additionally, anyone who is unmotivated, non-compliant and/or has poor care partner support may have difficulty managing the storage and delivery of the cassettes and the operation of the pump. Finally, the medication is expensive and health coverage may be an issue in some areas.

While not a solution for everyone, Duopa can be transformative for people experiencing frustrating "on/off" fluctuations who do not want, or are otherwise not good surgical candidates for DBS. People who have suffered from severe motor fluctuations may find this therapy allows them to maintain independence and substantially improve their quality life. Thus, Duopa should be considered as a viable option amongst the other potential therapies for advanced Parkinson's.

223

called a neurostimulator. These impulses can have a positive effect on brain activity that is involved in controlling movement and can improve tremor, stiffness, slowness, dyskinesia, medication wearing "off" and some types of walking problems.

WHEN TO CONSIDER DBS AS A TREATMENT OPTION

1. My symptoms still respond well to levodopa, but my Parkinson's medications are not lasting from dose to dose.

2. Parkinson's medication is unable to control my tremor.

3. My "off" time is not controlled with Parkinson's medications.

4. Dyskinesia is limiting my activities and has become bothersome.

5. I am having intolerable side effects from Parkinson's medication.

6. My mind is still sharp and I am not having hallucinations.

7. My mood is not depressed or anxious.

8. I can live with an implanted device in my brain and body.

9. My family is supportive.

10. I can perform most of my daily activities when my medications are working and have a lot of difficulty when the medications are not working.

For a more comprehensive self-assessment, complete the **Deep Brain Stimulation Self-Assessment** worksheet in **Worksheets and Resources**.

BE INFORMED: *It is very important to understand how stimulation will affect your specific symptoms before considering DBS surgery, as well as what stimulation can and cannot help when living with Parkinson's.*

As a general rule, a properly placed and appropriately programmed brain stimulator will mimic a person's best medication "on" state. This is the state that results from an optimal medication regimen. Stimulation can increase "on" time, decrease "off" time and reduce the severity of your "on/off" fluctuations. Dyskinesia typically improves over time, either as a result of medication reduction or as an effect of stimulation.

> ❝ *I started thinking about DBS six years after diagnosis. I'd noticed my tremor was increasing, and I was up to about 10 pills per day. I was concerned about having more of the side effects of the medication, dyskinesia and such."*
> — JOHN

Hear more about John's experience with DBS surgery: 🎥 **dpf.org/john**.

The implanted hardware consists of a thin wire implanted into the brain, which connects to an extension wire that then connects to a neurostimulator (sometimes called a battery or pacemaker). The neurostimulator generates electrical impulses that travel through the wires to a specific area of the brain. The neurostimulator battery is implanted just beneath the skin in the upper chest and connects to the wires that are implanted into the brain. At the end of the wire in the brain, there are multiple electrodes stacked in tandem that allow the stimulation to be transferred precisely into the brain tissue. The neurostimulator battery must be surgically replaced before the battery expires, typically every three to six years, depending on electrical settings. Rechargeable neurostimulators are also available and last more than five years. People who have rechargeable models charge their neurostimulators weekly. The neurostimulator is programmable using an external device that operates via radio signals in a manner similar to that of a heart pacemaker. Several programming sessions are needed to optimize therapy for each person and it can take up to six months for stimulation and medications to reach optimal performance. Over time, the neurostimulator system continues to control tremor, stiffness and slowness very well. Regular contact with a neurologist or DBS programmer who is skilled at adjusting your settings is key to success in reducing your symptoms.

> " *I don't understand why people say they want to keep waiting to start medications or treatment or consider DBS until they 'get bad enough.' Bad enough for what? I see that you're struggling. How bad do you have to be to want to get better?"*
>
> — JILL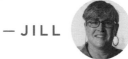

Hear more about Jill's experience with DBS surgery: 🎥 **dpf.org/jill**.

Some well-noted advantages of deep brain stimulation include:

- Reduction in tremor.
- Less dyskinesia and other motor fluctuations.
- Surgery can be performed on both sides of the brain to benefit symptoms affecting both sides of the body.
- The wires can be removed and the neurostimulator turned off if needed.
- DBS does not preclude other future treatment options.
- Stimulation provides continuous benefit and is not typically turned off.
- The user remote control allows you to adjust stimulation at home, as prescribed by your neurologist.
- The stimulation settings can be adjusted if needed.
- Stimulation-induced side effects are temporary and can be reduced or eliminated by adjusting stimulation settings.

WHAT TO EXPECT DURING THE INITIAL EVALUATION

Evaluation for DBS usually includes an examination by a movement disorder specialist and a neurosurgeon specializing in surgery for movement disorders. Most individuals are examined in the morning before taking any Parkinson's medications and then again after taking the first morning dose, a procedure referred to as "on/off" medication testing.

DEEP BRAIN STIMULATION FOR PARKINSON'S: A SURGEON'S PERSPECTIVE

By Kara Beasley, DO

Deep Brain Stimulation (DBS) is the surgical implantation of an electric wire deep in the brain with connection to a battery in the chest wall to treat Parkinson's, as well as other movement and psychiatric disorders. DBS was first approved by the FDA for Essential Tremor in 1997 and for Parkinson's in 2002. Since that time, more than 200,000 people have been implanted with these devices worldwide.

Essentially, DBS functions to provide electrical stimulation to the circuit in the brain that is malfunctioning in Parkinson's and bring it back into a more normal state. DBS is effective in treating the cardinal motor symptoms of Parkinson's, including tremor, stiffness (rigidity) and slowness (bradykinesia). DBS does not treat the non-motor symptoms of Parkinson's, such as drooling, constipation, softening of the voice or balance difficulties.

While DBS is not a cure for Parkinson's, there is overwhelming scientific evidence that proves for those who are good candidates for the procedure DBS is not only safe, but that it is often better than the best medical therapy alone in treating Parkinson's. There are studies that reveal DBS improves quality of life, including bodily discomfort, reduces social isolation, allows medication decreases that reduce or eliminate side effects and most exciting, improves mortality. In my work as a DBS surgeon, I have seen that DBS helps people with Parkinson's live better and longer than with medication alone. DBS is effective long-term. While your Parkinson's symptoms will continue to progress, you will continue to see benefit from stimulation, and the stimulator can be adjusted repeatedly, as needed, to maximize benefit.

That said, DBS is not for everyone.

There is a window for DBS. The ideal candidate is healthy enough to undergo surgery (regardless of age), who still has a good effect from medications (even if medications are less predictable, less effective or cause too many side effects) and who does not have too much cognitive decline. To determine whether you are a candidate, you will require an evaluation by your neurologist that includes "on/off" testing, described in the "What to Expect During the Initial Evaluation" portion of this DBS section.

It is vitally important that you and your doctors discuss your goals for DBS and establish reasonable expectations for what might or might not improve for you before you opt for DBS. Remember, YOU are a critical part of your treatment team!

While I admit that performing these procedures every day means I'm more accustomed to brain surgery than most, DBS is a minimally invasive surgical procedure. It involves a pre-operative MRI scan, usually performed under sedation, which is then used by your treatment team to plan exactly how to get from the outside to the target deep in the brain, while avoiding crucial brain structures. Then, on the day of surgery, the wire or "lead" is implanted through a hole in the skull the size of your thumb. When the lead is in the correct spot (target), it is locked into place and coiled under the skin. This procedure requires a night in the hospital, and Parkinson's symptoms will usually improve for a short period of time. This is called the "lesional effect" or "honeymoon effect" and is temporary. Then, one week to one month later, the lead is connected to a battery or "generator" implanted in the chest wall like a pacemaker. Once this is complete, the device is fully implanted. The last step is an ongoing process called programming, in which your neurologist will use a magnetic device to "turn on" the electricity and "turn off" your symptoms.

There are currently two types of DBS leads on the market. There is the traditional lead that delivers a circumferential ball of electricity, and a there is a "steerable" lead that allows the programmer to direct the electricity in a certain direction to minimize side effects. There are several techniques for placing DBS leads. The choice of technique depends on the discretion of the surgeon, his or her comfort with various techniques, as well as a discussion about your own goals and concerns.

The most common surgical technique is "awake DBS" surgery, in which you are sedated for the placement of a rigid frame or a tower known as "frameless" DBS. Both these devices are affixed to the skull, but the frameless device allows the head to move, whereas the frame secures the skull to the surgical table. Regardless of the frame or frameless, you continue under sedation until after the surgeon drills the thumb-sized hole in the skull. The sedation is then turned off, and the surgeon places a "microelectrode" in the brain while you are awake, but comfortable, "listening" to single brain cells on the way down to the target. The brain itself has no pain receptors, so this part of the surgery is very well tolerated; in fact, you might even find it interesting to hear your brain "talk." Each part of the brain has a different electrical sound and the surgeon will use these sounds, along with your own movement to ensure the target has been reached. Once he or she has reached the target, the actual lead is implanted in the same place and tested for how effective it is in improving your symptoms. As well, the team will be careful to look for any side effects from the stimulation that might occur from electricity "overflowing" into other structures in the brain. Once the lead is in the perfect spot, it is secured and coiled under the skin. The frame or frameless tower is removed and a small dressing is placed on the skull. Most people spend one night in the hospital and go home the next day. The advantage to this awake DBS technique is that the surgeon and treatment team can be sure that the lead is in the exact right spot, thanks to your brain's responses while awake.

The alternative technique for placing the lead is to place it while you are asleep, known as "asleep DBS" surgery. This is performed under general anesthesia. The frame or frameless tower is placed in the same fashion as the awake DBS surgery, but the microelectrode recordings and testing are not conducted because the brain is "asleep." Some surgeons use a robot to place the lead more precisely in this technique. To ensure that the lead is in the perfect spot, the surgeon will then use a CT scan or MRI in the operating room to see where the lead is placed and compare it to the precise pre-operative plan. The advantage to this technique is that you are asleep during the entire surgery, but the disadvantage is that no testing for efficacy or side effects can be performed while you are in the operating room.

Regardless of the technique used to place the lead, the generator (battery) placement is the same and is performed one week to one month after the lead implantation. During this procedure, you are placed under general anesthesia, and an extension wire is tunneled under the skin to connect the lead, which was implanted in your brain to the battery that is surgically placed in your chest wall. This battery will typically last three to five years and then requires replacement. There is a rechargeable battery available that lasts seven to nine years and requires recharging every few days, similar to charging your cell phone. The choice of device and battery options should be discussed with your surgeon before implantation.

Once the battery is in place, you will return to your neurologist, who will optimize stimulation settings for your device, which you can read more about in the "Expectations and Long-Term Maintenance" portion of this DBS section.

While risks and complications with DBS implantation are rare, every surgery has them. Risks include bleeding or stroke, infection, lead breakage, lead movement, failure to improve, the lead ending up in the wrong place and negative side effects of stimulation. It is important that you and your care partner talk to your surgeon about these risks and understand them fully, including which are correctable, before undergoing DBS.

If you have read this article and are excited about the possibilities of DBS, be your own advocate. Start by talking to your neurologist about whether DBS is right for you. Do your own research, prepare your questions and seek out a surgeon who specializes in DBS to get your additional questions answered.

Your neurologist will ask you which symptoms are bothersome enough to merit the risk involved in undergoing brain surgery. Unmet expectations can lead to dissatisfaction, despite successful surgery. A thorough evaluation including "on/off" testing is the first step in making sure your expectations align with the expected benefit from DBS, since your response to levodopa is the best predictor of your response to DBS. If speech, balance or walking do not improve with medication, DBS is not likely to improve these symptoms. This is crucial to evaluate as many people seek DBS for speech, balance and walking problems and if medication is not helpful for these symptoms, then DBS is unlikely to help them either.

Many people wonder how DBS can help symptoms that vary significantly from one person with Parkinson's to another. For an individual, DBS should improve the same symptoms that his or her Parkinson's medications improve. Not all Parkinson's symptoms respond to medication, and those same symptoms are not likely to respond to stimulation. An exception to the rule is tremor, which is not always well controlled with medication, but responds very well to DBS. You can use the **Deep Brain Stimulation Self-Assessment** in the **Worksheets and Resources** section to prepare for a conversation with your doctor about whether or not you are a good candidate for the surgery.

The following standardized evaluation protocol has been established after years of experience by the leaders in DBS:

- **"On/off" medication testing.** After establishing that your expectations are consistent with the expected outcome from DBS, you will be examined by your neurologist after not taking your Parkinson's medications for 8 to 12 hours. Immediately after the first exam, you'll be given Parkinson's medications and will wait in the clinic until the medication reaches its maximum effectiveness, at which point the exam is repeated. The "off" medication exam is then compared to the "on" medication exam. The neurologist will analyze which Parkinson's symptoms improved and which did not with medication. "On/off" testing is very important for both you and your neurologist to determine the expected individualized benefit that can be obtained from DBS. The caveat is that you must be already taking optimal doses of medication before your exam and must be in a typical "off" state for the initial "off" examination. Otherwise, the "on/off" testing may not truly reflect the severity of your symptoms and surgery may not be offered.

- **Neuropsychological testing** is performed to determine whether any significant thinking or mood-related problems exist that could increase your surgical risk or worsen thinking problems after surgery. More importantly, the testing provides you and your family with a baseline. Without a pre-surgery neuropsychological evaluation, there is no basis from which the DBS team can inform you about the cognitive risks of the surgery and no reference point if your cognition changes post-procedure.

- You will have **a brain MRI before surgery**. Inform your DBS team if you are claustrophobic, as sedation requires an extra step in ordering an MRI. If you cannot have an MRI because of metal in your body or a heart pacemaker, inform your DBS team right away. Your doctor will direct an alternative method, based on your specific situation.

- **Rehabilitation evaluation** will provide additional information about your speech, mobility, strength, fall risk, dexterity, joints, posture, fitness and stamina prior to DBS. The body can improve quickly after DBS is programmed, and rehabilitation specialists can prepare you ahead of time to reduce risk of injury and maximize your benefit after surgery.

- A **wrap-up appointment** with your neurologist is very important prior to surgery. This appointment will help you understand the results of the entire work-up, expected surgical outcome, any unusual risk factors, as well as give you a chance to ask detailed questions and understand recovery, restrictions and long-term care. This appointment is standard practice prior to major surgery. Meeting the person who will be adjusting your stimulation additionally ensures that you and your family understand the expected time commitment for follow-up care. Writing down your questions prior to this appointment is very important and helps you to stay focused on getting the answers you need before surgery.

- **Which device will be implanted?** This discussion has taken on new significance now that there are multiple, FDA-approved DBS therapy systems. Device options are likely to continue to increase as technology advances. You and your DBS team should decide together which device is best for you, as clinical expertise, long-term care and device characteristics may vary depending on the selected hardware.

When to consider DBS is one of the top questions people with Parkinson's have for doctors. As DBS techniques, qualified teams and risk mitigation improves, what was once considered a last resort is now simply another option in the neurologist's toolbox when symptoms negatively impact quality of life, despite dopamine replacement medication. The FDA approves DBS as a treatment option after symptoms have been present for at least four years. The decision to pursue DBS should always be your own. Weigh the potential risks and benefits, discuss them with your family and never feel pressured by advertising, research studies or someone else's personal experience with DBS, whether good or bad.

WHAT TO EXPECT DURING THE SURGICAL PERIOD

The surgeon and hospital admissions staff will prepare you for your surgery. Be sure to take the opportunity to ask questions and discuss medications, as well as confirm which medications (prescribed and over-the-counter) should be avoided prior to surgery. Either your neurologist or neurosurgeon will advise you on how and when to "hold" your Parkinson's medications before surgery. You likely will be required to obtain surgery clearance from your primary care physician. If you don't have a primary care physician, the surgery may be delayed until your general medical health is evaluated and determined to be stable prior to surgery. For instance, diabetes and thyroid conditions that are not well-treated will delay surgery until they have been adequately treated.

Surgery is often done in two stages. The first stage is implantation of the wires (leads) into the brain. A targeting system is required for the surgeon to locate the area to implant in the brain. Two systems are available and include a metal frame that is secured to the head the day of surgery, or tiny screws may be placed in the scalp a few days prior to surgery. Individual surgeons each have a preference on how much hair is shaved (full head or small patches) and the shape of the incision. If this concerns you, ask your neurosurgeon about how much hair they will remove.

Most often, you will be sedated (asleep) during the surgery until the point during the procedure when the surgeon actively tests the effect stimulation has on reducing tremor, stiffness and slowness while you are on the operating table. Being awake during this part of the surgery is not painful and provides the surgical team with clarity on precisely where to position the wire. Stimulation is typically turned on to record improvement in your symptoms and at what stimulation power causes side effects. This information is very helpful for the healthcare practitioner who later adjusts the stimulation. Anesthesiologists are present to quickly wake you for testing and then quickly return you to a sleep state for the final implantation of the wire. In some situations, the surgeon may determine that you should not be awakened during the surgery. This approach should be discussed with you and your family prior to scheduling the surgery. All surgical risks will be reviewed with you prior to surgery.

> *It was comfortable, and I could hear them talking and what they were doing. You feel pressure and hear the drilling, but there's no sensation; they use the anesthetics. Once the surgeon implants the wires, then the neurologist tests the wires and creates this ethereal feeling while they run these sounds for them to assess if they had placed the leads exactly correctly to impact my symptoms."*

— JOHN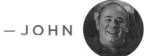

Implantation on both sides of the brain is typically required to control the symptoms on both sides of the body. Sometimes, only one side of the brain is implanted at a time. After the wire(s) are implanted, you may experience what is often called the "honeymoon period," with an improvement in your symptoms for a few weeks after surgery, despite the fact that stimulation has not yet been turned on. It is very important to call your doctor during this time if you think your medications should be adjusted, as the beneficial effects can wear off suddenly. Abrupt decrease in your medication can cause depression, anxiety, apathy, confusion, insomnia, swallowing and speech problems, falling and suicidal thoughts.

The second step involves the surgical insertion of the neurostimulator battery under the skin (usually below the clavicle or collarbone). This is typically done one to three weeks after your first surgery as an outpatient procedure. Your surgeon may restrict driving and lifting until after your chest has healed from the neurostimulator insertion.

After the neurostimulator batteries are implanted, the stimulation system can be turned on and programmed. Initial programming may take a few hours while you are in the medication "off" state. Each of the electrodes is tested to determine which one provides the greatest benefit. Once the stimulation settings are set, the amplitude may be turned up gradually as your brain becomes accustomed to the stimulation. The maximal improvement in symptoms typically does not occur immediately, and it can take six months to a year to see the full benefit of the procedure. While the amplitude is increased, some people report that the improvement wanes after a week or two until the stimulation power is high enough to maintain the improvement. This is the most difficult time for many people, because they are anxious to have stimulation settings optimized. Once the final settings are achieved, however, stimulation settings change very little over time.

> *Programming requires a give-and-take and I need to clearly describe the feelings I have so my programmer can help optimize my settings."*

— JILL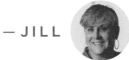

You will receive your own remote control that can be set to either simple or complex mode. In simple mode, you can determine for yourself whether stimulation is on and can power stimulation on and off to check the battery level. Your doctor or DBS programmer can activate complex mode if stimulation needs to be adjusted at home. The remote is easy to use and comes with an instruction book. Your DBS programmer also will discuss with you how to operate the remote. Hear from co-lead author of this manual and DBS programmer, Sierra Farris, more about programming: 🔊**dpf.org/DBS-programming**.

STIMULATION SIDE EFFECTS

Stimulation side effects are temporary and vary depending on where the wire is placed. Stimulation-induced side effects are expected and help determine optimal stimulation settings. These side effects are reversible and occur when the stimulation expands beyond the intended area and can include tingling, numbness, heaviness, swallowing and/or speech problems, muscle contractions, vision changes, dizziness, nausea, sweating, anxiety, worsening slowness, worsening gait and balance problems. Some side effects may not abate after you leave the clinic, so it is important to report any side effects while your DBS team is adjusting your stimulation settings. Typically, reducing stimulation power will alleviate stimulation-induced side effects.

EXPECTATIONS AND LONG-TERM MAINTENANCE

DBS is by no means a cure, although it can restore a remarkable amount of function quickly. Tremor, slowness, stiffness, dyskinesia and some walking problems related to Parkinson's typically respond well to DBS for many years. Most people will be able to reduce their medication. Living with DBS requires long-term maintenance and includes battery and system checks at least every six months, depending on neurostimulator settings and travel distance from the clinic. Arc welding and therapeutic ultrasound (also called heat ultrasound or diathermy) are not permitted after implantation of the neurostimulator system, due to risk of stroke, coma and death.

Depending on which DBS system is implanted, an MRI may be performed if all the safety parameters are met and the radiology department has the appropriate imaging machine. There is risk of damage to the brain or damage to your DBS system if these safety measures are not met. For maximum safety, talk with your neurologist or programmer prior to making the decision to proceed with a MRI scan. Have a DBS system safety check, and review your system's safety checklist to understand and be informed about risks and safety. Many times, an alternative test to MRI can be ordered if your neurologist has any safety concerns.

You must also understand which symptoms DBS will not improve. There is tendency for people to expect incremental increases in stimulation to continue to improve symptoms that progress over time. However, remember that DBS will not improve symptoms that do not improve with levodopa, such as worsening swallowing, speech, balance and gait freezing.

You'll also want to monitor the skin around the hardware and report any unusual changes to your doctor. Routine DBS system check-ups are recommended for battery replacement and especially if you have recently fallen or have had an accident.

When DBS Isn't What You Expected

Dissatisfaction with DBS can occur at any time, including during the initial "honeymoon period," during the active adjustment stage and most commonly, during the long-term maintenance stage. If you feel dissatisfied, it is important to discuss with your neurologist why you feel DBS has not worked out as well as you had expected. This circles back to the first step when considering DBS: discussing expectations. This is crucial to avoid feeling like you didn't get the results you thought were promised. For example, if you think you want DBS surgery in order to improve your handwriting, but your handwriting will not improve, of course, you don't want to have DBS. Handwriting is a complex function and can be diminished because of tremor, stiffness, slowness or muscle cramping. Although DBS can improve all those causes of poor handwriting, the function of handwriting itself might not ever be what it was before Parkinson's.

A less common, but still possible, cause of dissatisfaction is related to poor programming of the stimulation settings or damaged implanted hardware that doesn't function properly. Investigating technical problems requires knowledgeable and highly experienced healthcare providers. If a problem is identified, stimulation settings and damaged hardware are correctable.

233

“ *DBS has been a lifesaver for me, but it hasn't helped every aspect of Parkinson's. My cognitive function has slowed down and it continues to slow down. I'm not the go-getter I used to be, either.”*

— JILL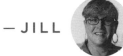

Lastly, dissatisfaction can occur when symptoms progress, despite DBS. As you read these words, please say out loud to yourself: "DBS is not a cure." DBS does not prevent the symptoms of speech, walking, balance and swallowing from progressing over time. However, several long-term outcomes studies show that when comparing people living with DBS versus those without, DBS does improve quality of life for many people living with Parkinson's.

What becomes increasingly important as symptoms change is to remember the crucial role that rehabilitation plays. The next section reviews other therapies that are a mainstay in the treatment of Parkinson's in early, middle and late stages and are an essential companion to any surgical therapy.

By The Jeff and Diane Ross Movement Disorders Clinic in Toronto, Ontario

Living with Parkinson's can be challenging and overwhelming. When first faced with a diagnosis of Parkinson's, it is easy to focus on the complex medical management of the disease, that very often the complementary approaches to managing symptoms and optimizing health are overlooked.

Parkinson's is a multifaceted disease that can affect many parts of your body and can impact each person in unique ways. Since symptoms can include movement and walking concerns, speech and swallowing difficulty, bowel and bladder problems to emotional and cognitive challenges, it is crucial that you know and take advantage of the complementary therapies that will help tackle the problems that you are experiencing. Remember, complementary therapies are exactly that: complementary. They are used to enhance, not to replace, traditional medical and surgical therapies recommended by your doctor.

To start with, having a great team is half the battle. Establishing an "A-team" of healthcare providers can help ensure that you receive comprehensive and holistic care. Your A-team equips you with knowledge, as well as helps you to access the support you need, when you need it. This team can

COMPLEMENTARY THERAPIES

A common misperception is that complementary therapy, designed to be used in conjunction with traditional medication and surgical therapies, is not helpful until your symptoms are advanced. **Rehabilitation is effective at all stages of Parkinson's. In fact, the earlier rehabilitation is started, the better!** Rehabilitation therapists can include physical, occupational, speech and swallowing, art, music and recreational therapists.

After you read this chapter, turn to the **Worksheets and Resources** section to explore how the therapies described here can help you with your own symptoms. If you understand what therapies are available to you and what they can do, you can ask your doctor for a prescription for the help you need. This is especially important for people who do not have centralized Parkinson's resources in their area and are assembling their own wellness team from various specialists within their community.

> **BE ACTIVE:** *Rehabilitation therapy can improve quality of life by focusing on independence, physical conditioning, movement abilities, home and community safety, prevention of injury, ability to perform daily activities, communication, socialization, creativity and education.*

be comprised of a wide spectrum of coordinated professionals, including Parkinson's nurse specialists, physical therapists, occupational therapists, speech language pathologists, technologists, dietitians and emotional well-being professionals. Knowing the role of the various professions will help you identify which profession to seek out, depending on your Parkinson's symptoms.

It is important to bear in mind that expert medical care, combined with expert allied health interventions, promises to be the best formula to help you live well with Parkinson's.

So, what do these professions all do, and what can they offer?

Parkinson's Nurse Specialists. Parkinson's nurse specialists are an integral part of your team. They help bridge the gap and coordinate services between your neurologist, pharmacist and your other healthcare providers in the community, home and aged care facilities. They have the expertise and understanding to educate you on the often-complex medical management, including medication timing and regimes. Nurse specialists are also very familiar with the supports and programs in the community and are often the first to identify other professionals who may be important to involve in your own customized wellness team.

Physical Therapists (PTs). In Parkinson's, the cardinal motor symptoms include changes in balance, walking, slowness, tremor and rigidity. As such, physical therapy is an important complementary therapy to include in your care plan. PTs are trained to help improve bed mobility, walking mechanics (which may involve prescribing a walking device if needed or providing cueing strategies to manage freezing of gait), address balance and postural instabilities and provide education on fall prevention.

In addition to addressing your current mobility challenges, physical therapists play a role in symptom prevention through the supervised implementation of appropriate exercise. Research is increasingly emerging to demonstrate that vigorous physical exercise has a neuroprotective effect on the brain and can help to preserve movement, mood and cognition. Establishing a comprehensive sustainable exercise regimen consisting of strength, aerobic, balance and posture and stretching exercises is crucial. A physical therapist can help you get started!

When you first meet with a PT, you will be assessed according to your current fitness levels, identify areas for improvement and take into consideration any medical risk factors when establishing an exercise program tailored to you. To continue with your exercise regimen, some find it beneficial and more cost-effective to exercise with a personal trainer, find enjoyment in joining group fitness classes or follow a self-directed exercise plan. No matter how you schedule exercise into your day, it is important that the exercise you choose be fun! Depending on your interest and goals, Nordic pole walking, boxing, tai chi, yoga and dancing are a few you can choose from. The following are some key resources on programs that may pique your interest:

- **Dancing.** The rhythmical nature of music and dance allows you to use alternative brain pathways to create fluid movements. Dance for PD (danceforparkinsons.org) is a great resource to find classes near you.

- **Nordic walking.** Studies show that incorporating poles into walking can improve motor skills, coordination and gait quality. Urban Poling is a good reference to learn more about Nordic poles and to find classes in Canada (urbanpoling.com).

- **Boxing.** Boxing is a great form of exercise that can improve agility, speed, footwork, balance and hand-eye coordination. Rock Steady Boxing is an organization that offers non-contact boxing programs to individuals at any stage of Parkinson's (rocksteadyboxing.org).

- **Parkinson's-specific exercise classes.** Search online for local classes, or look for online exercise videos that you can do in the comfort of your own home. ParkinsonNet (parkinsonnet.info) is good resource to find the most up-to-date exercise guidelines for individuals with Parkinson's.

235

- **LSVT BIG program.** This is an evidence-based exercise program designed for people with Parkinson's. You can search for LSVT certified clinicians on their website (⟳ **lsvtglobal.com**).
- **Assistive Technology Clinic.** Provides integrated medical, rehabilitation and technology programs to people living with Parkinson's and other neurological conditions in Toronto and surrounding areas (⟳ **assistivetechnologyclinic.ca**).

OCCUPATIONAL THERAPIST (OTs)

At times, daily activities in the workplace, home or community can become more challenging, whether it is because of loss of hand dexterity, reduced upper extremity mobility or cognitive changes. Occupational therapists can offer suggestions for adaptive equipment and strategies to help you to continue to independently perform your daily activities. This can include training on activities such as dressing, self-care and meal preparation, to more precise activities like handwriting. Depending on what your needs are, adapted utensils may be helpful. A relatively recent advancement in adaptive technology is the introduction of the Liftware spoon—a self-leveling utensil designed to cancel out tremors. Other options for writing aids, like adapted pens or computer technology may be explored. OTs can also assist in mobility equipment like canes, walkers or wheelchairs, if necessary.

One of the invaluable features of including an occupational therapist in your team is their role in providing home safety considerations and driving assessments. They can personally visit your work or home and screen for any safety concerns in your environment and provide suggested modifications to specifically address your needs.

SPEECH-LANGUAGE PATHOLOGIST (SLPs)

Speech-language pathologists are professionals who specialize in helping with communication and swallowing changes that can occur with Parkinson's. Common communication issues that may arise include having a quiet voice, "slurred" speech, difficulties with memory or finding the right words to express yourself. A SLP can provide customized therapy to address these issues, or they may recommend a specific voice strengthening exercise program. In some cases, SLPs may suggest augmentative and alternative communication (AAC) or devices that supplement natural speech, such as a voice amplification system (a portable speaker system that amplifies voice volume). For individuals experiencing swallowing challenges, SLPs are also responsible for assessing your ability to eat and drink safely and efficiently. They will often work closely with a registered dietitian to help you establish healthy eating, swallowing and nutritional habits.

DIETITIANS

With Parkinson's, your diet is especially important when trying to avoid drug interferences and managing the effects of Parkinson's symptoms like constipation, lowered energy levels, weight loss, lightheadedness and sleep disturbances. If these are concerns that you are experiencing now, adjusting your diet can be something under your direct control that can alleviate some of these issues. A dietitian is a good resource to guide your dietary changes based on the particular concern. For example, it may be beneficial to increase your salt intake to manage lightheadedness, as blood pressure may be low; or increase your soluble fiber consumption and add fluids to manage constipation.

Of particular importance is the interference of protein with drug effectiveness. For certain medications like levodopa, the timing of each dose and protein intake is critical to ensure optimal performance of the medication. As you can see, this can all become quite confusing, especially the questions like, "How should my meals be scheduled around medication timing?" and, "What foods should I be including or avoiding?" A consultation with a knowledgeable Parkinson's dietitian can help you get on track. There are many websites that can help you understand the impact of diet on Parkinson's and offer suggested meals and recipes. Living well with Parkinson's (⟳ **livewellwithparkinsons.com**) has a great selection of educational videos on diet and nutrition.

236

EMOTIONAL WELL-BEING SPECIALISTS/COUNSELING

Some of the most underappreciated aspects of Parkinson's are the non-motor symptoms, such as fatigue, sleep difficulties, anxiety, depression and apathy. Many of these symptoms have a direct influence on mood and emotions. Although a multidimensional approach, comprised of managing medications, introducing regular exercise and improving diet can help mitigate these issues, sometimes there is a need to introduce a counselor into the care plan. Whether it is individual counseling or group counseling as in the case of support groups, counselors can help you and your family by addressing your concerns, providing insight, identifying coping strategies and sharing the experiences of others who face similar struggles. The earlier these concerns are addressed, the sooner you can return to staying positive, minimize caregiver burden and lessen the psychological impact of living with Parkinson's.

OTHER ALTERNATIVE THERAPIES

There are a number of alternative modalities that have existed for many years, which are now being introduced as potential therapies for individuals with Parkinson's. The common alternative modalities that have gained popularity in Parkinson's include acupuncture, energy therapies such as Reiki, Alexander technique or biofeedback stimulation technology.

It is important to be aware that these alternative modalities are intended to relieve aspects of Parkinson's symptoms and are not a "cure." These are for symptom management. Acupuncture, for example, has been shown to positively influence symptoms that are often similar to those experienced by individuals with Parkinson's. In particular, acupuncture has been indicated for managing fatigue, improving mood and regulating digestive complaints.

When pursuing these alternative therapies, keep in mind that there is very little scientific evidence to support or refute their use in the treatment of Parkinson's. If you are uncertain whether a particular therapy may benefit you, discuss these options with the doctor who knows you best. He or she can help you weigh the associated risks versus benefits.

Remember, you will always be your own best advocate. You are more in control than you realize. Staying well informed on new and alternative therapies, discussing these therapies with your primary doctors and requesting referrals to the practitioners who you know will benefit you as your symptoms evolve, is the best way to stay in control and enjoy the best possible quality of life. Although Parkinson's is a progressive condition, exploring your therapeutic options and knowing how to access them can help ensure that you live well with Parkinson's.

The content of this article is used with the express permission of Pearl Gryfe, Clinical and Managing Director of the Assistive Technology Clinic. The article authors would like to acknowledge the contribution of the entire team at the Jeff and Diane Ross Movement Disorder clinic, Toronto, Ontario: Dr. Galit Kleiner, MD; Dr. Anita Madan, MD; Karen Hall, OT and Clinic Manager; Ilyssa Abalajon, RN; Lacey Gore, RN; Christine Master, RN; Rose Kim, PT; Christina Samy, PT; Kara Bagnulo, S-LP; Stephanie Wong, S-LP; Nicole Shuckett, RD; Karen Fox, SSW; Pearl Gryfe, Clinic Director.

237

PHYSICAL THERAPY

Physical therapy works to restore and maintain the body's functional performance. In general, the physical therapist evaluates and treats problems related to movement and musculoskeletal problems. Since balance, walking (including freezing of gait), slowness and rigidity are the main motor symptoms of Parkinson's, physical therapy is an important part of your treatment. Fatigue, poor leg power and stamina are common symptoms that limit daily activities. Physical therapists are trained to have the greatest understanding of the factors that improve or deplete muscle energy. Look for physical therapists who specialize in neurological conditions like Parkinson's.

BALANCING LIFE, EXERCISE AND FUNCTION FOR OPTIMAL HEALTH

By Mike Studer, PT, MHS, NCS, CEEAA, CWT, CSST

As a physical therapist with over 25 years of experience, I have witnessed a transformation in our understanding, management and hope when it comes to Parkinson's. Most people living with Parkinson's seek physical therapy to help with balance, fall prevention and walking. In contrast with even 15 years ago, we now have the research-based tools to modify the effects of Parkinson's and to actually *improve* safety and mobility for daily life.

Some of the most common walking and balance challenges that I address include:

- Short steps, or shuffling (festination)

- Difficulty changing directions

- Difficulty keeping balance while rising to stand or sitting down from standing

- Halting, hesitating or "freezing" while walking

- Involuntary movements of the body, arms or legs (tremor or dyskinesia)

Clearly, there is a purpose to walking: to move safely and efficiently from one place to another. Often, people facing walking and balance challenges choose to reduce their walking in an effort to avoid injuring themselves in a fall. While this may seem like an effective

238

" *I fall a lot. However, physical therapy and exercise, especially working out in the pool and boxing, have all helped me understand falling and how to catch myself."*

— BRIAN

The initial evaluation might include testing for muscle range of motion, muscle strength, degree of rigidity, walking, balance and posture. The evaluation will include an assessment of turning, standing, sitting, lying down, rolling over and getting up out of a chair and from a lying position. Physical endurance also can be measured by the physical therapist. If a walking device, such as a cane, walker or wheelchair is needed to maintain safety and independence, the therapist will evaluate for the most appropriate device and provide instructions for proper use. The actual therapy can include any or all of the following:

- A home exercise program tailored to you, your Parkinson's and your current level or abilities

- Balance training and posture exercises

- Stretching and strengthening exercises

- Conditioning or endurance exercises

- Footwear assessments

- Strategies for fall prevention

- Instruction in "safe falling" to the floor and proper techniques for getting off the floor

- Techniques to lessen freezing of gait

- Walking aid training (walkers, wheelchairs, lift belts)

- Home assessments for safety and adaptive equipment

- Treatment of any joint, back, neck or muscle pain and problems

- Care partner training for in-home therapy exercises and transfers

strategy, it can lead to more weakness, and therefore, a greater risk of falling, due to the combination of a movement disorder plus weakness plus fear. This can limit people in moving even from a bed to a wheelchair and cause them to consider giving up walking altogether. So, what is the solution?

HOPE AND EXPECTATIONS

While there is no single physical therapy solution that suits everyone with Parkinson's, there is certainly increasing hope. Research-based evidence tells us (and my personal experience supports this) that people with movement disorders at any level of ability *can* help themselves and can improve even further through therapy. Rehabilitation professionals working with people with Parkinson's have now come to *expect* to make a positive difference that lasts.

Some of the most well-researched techniques in rehabilitation for gait and balance issues specific to Parkinson's include these categories:

- **High-intensity exercise.** In this category, we practice activities that require speed (treadmill or fast walking), power (strength applied quickly in time, such as a fast effort to "jump up" to standing) or excursion (often referred to as "big" movement, with exaggerated motion of larger scale by arm swing or step length).

- **Agility training.** Tasks that involve a rapid alternation of movement, such the efforts of a combination "right-left-right" as in boxing, or as in the footwork in dancing. It even can include efforts to step around barriers or obstacles, as in hopscotch.

- **Combining auditory or music conditioning.** Adding music to one's exercise routine or moving to a pace set by a particular beat.

- **Concentration-focused.** Efforts to rebuild distraction tolerance and the automatic nature of some routine tasks. Research has proven that people with Parkinson's can preferentially lose, but also *improve*, their ability to move with distractions. Walking, dressing, getting out of bed and brushing teeth are but some examples of life's automatic movements, thanks to years of repetition. However, Parkinson's can interrupt automatic access without sufficient rehabilitative training, putting you at risk for falling when distracted during these and other routines.

- **Compensatory.** Identifying and prescribing the right adaptive equipment/assistive devices to best serve your needs of remaining safe and active (walkers and canes, some of which are equipped with visual or auditory cues in the form of laser lines, metronomes or music)

PERSONALIZATION FOR SUCCESS

The best rehabilitation is personalized for you. Your symptoms, your preferences and the things that you respond to best add up to the right physical therapy approach. Additionally, your therapy should be based on research specifically shown to be effective for Parkinson's. This research tells us to use more repetitions, practice daily, include general exercise, as well as activity focused on balance and to make it fun! When movement and exercise are fun, we work harder and receive more benefits from our efforts. Research also tells us that participating vigorously in something that is enjoyable causes the brain to release dopamine – that's right, the very same chemical that Parkinson's limits!

There are also things that you can do at home to continue to improve your walking and balance skills. Ideally, you'll first visit a physical therapist with experience in and a passion for movement disorders so that you can receive a personal examination that includes measurements of your abilities. Having a personalized baseline with measurements and data that you can work to improve over time can be very inspiring. Often tracking progress gives people more drive to work on home exercises with greater effort and regularity. Ask your physical therapist to build an individualized program so that you can re-measure your abilities at intervals and see your progress. If you are limited in your search or access to physical therapy, consider selecting activities from the table below, remembering to include repetition, daily practice and to choose activities that are fun for you.

239

Home Therapy for You and Your Care Partners

1. **Sitting to standing repetitions.** Practice a few repetitions of standing up FAST, then do some VERY SLOWLY, with control.

2. **Standing still with your feet together.** Practice this with your body near a bed or with a care partner if this is challenging.

3. **Big step forward, big step back.** Stand with your back to a chair or bed. Take one BIG step forward, and return back to the starting position. Then, switch legs. As you become more comfortable, you could increase the speed and the length of steps.

4. **Walk short distances with weights around your ankles.** Try 3-lb. or 5-lb. weights, and walk with guidance from a care partner or potentially, a cane or walker to begin. Slowly increase the time spent by a few minutes at a time. FOCUS on lifting your feet up (not shuffling).

5. **Change directions.** Walk with turns, forward-backward walking, etc. Walk in your home, preferably in a hallway. Start out moving forward. Turn around midway down the hall the first time. Then, make it more complicated, and take a few steps sideways or backward. This can be challenging. Take extra caution as you begin, enlisting help from your care partner, as needed.

6. **March in place with "high knees."** This can be done in sitting or standing. Exaggerate your movement and extend your time as you become stronger.

7. **Full-circle turnarounds.** With assistance, stand in a hallway, and turn a full circle.

8. **Standing still, or sitting to standing, with eyes closed.** Stand in one place and practice balancing, with your eyes closed. Try standing up from a seated position with your eyes closed. This is another challenging exercise. Start with assistance and use caution.

Exercises should be chosen based on individual need, ability to safely perform and availability of care partners.

240

SAFETY FIRST

All exercises practiced for the first few times can be challenging, if not dangerous, if misprescribed for your situation. Some tips to ensure that your efforts to improve your balance and mobility do not result in an injurious fall include:

- Ask for and wait for help EVERY time you try a new exercise

- Limit distractions when trying new balance exercise challenge

- Use smaller ranges of motion to begin your first few trials each time you exercise

Finally, consider your overall activity level and general fitness. If you feel limited in your ability to walk for long periods (more than six minutes at a time), consider using a walker or walking with a care partner to enable you to go farther safely, several times per week. Be consistent and exercise regularly, so that you will increase both your stamina and balance.

OCCUPATIONAL THERAPY

Occupational therapy (OT) can help people with many parts of their everyday activities at work, home and play. For example, OT can work on upper arm and hand strengthening and coordination because the arms are involved in performing many activities of daily living, such as household chores (washing dishes, vacuuming, dusting), personal grooming (brushing hair, washing face, shaving), driving, etc. OT can also focus on endurance and strength to help you move from a chair to standing, to bed, to the toilet, etc. Your occupational therapist can additionally help you with a wide range of daily activities, from dressing and eating, to overcoming freezing problems at home or in the community, to installing and using adaptive equipment.

" Occupational therapy has helped me a lot with fine motor skills, like handwriting. My fine motor skills are terrible, so I have a box I made up with things like a deck of cards, a small ball I squeeze with my hands, a medicine bottle with some money in it, scissors, an adult coloring book with colored pencils, a clothespin, a rubber band, etc. I play with all these supplies when I'm watching TV or sitting around to practice and improve my fine motor skills."

— LINDA

Hear more about how occupational therapy has helped Linda: 🎥 **dpf.org/linda**.

Occupational therapy can include any of the following:

- A home exercise program
- Treatment for arm and shoulder strength problems, hand dexterity and handwriting difficulty
- Endurance and strength training

DRIVING

Occupational therapists have training in the areas of visual-perception skills, cognition and movement that uniquely qualify these professionals to assess the skills required to safely operate an automobile. A driving evaluation can help you and your family determine whether driving is safe for you. Sometimes special recommendations are given, such as:

- Recommending special equipment to assist in steering, speed control and visual scanning.
- Using a driving simulator to improve lane control, turning, braking or any other driving weakness you may demonstrate.
- Recommending alternative driving schedules and routes.
- Practice to improve your ability to recognize threatening situations.
- Practice to eliminate bad driving habits.

WARNING SIGNS OF A HIGH RISK DRIVER

Talk to your doctor if you or your loved one has any of the following warning signs:

- Vision changes, significant movement slowing, anxiety or confusion
- Falling asleep while engaged in activity
- Driving well below the speed limit
- Problems staying in their own lane
- Last-second stops
- Risky left turns
- Making turns that are too wide
- Failing to yield properly
- Problems checking the blind spot before changing lanes
- Unexplained dents in the car
- Difficulty parking or backing up
- Failure to use turn signal
- Recent traffic tickets or accidents
- Ignoring traffic signs or signals

242

- Motor biofeedback, stress management and relaxation techniques
- Dressing, hygiene, performing daily chores, meal preparation
- Performing transfers (bed, tub, toilet, wheelchair)
- Improving mobility, task efficiency and safety
- Use of adaptive equipment or aids (grab bars, commodes, tub seats)
- Occupational and work-related concerns
- Home assessments for safety
- Driving assessment
- New methods of performing the tasks of daily living to preserve energy and reduce fatigue
- Identifying problems with movement freezing and the environment
- Medication and time management
- Cognitive therapy
- Care partner education and training
- Non-motor symptom treatment: dizziness, sleep, hygiene, bowel and bladder management, apathy
- Nutrition and food preparation
- Overall disease management

" *I recently gave up driving and it's been really hard. I still have tears about it. I was having such dystonia that I would get paralyzed. I also have a lot of anxiety, and I was so afraid I would get one of those attacks while I was driving. I didn't want to be in the position where I could hurt someone else. Plus, all my medications may cause drowsiness, so I decided to be proactive and admit that I have a problem and need to stop driving."*

— LINDA

Hear more about Linda's experience giving up driving: 📹 **dpf.org/linda**.

OCCUPATIONAL THERAPY FOR PEOPLE LIVING WITH PARKINSON'S

By Cynthia Raczko, OTR/L

Occupational therapy (OT) is the only profession that helps people across the lifespan to do things they want to do through the use of therapeutic activities (occupations). Occupational therapists enable people of all ages to live life to its fullest by helping them promote health and prevent or live better with injury, illness or disability.

OT interventions focus on adapting the environment through modifications, modifying the task, teaching a skill and educating the person, care partner and family in order to increase participation and ability to perform daily activities. OT is practical and customizable, focusing especially on activities that are important and meaningful to each specific person.

OT encompasses several different areas:

- **Activities of Daily Living (ADLs).** These are the basic self-care skills of eating, dressing, grooming, bathing, toileting and toilet hygiene, personal care devices (contacts, glucometers, hearing aids, etc.).

- **Instrumental Activities of Daily Living (IADLs)**. These include the care of others, care of pets, financial management, driving and community mobility, health and medication management, meal prep and clean up, religious and spiritual activities, shopping, safety and emergency maintenance, etc.

- **Functional Mobility.** This includes getting around your home and environment to perform your daily activities, transfers to bed, toilet, bathtub/shower, couch, recliner chair, wheelchair, car, etc.

- **Adaptive Equipment.** This includes long handle utensils to reach your feet or back, tremor management eating utensils, non-skid mats, button hook, lidded cup with straw, scoop dish, adaptive pen, etc.

- **Work Activities.** This includes work station set-up/ergonomics, adaptive devices to make it easier to perform work tasks (tremor management software/keyboard cover, adaptive mouse, Dragon Speak software, etc.).

- **Cognition.** This includes activities to stimulate cognitive function to maximize performance (memory and organizational strategies, visual-spatial skills, divided attention, etc.).

OT Helps People at All Stages of Parkinson's, in All Areas of Life

Here is an overview of how OT can help improve your quality of life throughout the progression of Parkinson's:

In early Parkinson's, tremor and other movement symptoms are mild and typically affect one side of the body. OT during this time can address:

- **Bathroom.** Use night lights, grab bars in the shower and around the toilet, wipe up any water immediately to prevent slips and falls, patch leaks to prevent water on the floor, use a rack to position items conveniently in the shower.

- **Bedroom.** Keep eyeglasses within reach of bed, use lamp next to bed, secure cord to prevent trips and falls, keep a clear path for walking free of clutter for walking around the room, use a portable commode to reduce walking at night.

- **Kitchen.** Arrange cupboards and drawers for safe and easy access to all items, remove throw rugs to prevent trip and falls, sweep often and wipe up spills immediately, don't use a chair as a step stool, have someone else reach things in high places for you.

243

- **Living Area.** Flat and sturdy walkways, remove throw rugs, use tall chairs with armrest to help with transfers, keep a straight path that is free of furniture, use longer cords on ceiling fans and lights.

- **Community Support Groups.** Provide resources for Parkinson's support groups and social activities, equipment lending closets, Parkinson's exercise classes (such as dance, boxing, biking, large amplitude exercises like LSVT BIG and PWR Moves).

- **Exercise Training.** Upper body exercises for tremor management and fine motor activities, large amplitude exercises like LSVT BIG and PWR Moves.

- **Tremor Management Strategies.** Can be used with handwriting, computer use, activities of daily living (ADLs), instrumental activities of daily living (IADLs).

As Parkinson's progresses, tremor, rigidity and other movement symptoms impact both sides of the body and posture and walking are also affected. OT during this stage can address:

- **Dressing.** Stretch to warm up before dressing. Allow plenty of time to get ready before going out into your community. Use adaptive equipment to make dressing easier, such as a long handle shoe horn, elastic shoe laces, button hook, Velcro closures on shoes and clothes, etc.

- **Toileting.** Use a regular schedule to help prevent accidents. Use pads, briefs and/or panty liners to help with incontinence. Use plastic or washable pads for bed.

- **Exercise Training.** Continue large amplitude exercises as you are able.

As Parkinson's continues to progress, symptoms include loss of balance and slowness of movement, and falls are more common. Though the person living with Parkinson's is still fully independent, symptoms significantly impair activities of daily living such as dressing and eating. To help during this time, OT can address:

- **Eating.** Use of adaptive equipment (tremor-reducing spoon, lidded cup with straw, scoop dish, etc.), positioning to stabilize arms and decrease distance from table to mouth are strategies that help maintain independence.

- **Dressing.** Sitting in chair with arms to put on pants, socks/shoes, avoid leaning over to feet, use adaptive equipment to reach feet (long handle shoe horn, elastic shoe laces).

- **Bathing.** Transfer training, grab bars, tub chair/bench for safety, long handle sponge to reach feet and back.

- **Toileting.** Use grab bars around toilet, tall toilet or commode chair.

- **Exercise Training.** Continue large amplitude exercises as you are able.

In later of Parkinson's, symptoms are severe and very limiting. Tremor may be less, but rigidity and freezing can profoundly affect your quality of life. While it's possible to stand without assistance, movement may require a walker. OT during this phase can address:

- **Bathroom.** Adaptive equipment may include roll in shower chair, toilet lift, bidet.

- **Functional Mobility.** Use equipment to help with mobility. This may include bed cane, transfer pole, bed rails or even a hospital bed. Sit to stand transfer can be made easier using an electric lift chair.

- **Exercise Training.** Continue large amplitude exercises with assistance as you are able.

In late Parkinson's, symptoms are the most advanced and debilitating. Leg stiffness may make it impossible to stand or walk. People may need a wheelchair or be confined to a bed and need round-the-clock care. OT during this time can address:

- **Care Partner Training.** Teach the care partner how to use proper body mechanics with moving person with Parkinson's in bed, in the bathroom, slide board transfers, lift equipment, active assistive/passive range of motion to arms and legs.

SPEECH-LANGUAGE AND SWALLOWING THERAPY

A speech-language pathologist evaluates and provides treatment for disorders of speech, voice, language, cognition and swallowing. Once an evaluation is completed, a specific plan of care is developed for your unique needs. Speech therapy is more than just speech; it is about communication. Remember that 70% of communication is non-verbal. People rely on facial expression, change in tone, body language and actual word meanings to communicate. The main goals of speech therapy are to improve someone's ability to communicate effectively, improve communication in social interactions and increase the safety of someone's swallowing skills. Discover the best time to begin speech therapy for Parkinson's: ◼️ **dpf.org/begin-slp**.

> ❝ *I went to speech therapy because I was getting really weak in my voice. After the initial SpeakOUT! program I did with the Parkinson Voice Project, I joined their Loud Crowd, which gives you ongoing maintenance and accountability. It forces you to do your exercises and continue practicing, which I need.*❞
>
> — LINDA

WHY WOULD I BE REFERRED TO A SPEECH-LANGUAGE PATHOLOGIST?

The following speech and swallowing changes can occur during the course of Parkinson's and are reasons for a referral to a specialist:

- Soft voice
- Slurred or mumbled speech
- Rapid or run-on speech
- Stuttering
- Decreased facial expression (facial masking)

Let this be a guide as you begin exploring how OT can help you, and be sure to consult with your wellness team before trying these tips. To find an occupational therapist to address your needs throughout all the stages of Parkinson's, contact your primary care physician or neurologist for a referral.

245

THE BENEFITS OF SPEECH-LANGUAGE THERAPY IN PARKINSON'S

By Michelle Underhill, MA, CCC-SLP

Most people living with Parkinson's experience difficulties with communication and swallowing. These challenges may show up as a quiet voice, unclear speech, trouble finding words, avoidance of certain foods or liquids, frequent coughing or clearing the throat. How many of the following statements relate to you?

- People often ask me to repeat what I said.

- I run out of air quickly.

- I find myself talking less and less.

- It's not my voice that's the problem, it's their hearing!

- I used to have a beautiful voice. Now...not so much.

- I start talking, then get stuck on a word. It's awkward and uncomfortable.

- I cough more when I'm eating than when I'm not eating.

- I can't seem to swallow enough to keep my mouth clear. There's too much saliva!

- I don't eat _____ anymore. It's too difficult to get down.

- Sometimes my mouth is so dry I can't swallow. Nights are rough.

WHEN SHOULD YOU SEE A SPEECH-LANGUAGE PATHOLOGIST (SLP)?

If you answered affirmatively to any of the above statements, establishing a relationship with a SLP will help you discover strategies to improve your function. Additionally, if you have recently been diagnosed, undergoing an evaluation with a SLP can provide you with valuable information, which you may use for comparison in the future. This is a perfect time to learn strategies to maintain your vocal strength, articulation and swallowing safety.

When you meet with the SLP, share your specific concerns, situations that create problems and observations others have shared with you. From there, the SLP will conduct an evaluation targeting your personal difficulties and complete a comprehensive speech-language pathology assessment.

Your evaluation should include an interview, a review of your medical history and assessments of your speech, language, voice, swallowing and cognition (thinking and memory). These assessments may be informal (discussion, observation, self-reports), or they may be formal (standardized tests). Your SLP will consider your results against normative data for your age to assist in determining which outcomes are considered "within normal limits" and which results fall outside of that range. Your evaluation may include the following:

- Listening to your speech and articulation, observing the coordination, strength and motion for your tongue, lips and cheeks and evaluating your breathing.

- Conversation with you, and perhaps someone you bring along to the evaluation, to determine how well you are able to express your thoughts and understand what others say.

- Measurement of your voice for loudness, endurance, quality and respiratory support. You may be asked to breathe into a device that measures your lung capacity. Recordings of your voice may be taken to compare with future status.

- A hands-on evaluation of your swallow as you eat and drink various items. This is called a clinical swallow examination, and is helpful in determining your current status and if additional, more invasive testing is needed. Your SLP will ask you to move your face, mouth and head to check overall function and ability. The SLP will also gently place their hand along your throat while you consume foods and liquids, and may feel other aspects of your neck and face.

- Screening or evaluation of your cognitive abilities. The SLP is checking your attention, information processing, memory, problem solving and decision-making.

WHAT DO SPEECH THERAPY SESSIONS LOOK LIKE?

Your speech therapy treatment should:

1. **Address your specific areas of need:**

    a. "I have to repeat myself most of the time."

    b. "I miss drinking coffee with my friends, but it's embarrassing to cough and sputter."

    c. "My kids can't hear me on the phone."

2. **Reflect your personal goals for improvement:**

    a. "I want to speak so others can hear and understand me."

    b. "I want to swallow pills more easily."

    c. "I want to find the words I need when I am talking."

3. **Change with you as you change:**

    a. Increase the level of challenge to continue improving your voice as it becomes stronger and louder.

    b. Return to enjoying foods and drinks you love using learned tips and tricks.

    c. Educate your family and friends to adjust interactions to promote your success.

There are many therapy strategies to improve communication and swallowing. Your SLP will determine which approaches are most appropriate for you, but until you are able to connect with a SLP, you might consider implementing these techniques:

- **Speech.** Speak LOUDLY. Place a sucker inside your cheek and practice speaking to help you to articulate more clearly. When others have difficulty understanding you, restate your information in a shorter sentence or use different words.

- **Language.** If you didn't understand what was said, ask for repetition or more information. Express your thoughts and ideas to your loved ones and friends – they want to hear what you have to say! When you struggle to find a word, describe it in other ways (what it looks like, where you use it, etc.). Keep talking...the word you want may come to you, or it may occur to your conversation partner.

- **Voice.** Be louder than you think you need to be. If you are comfortable, you are probably too quiet. Breathe! It is easier to be loud and clear when you have air in your lungs to support your voice. When you are loud, the quality of your voice tends to improve.

- **Swallowing.** Whether you have too much saliva in your mouth or not enough, try sucking on lemon candy, small suckers or chewing gum. Yes, this will create more saliva, but it will also help you to swallow more frequently. The more you practice swallowing, the more those muscles receive exercise.

- **Cognition.** Think about how you prefer to learn information. Do you have to hear it? See it? Feel it? If you need to see something to remember it, make a mental picture in your mind when you want to commit something to memory. Write a note or say it out loud. Find mental challenges that take you outside of your comfort zone, but in which you can still achieve success. Look for activities that require new learning, mental effort AND bring you enjoyment.

During the course of your speech therapy, you will need motivation, diligence and a willingness to complete exercises and strategies outside of therapy sessions. Your SLP will help you achieve greater health, and your newly-learned knowledge and strength will benefit you now and into the future.

An annual evaluation is recommended and may or may not be followed by therapy, depending upon your needs at the time. Continue with your personal strategies and exercises each day. You may find that you prefer to stay in regular contact with your SLP for maintenance therapy to stay on top of any changes you are experiencing.

HOW CAN I FIND A SPEECH-LANGUAGE PATHOLOGIST?

It is important to find a SLP who is trained in evaluating and treating people living with Parkinson's. All SLPs have education in general speech-language evaluation and therapy, but when possible, having someone on your team who treats adults and who is familiar with the unique aspects of Parkinson's is to your greatest benefit. SLPs in the US are certified by the American Speech-Language-Hearing Association (ASHA). You can search for a speech-language pathologist by state and city at **ASHAcertified.org**. Look for similar organizations in your home country.

You have more control of your communication and swallowing than you may believe. Seek out a speech-language pathologist to help you find the tools to live well today.

- Drooling or needing to clear the throat frequently

- Swallowing difficulties, such as difficulty swallowing pills, swallowing several times with each bite, coughing while eating or sensing food is stuck in the throat

- Coughing and throat clearing due to aspiration (food or saliva getting into the breathing tube or lungs) while eating and drinking fluids

TREATMENTS AND STRATEGIES FOR IMPROVING SPEECH AND SWALLOWING

- Speech exercises to improve speech volume and intelligibility

- Cognitive strategies to improve speaking and language function

- Counseling about communication, impact of body and facial expression

- Understanding the impact of facial expression and speech changes on communication and relationships

- Instruction on proper neck and body positioning while swallowing

- Recommendations for dietary changes based on swallowing abilities

- Improvements to eating habits leading to safer eating and weight control

- Care partner instruction on the Heimlich maneuver

Find and practice speech exercises to help you overcome a variety of Parkinson's-related challenges: ■ **dpf.org/speech-exercises**.

Sometimes a modified barium swallow is needed to diagnose swallowing problems. This is a radiology procedure that can visualize the passage of food or fluids from your mouth to your stomach. This test can determine whether food or fluids are entering into the lungs, called aspiration.

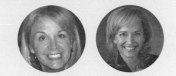

By Lorraine A. Ramig, PhD, CCC-SLP and Cynthia Fox, PhD, CCC-SLP

" *If I have no voice, I have no life.*"

This statement reflects the devastating impact that a speech and voice disorder can have on quality of life in a person with Parkinson's. This person is not alone. Research shows that 89% of people with Parkinson's will experience speech and voice disorders. Reduced loudness, monotone, breathy and hoarse voice quality and imprecise articulation can occur at all stages of the disease. As a result, many people report that they are less likely to participate in conversations and lose confidence in themselves.

There are several reasons why people with Parkinson's have speech and voice disorders. One reason is that the bradykinesia (slow movement) and hypokinesia (small movements) accompanying Parkinson's can reduce movement in the speech production system. This can affect the respiratory system (reduced breath support), larynx/voice box (reduced vocal loudness) and articulation (reduced clarity of speech).

In addition, people with Parkinson's are often not aware that their speech is getting softer and more difficult to understand. When "soft speaking" people with Parkinson's are asked to speak louder, they will often reply, "No, my voice is not too soft! My spouse complains all the time, but he/she needs a hearing aid!" Furthermore, if they are encouraged to bring their voice to normal loudness, they will often complain that they feel as though they are talking too loudly or shouting, even though they are perceived by listeners to be speaking normally.

Most people with Parkinson's can respond to a request to "speak louder!" and their speech will improve quite a lot, but it is difficult for them to increase their loudness on their own without being reminded.

Given these challenges, it is not surprising that historically speech and voice disorders in Parkinson's were difficult to treat. In fact, the conventional wisdom was that speech treatment was not successful in Parkinson's and that improvements in the speech treatment room disappeared on the way to the parking lot.

249

YOU CAN MAKE LASTING IMPROVEMENTS TO SPEECH AND VOICE

Today people with Parkinson's can make lasting changes in their speech and voice that significantly improve their functional communication. More than 20 years of published evidence exists for the short and long-term efficacy of Lee Silverman Voice Treatment (LSVT LOUD), named for a woman with Parkinson's. This research-based treatment protocol was designed to specifically address the motor, sensory and learning challenges faced by people with Parkinson's when working to improve their speech and voice.

Lasting improvements have been documented after treatment in a range of characteristics, including vocal loudness, breath support, voice quality, intonation, speech articulation and speech intelligibility.

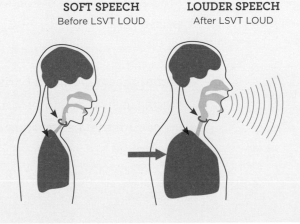

SOFT SPEECH
Before LSVT LOUD

LOUDER SPEECH
After LSVT LOUD

LSVT LOUD has been documented to improve vocal loudness, breath support, voice quality, intonation and speech articulation (Mahler et al., 2015). The goal is always healthy vocal loudness.

Speech treatments for Parkinson's have historically been focused on articulation and speech rate and have been given at a low-intensity dosage (e.g., one or two sessions per week for some period of time). LSVT LOUD takes a very different approach, focusing on the singular target of increasing *vocal loudness* to normal levels and delivering the treatment in an intensive, high effort manner.

Treating vocal loudness has been documented to make changes across the entire speech production system and improve functional communication.

This figure shows the changes from soft speech, before LSVT LOUD (left) to louder speech, after LSVT LOUD (right) observed in people with Parkinson's. Although the "speak loud" concept may appear simple on the surface, a trained speech therapist is necessary to help people with Parkinson's improve loudness in a healthy way.

Because LSVT LOUD is given in an intensive, high effort mode, it is consistent with studies on motor learning and neuroplasticity. After 16 one-hour sessions of treatment over the course of just one month, speech production is significantly improved.

During treatment, patients also learn how to maintain and advance their speech and voice improvements after they complete treatment through follow-up classes and home exercises. The goal is enhanced, functional speech production that continues through the years.

OBTAINING A REFERRAL TO A SPEECH THERAPIST

It is recommended that all people with Parkinson's be referred for a speech evaluation as soon as possible, upon diagnosis. The evaluating therapist can establish baseline speech performance data, determine the need for treatment and help choose the best treatment for specific symptoms.

Speech and voice symptoms may be subtle at first, and people often fail to notice changes or deny any concerns, but we know that by diagnosis, the neuropathology already is anything but "early." A speech therapist can "unmask" subtle and hidden deficits and educate people with Parkinson's on the best time to start therapy. Still, it's never too late for evaluation and treatment. People in later stages can gain benefits as well.

Swallowing problems can also occur in people with Parkinson's and there may be subtle, early changes that a speech therapist can detect. When eating or swallowing difficulties occur, ask the doctor for a referral to a speech therapist for a swallowing examination.

It is important to recognize that while hoarseness is a symptom of Parkinson's, it can also be a symptom of other serious disorders, including gastric reflux disease or laryngeal abnormalities. Only an examination of the vocal folds (laryngeal exam) conducted by an otolaryngologist (ear, nose and throat doctor) can confirm the diagnosis.

FINDING A SPEECH THERAPIST

Speech therapists work at facilities including hospitals, out-patient rehabilitation centers, university clinics and private practice offices. Research has also documented that some speech therapy can be successfully delivered online to your home or office (e.g., telemedicine) and that software can support your independent practice during and after treatment.

There are several referral sources for finding speech therapists that are experienced in using evidence-based speech treatment for Parkinson's, including The American Speech-Language and Hearing Association (ASHA, ⌨ **asha.org**) and LSVT Global (⌨ **lsvtglobal.com**).

Communication is a key element in the quality of your life and can help you maintain confidence as you deal with the challenges of Parkinson's. Speech therapy is increasingly viewed as an intervention that can greatly enhance speech and overall quality of life. You have the power to improve and maintain effective communication so that your family and friends can hear and understand all that you have to say.

CREATIVE THERAPISTS

Music therapists use music to help with movement. Music naturally drives movement, whether it is a simple tapping of the foot, drumming or dancing. Musical rhythms can help with walking, freezing, coordination and exercise. Music taps into our emotions in a way that improves movement (such as the natural flow and coordination that happens with dance), adds enjoyment (can increase the release of dopamine), creativity and rhythm, and keeps exercise fun.

> *" My piano and my bicycle are my psychiatrists."*
>
> — BRENDA

An art therapist uses art and creative expression as a healing tool to express our inner self and emotions. Art and creative activities help keep your mind active and strong, which is important as we age. It is a different way to express yourself, and this can be helpful for people who are not comfortable talking about their feelings or who have difficulty expressing themselves due to thinking or speaking problems. Expressing your emotions, struggles, strengths, weaknesses, desires, grief, joys and pains through art helps you work through issues and gain a deeper understanding.

A recreational therapist can help you stay active in hobbies and play. Hobbies and play are important parts of enjoying life. A recreational therapist can show you different ways to modify or adapt activities so you can stay involved with your favorite activity or find a new activity that fulfills your life.

Some people with Parkinson's may struggle with feelings of apathy and then tend to withdraw from activities and events. It is especially important to maintain or add well-balanced leisure activities to your lifestyle. It is important to choose activities that are fulfilling physically, mentally and socially. Find activities, such as arts and crafts, cooking, drama, sports and games, etc., in each of these areas that make you feel good and are fun.

■ WHAT TO KNOW ABOUT HOSPITAL STAYS AND EMERGENCY ROOM VISITS

Hospital stays for people with Parkinson's — whether planned or unplanned — require special consideration. Discuss your medication needs with your nurses right away. You can request an "Aware in Care" kit, designed for people with Parkinson's to use before, during and after a hospital stay at ⤤ **awareincare.org**.

Bring the **Daily Medication Log** in the **Worksheets and Resources** section to provide a complete list of your medications, dosage and the time of day that you take them. Be sure your hospital care team understands that **all Parkinson's medications must be given on time**. Ask if you or your family can keep medication at your bedside to ensure it's given on time. Parcopa or dissolvable carbidopa/levodopa can be used if you are not able to swallow or able to eat. You can use the **Prepare for Your Hospital Stay** and **Medical Summary for Your Doctor's Appointment** tools located in the **Worksheets and Resources** section to capture this and other information in one place. Download and print a copy of these tools at ⤤ **dpf.org/worksheets**.

Bring the **Current Symptoms Summary** with you to help describe your symptoms to your hospital care team, as they may not be familiar with such problems as dyskinesia, "on/off" fluctuations and freezing of gait. Be sure to let them know how your movement and abilities change during the medication's "on" or "off" state. This also helps the hospital care team understand why it is so important for you to get your medications on time.

Your motor symptoms can worsen when you are coping with a medical illness in addition to your Parkinson's, so you might not be able to move as well and might find some symptoms, such as tremor, dyskinesia and freezing, worsen during your hospital stay. In a similar fashion, confusion and hallucinations can occur or worsen in the setting of medical stress, or as a result of new medications, such as narcotics for pain, or sedatives for sleep, anxiety or agitation.

BE ACTIVE: *Ask your doctor if you can receive physical therapy during your stay, if appropriate, and afterwards to avoid unnecessary physical decline and complications.*

Ask for a physical therapy, occupational therapy, swallowing evaluation or speech therapy consult as illness and prolonged bed rest can weaken your body and affect daily activities. Also consider asking to see a social worker, especially if you have questions about community resources, special needs after discharge or changes in living arrangements. Chaplain services are available in most hospitals and are there to support you, no matter what your spiritual needs or beliefs.

Ask your doctor for rehabilitation after discharge, as you may be weaker due to your illness. If you have had a serious illness or surgery, ask your neurologist and doctor about inpatient (hospital-based) rehabilitation or home health services that may include social work, nursing, dietary or rehabilitation services.

QUESTIONS TO ASK BEFORE DISCHARGE

- Have your neurologist and primary care physician been notified of your condition while in the hospital?
- When should you see your primary care physician?
- Should you receive additional rehabilitation, such as physical therapy?
- What important tests, procedures or new diagnosis have you received?
- What medications have been changed and why?
- How do you get a copy of the hospital records sent to your doctor?

MEDICATIONS TO AVOID

Some medications can worsen motor symptoms of Parkinson's, including slowness, stiffness, tremor and dyskinesia. These drugs, listed below, are used to treat psychiatric problems such as hallucinations, confusion or gastrointestinal problems, such as nausea. The stress of your illness, hospital stay or new medications can increase your risk of hallucinations or delirium while hospitalized. New onset delusions, paranoia and agitation signal to the medical team that a longer hospital stay or skilled nursing is required before going home. Common anti-hallucination medications to be avoided are listed by generic or chemical name followed by the trade name.

ANTI-HALLUCINATION MEDICATIONS TO AVOID

The anti-hallucination medications quetiapine (Seroquel), clozapine (Clozaril) and pimavanserin (Nuplazid) can be used with Parkinson's. Of these, Nuplazid is the only anti-hallucination medication approved for Parkinson's.

The following should be avoided:

- Aripiprazole (Abilify)
- Chlorpromazine (Thorazine)
- Flufenazine (Prolixin)
- Haloperidol (Haldol)
- Molindone (Moban)
- Perphenazine (Trilafon)
- Perphenazine and amitriptyline (Triavil)
- Risperidone (Risperdol)

253

- Thioridazine (Mellaril)
- Thiothixene (Navane)

ANTI-NAUSEA MEDICATIONS TO AVOID

Serotonin (5-HT3) antagonists work to block the effects of serotonin in order to reduce nausea and vomiting and do not worsen symptoms of Parkinson's. Ondansetron (Zofran), dolaseton (Anzemet) and granisetron (Granisol) are acceptable alternatives to the list below. Older and cheaper anti-nausea medications block dopamine, therefore, worsening Parkinson's symptoms.

The following should be avoided:

- Metoclopramide (Reglan)
- Phenothiazine (Compazine)
- Promethazine (Phenergan)

MEDICATIONS TO AVOID IF YOU TAKE RASAGILINE (AZILECT) OR SELEGILINE (ELDEPRYL)

- Pain medications meperidine (Demerol), tramadol (Ultram) and methadone
- Antispasmodic medication (Flexeril)
- Dextromethorphan (cold medication) and ciprofloxacin (antibiotic)

Note: This is not a complete list of medications to avoid. If you have questions about other medications, ask your pharmacist or doctor.

254

HOSPITAL TIPS FOR INDIVIDUALS WITH DUOPA OR DEEP BRAIN STIMULATION

Be sure your doctors and nurses are informed about your enteral suspension (Duopa/Duodopa) or DBS. In most cases for DBS, MRI and diathermy cannot be performed without risk of serious injury to you. Use the **DBS Medical History** form in the **Worksheets and Resources** section to provide your hospital care team with the appropriate information about your DBS in the event that a surgery or procedure must be performed.

MEDICAL ALERT BRACELET

Wear a medical alert bracelet if you have serious medication, latex or tape allergies or if you have a surgical implant. If you have a stoma for enteral suspension (Duopa/Duodopa) or DBS, include the manufacturer's phone number on the medical alert bracelet in case of emergency.

■ PARKINSON'S AND THE FAMILY

When you are diagnosed with Parkinson's, your thoughts may naturally focus on your own health and prognosis. It's *you* who is living with this news, *you* who will need to take medications, *you* who will need to make adjustments and *you* whose future plans are most impacted.

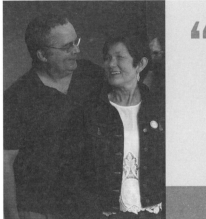

> 66 *This past year, I went through breast cancer and Brian became my care partner. Switching roles gave us a new level of respect and understanding and we try to practice that for each other throughout each day. We get new curveballs thrown at us all the time, but we have a strong foundation of respect."*
>
> — LILY

Yet, Parkinson's inevitably affects more than just the one who has been diagnosed. The changes Parkinson's brings with it alter the lives of spouses, partners, children, grandchildren and friends, too. Care partners, especially, can think that they need to be a rock for the person living with Parkinson's, neglecting their own needs in the process. Parents living with Parkinson's struggle with how to talk about diagnosis and symptoms when there are young children living at home. Adult children of people living with Parkinson's who no longer reside at home wrestle with how to stay involved and connected when they are not living the daily reality of Parkinson's.

In the following pages, a variety of experts and veteran Parkinson's families share their experiences and advice for adapting to changes, strengthening relationships and addressing topics about living well with Parkinson's related to care partners, children and families.

> 66 *Some people said all the wrong things. In the end, we made many new friends who did not know Davis before Parkinson's. That has helped him and me tremendously."*
>
> — CONNIE CARPENTER PHINNEY

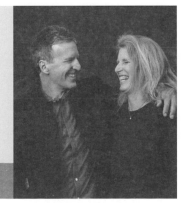

255

HOW PARKINSON'S AFFECTS THE FAMILY

By Nancy Bivins, LMSW

A Parkinson's diagnosis leaves each family member with his or her own set of questions: Will my husband be able to continue working at his job's required level of speed and accuracy? How will this affect our relationship as a couple? Will we have to give up our plans to travel? When will we tell our friends? Is Dad going to be able to go on our annual fishing trip? Can Grandma get down on the floor and play with us?

One of the most immediate changes for loved ones is that people in the healthcare field almost immediately begin referring to you as the caregiver or care partner. You probably think of yourself as the spouse, the partner, the daughter, the son, the grandchild, the sibling, the friend, but suddenly, your identity now also includes care partner.

The term, "care partner," refers to the person that most closely accompanies his/her loved one with Parkinson's. Though you don't have Parkinson's yourself, you certainly are living with it. Exactly how the future with your special person will unfold is unknown, because everyone's journey is different. What is universally important is taking steps to acknowledge the impact your loved one's condition has on you and taking steps to protect and preserve your relationship as well as your health.

KEEP THE LINES OF COMMUNICATION OPEN

One of the most critical components to a good Parkinson's journey is maintaining ongoing, open dialogue. Communicate regularly with each other about both of your health, your concerns and your perspectives. The renowned social scientist, Virginia Satir, developed a template to facilitate such conversations for couples called *The Daily Temperature Reading*. She offers five communication tools:

1. Share **appreciation** for the other person. The more specific this communication, the better. Instead of saying, "You're a good help," say, "Thank you so much helping me weed the garden."

2. Share **new information**. This could be a change in plans, gossip, a fear, something of interest — anything that helps your loved one keep up with what is going on in your life.

3. Share a **puzzle**. Instead of assuming you know the answer, ask: "Why did you choose not to go to lunch with Bob?"

4. **Pair a complaint with a suggestion.** For instance, "Yesterday you said…, but I would appreciate it if you would instead say…" Listen to the words, but also listen to the emotions behind the words. If the two are not congruent, address the emotion you perceive: "You seem sad."

5. Share **wishes, hopes and dreams**. Invite each other into your wishes, hopes and dreams for this day, this year and your long-term future.

Talk to each other, share with each other and keep doing it. Remember that it is healthy for both of you to maintain a balance between giving and receiving.

LEARN AS MUCH AS YOU CAN

Parkinson's is a complicated and multifaceted condition, and although there are many symptoms, no one person will experience all of them. As you learn more, remember that each person's experience with Parkinson's is unique. Knowledge will help both you as the care partner and your loved one with Parkinson's be alert to Parkinson's symptoms that you might otherwise overlook. You'll be better able to communicate important observations to your doctor, and he or she will have a more comprehensive picture before recommending treatment. Knowledge will also give you a better understanding of the impact Parkinson's is having on your loved one. Hear from Scott about balancing being informed and staying grounded: 🎥 dpf.org/scott.

STAY SOCIALLY ACTIVE

People with many friendships are less likely to experience sadness, loneliness, low self-esteem and problems with eating and sleeping. Of course, friends and family do move away, pursue other interests and have their own health issues. With a little effort, though, we can all do better to maintain these connections. Because social isolation is a gradual process, it's possible to be in the midst of it and not even be aware of it. Isolation can affect you, your loved one with Parkinson's and the two of you together. Be proactive: invite people in, accept invitations for get-togethers or impromptu outings. Sign up for a class, or visit your local senior center. This advice applies to both of you.

Begin setting aside time on your calendar for yourself, and don't delay, whether you're the person living with Parkinson's or you're caring for someone who is. The key is to schedule this "me time" with the same degree of commitment you would if it were a medical appointment. Reserve this scheduled time to engage in activities that bring you joy. If something does not come immediately to mind, try something new. Discovering what energizes and refreshes you is critical for your well-being over time.

> ❝ *It can be hard to do, but you have to find friends or get a hobby or take a painting class – do something outside of everything that places demands on you.*"
>
> — SHERYL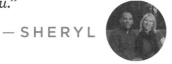

A support group is a great resource for care partners, whether spouses, children or friends of people living with Parkinson's. It's easier to share your concerns with a group that is facing similar issues. Keep in mind that not all support groups are created equal, so visit a support group at least three times before deciding to stay or to move on. If after your third visit you're not convinced that it's the right group for you, try a different group, but please don't give up! Great, lasting friendships are often forged in support groups. Don't miss out on the joy of making new friends.

REST OFTEN, GET HELP WHEN NEEDED

Since responsibilities are shared in a partnership, it is reasonable to expect that when the partner living with Parkinson's is no longer able to do something, the care partner will automatically assume the task. However, it is important to realize that some of these tasks might not be something that the care partner should take on. Just because you *could* do something, doesn't always mean that you *should* or even that doing so is the best option. Sometimes, better options include hiring someone, asking family or friends to help, adjusting your standard (i.e., mowing the lawn every two weeks instead of every week) or eliminating the job altogether (i.e., someone else can host the annual summer party). Listen as Dave explains how he's learning to take time to care for himself: ◼ **dpf.org/dave**.

Drawing realistic boundaries and sharing responsibilities are necessary if you are to have opportunities for adequate rest. Rest is not some kind of reward, only to be enjoyed when everything else is done! Rest is vital to your health as a person with Parkinson's and as a care partner. Research has revealed that sleep is as important to a person's well-being as diet and exercise, and yet it is often the first to suffer. When your schedule is demanding, don't sacrifice sleep and relaxation. If you are awake during the night, sleep in or nap during the day to recoup the lost rest. If your loved one with Parkinson's has significant nighttime needs, some care partners find success in hiring help in the home overnight. With this arrangement, the person living with Parkinson's is safe; his or her needs are met by the in-home care professional. This is a win-win: you wake rested, and your partner receives attentive care throughout the night.

Develop a relationship with a social worker knowledgeable about Parkinson's. Resource lists are helpful, but they cannot take the place of someone with whom you can have a conversation to assist you and your loved one in narrowing the field of options so you can develop a course of action best for you. There is no single "Parkinson's Plan." Your course and decisions will be unique. There will be changes along the way, and the social worker is the expert that can help you gather appropriate information to help you to make the best decision possible.

MAKE THE MOST OF TODAY AND EVERY DAY

Enjoy life, and live it to the fullest! Although Parkinson's will impact many different aspects of your life now, it is important to not let it become the central focus for either of you. I frequently hear people in the exercise classes at the Muhammad Ali Parkinson Center shouting with gusto, "I may have Parkinson's, but Parkinson's doesn't have me!" While this may sound simplistic, it's a critical idea for both people with Parkinson's and their care partners to take to heart and put into action.

PARKINSON'S AND CARE PARTNERS

CARE PARTNER HEALTH: A MEDICAL PERSPECTIVE

Not all experiences as a care partner are negative. In fact, being a care partner can be very rewarding.

STRESS AND STRAIN OF CARING FOR SOMEONE LIVING WITH CHRONIC ILLNESS

Caring for someone with a chronic, progressive condition can consume a lot of extra time and energy and impact your resilience to stress and illness. Several factors can contribute substantially to the stress of being a care partner. Understanding these factors can help you deal with care partner stress.

Stressors associated with chronic conditions typically consist of emotional, physical and financial factors that are directly related to the duties and responsibilities of the care partner. Poorly managed stress leads to strain. If not corrected, it can lead to burnout. Burnout occurs when the care partner is at the point of exhaustion. Burnout is a preventable consequence of unsupported caregiving. Care partners that are experiencing burnout are at risk for serious health problems, they can become overwhelmed and eventually may become ineffective in their care partner role.

Unfortunately, care partner strain is not often a concern during medical appointments, since time with the doctor is generally focused on the medical needs of the person with Parkinson's. Social workers and counselors have the expertise and knowledge about community resources to address care partner stress issues, but they may not be available in many medical clinics.

> " *I don't think my kids necessarily understand the weight that is on me. I don't want to dump on them, and there's no way to really tell them. It is hard that family doesn't necessarily understand the weight that I carry.*"
>
> — SHERYL

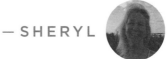

When social workers and counselors are not available to help, care partners can be proactive about their own wellness, using the same approach that this manual advocates for people living with Parkinson's. Learn more about care partner strain and take steps to limit or avoid factors that lead to burnout. Encouraging your partner to learn more about Parkinson's is one of these steps. Research has shown that when people with Parkinson's have a sense of control over their disease, care partner strain is reduced and well-being is improved.[1] This manual promotes a "take-charge" attitude and provides skills and education that enable the person

259

---

1   Wallhagen, M.I. & Brod, M. Perceived Control and Well-being in Parkinson 's disease. (1997). *Western Journal of Nursing Research*, 19(1), 11-31.

with Parkinson's to maintain control over the disease. This effort to live well will minimize the impact of Parkinson's on the health of the care partner.

> " *Finding the line between being a care partner and being a nag is something I have to think about. I try not to be motherly or add pressure, but be supportive. I help when I know he needs the help, but give him the dignity of doing things independently.*"
>
> — NANCY

COPING STRATEGIES ARE NOT CREATED EQUAL

Previous sections of this manual have discussed ways in which the diagnosis can affect the person with Parkinson's. *Equally important is the effect of the diagnosis on the care partner.* The diagnosis of Parkinson's elicits emotional reactions from the care partner, along with thoughts that can range from optimistic to pessimistic or combine elements of both. These emotional reactions can compound the initial strain that comes with the diagnosis. Most people deal with these reactions by using either emotion-based or problem-based coping strategies. Some people employ a combination of coping styles, but one strategy tends to prevail when stress gets high. People who use emotion-based coping strategies focus on finding a way to reduce their stress. They may choose avoidance, meditation, relaxation, exercise, religion or social support. People who use problem-based coping strategies are more likely to address the actual source of the stress. For example, they may seek as much information about Parkinson's as possible, soliciting opinions from multiple providers, searching for alternative or complementary therapies or focusing on disease symptoms and management.

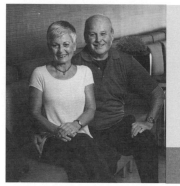

> " *The biggest thing I've learned is that you have to separate the woman you married who is living with Parkinson's from the issues you may have had with your spouse all along.*"
>
> — SCOTT

In situations involving chronic disease, problem-based coping leads to lower levels of distress. Reliance on emotion-based coping styles is associated with higher levels of distress,[2, 3] which is especially true when avoidance is the emotional coping style. Counseling can help you analyze your coping style early on, before helping to manage the symptoms of Parkinson's requires

---

2   Pakenham, K. I. Adjustment to multiple sclerosis: Application of a stress and coping model. (1999). *Health Psychology*, 18: 383-392.

3   Sanders-Dewey, Mullins & Chaney. Coping style, perceived uncertainty in illness and distress in individuals with Parkinson's disease and their caregivers. (2001). *Rehabilitation Psychology*, 46(4): 363-381.

more of your energy and time. Talking to a counselor can also better prepare you to cope when your loved one's symptoms worsen.

PARKINSON'S IN MY HOUSE

By Connie Carpenter Phinney, MS

Parkinson's entered our lives when our kids were small and Davis' career was thriving. But truly, it had been lurking and provoking us for years. Fatigue was the primary early symptom that affected our marriage and family, but Davis unwittingly was dealing with various symptoms. I remember nagging him to pick his feet up when he walked because he stumbled a lot. His voice softened, and TV producers asked him to better modulate his voice, but he couldn't seem to do it. The tremor emerged in the spring of 2000, and that is what finally got him to the doctor – or in his case, to many doctors.

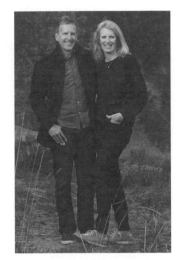

Diagnosis is traumatic. And for a while it felt like the bottom had fallen out of his world. Max Testa, his cycling team doctor from Italy, remarked that it would take him two years to adjust and adapt to this new challenge. He was right. But the neurologist who told him that he'd feel "as good as ever" was wrong. So, you get mixed messages from even the doctors, and in the end, how you respond to the diagnosis really depends on where you are in your life.

Once we settled into the new life – post-Parkinson's diagnosis – we did realize how lucky we were in one sense. Davis stopped traveling. He had been on the road working somewhere between 75 and 100 days of the year. This was far less compared to his previous life as a cyclist, when he was away more than 150 days of the year. But it was a lot for the kids and for me. So Parkinson's gave us one treasure: We got Davis back. He is a gifted father. It would have been a shame for him to miss so many of the fun years with the kids.

My dad told me an interesting thing one night when we were talking about the course of his life. He said that when my mom was diagnosed with multiple sclerosis, he lost his ambition. He wondered aloud if that was a bad thing. I asked him, "In what regard?" And he said that he was content with his family business and never had the desire to risk growing it. He thought maybe he could have made more of his life. I told him that he was the best dad imaginable, and that I was so grateful for that. While I knew he worked hard, he put his family first, and caring for us kids and my mom was his best work.

For me, when pressed, I can tell you that watching my strong man (Davis) suffer is tough; the diminishment of so many of his strengths is heartbreaking. It is our reality, and we accept it. There's a fine line between giving in and giving up. I think we strive to stay on the high wire every day. Some days, he has to give up some of what he's planned to do, but it's not

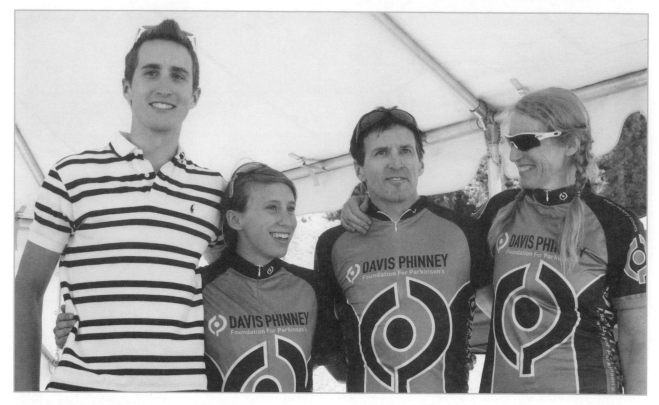

The Phinney family in 2009

like throwing in the towel. It's the rest required of a soldier who is preparing for another day. Together we soldier on. Some days feel more daunting than others, but we know good days will come.

On a daily basis, the hard part has been to keep Davis tasked. I could do it all, and people who know me can attest to this. If I did do it all, I'd probably start to feel angry and overburdened. I realized that Davis needed to be engaged in his daily life, and if he was going to stay home, he had better contribute. I give him duties and departments – cars, bikes, dishes, for example. Initially the Bike Camp business was thriving, and I still needed him to help with that. Physically, when he couldn't manage riding his bike, he could photograph our clients and provide slide shows or videos of the week long tours. I learned to parcel out tasks that he could do. Granted, the fog that he often lives in mentally and the weight of Parkinson's on him physically make every day challenging, and often we need to be spontaneous in terms of what he can do, day by day. I find that if we try to share the burden – if we share the weight of the load – then each of us feels better.

Perhaps harder still for Davis was life outside of the home. He was uncomfortable, self-conscious and tended to isolate himself. Going to the store was a chore. Luckily, our daughter Kelsey did not mind accompanying him, and her grown-up demeanor at a young age aided us greatly. I have always tried to bring the outside in, where we can control it best and where he is most comfortable. We even remodeled our house to make it more Davis-friendly: calming walls and spaces and comfortable chairs were keys to allowing him to live better. Enlisting the kids is really important, and both of ours have helped us a lot.

How you include your children in the dialogue of the disease is up to you. We've always been honest with our children, without overburdening them. That is a line you will have to tread. I think the difficult years for our kids were the med-cycle years, which were very uncomfortable for Davis and tended to make him very moody. In that case, it was especially important to talk about why Dad felt so uncomfortable and how that affected all of us. It's most important for the kids not to have to carry too much of the burden; not easily done if your kids are sensitive, but worth the dialogue to make it clear, all the same.

We had the opportunity to live in Italy for three years and to make the most of our Bike Camp business there. It was a good excuse to start fresh and to give the kids a chance to learn a foreign language and live outside of their culture. It bought us a lot of time to get adjusted to the disease, as well (we moved there two years post-diagnosis). We all thrived – primarily because we depended on each other so much. The family dynamic was strongest when we were united so closely, and every day was an adventure. Not everyone has this opportunity, but everyone does have the opportunity to rewrite the way they live. Parkinson's can give you a second chance in how you live your life. Surprisingly, Davis' Parkinson's opened doors that would have otherwise stayed closed because of the busy life he led prior to Parkinson's.

We try not to be defined by Parkinson's. Many things conspire to give me a rich life. Davis' sense of humor and world-view, our active kids, a few close friends and my close family all give me much more than a safety net. They are the fabric of my life. I'm not always happy about the omnipresent weight of Parkinson's, but then, neither is Davis.

We share many things – love of sports, physical activity, arts, books – and we constantly admire the world around us. Our children give us great joy, and we pay attention to them together. We share the burden of Parkinson's well, talk about it a lot, assess our family and business goals together and accept with grace both the good and the bad days.

We wake up in the morning expecting a good day. That's where it starts – every day.

CAREGIVER STRAIN: A MEDICAL SYNDROME

Strain and stress may not sound like medical conditions, but care partners need to be aware of caregiver strain, which is a very real medical syndrome requiring attention. Research identifies differences in how some people react to or experience caregiver strain. These differences are described in the sidebar on the following pages.

Being a care partner will bring many additional, unanticipated demands. Many people aren't equipped to manage the emotional, physical and financial demands of the care partner role. Caregiver strain occurs at all stages of Parkinson's and increases as the disease progresses over time.[4] Being aware of the reality and impact of caregiver strain is a first step in the journey of planning for how you will handle the weight of being a care partner, allowing you

---

4   Lyons, Karen S., et al. Pessimism and Optimism as Early Warning Signs for Compromised Health for Caregivers of Patients with Parkinson's Disease. (November/December 2004). *Nursing Research*, 53(6).

Stratifying Characteristics that Can Increase Caregiver Strain

Gender. Gender differences impact the strain of caregiving. Research finds that women are generally the sole caregivers and often feel guilty of not giving enough or of somehow being responsible for the Parkinson's disease.[8] This is especially true given the increased prevalence of Parkinson's in men compared to women. Women generally report twice the amount of caregiver strain that men report, perhaps because of an increased sensitivity to the declining health of the person with Parkinson's and to greater struggles with the physical demands of caregiving.

Age. Age also affects care partner strain and health. Younger care partners are typically less financially stable and are managing a full load of working and caring for children. This can drain their time and energy resources.[9] The younger the care partner, the greater the negative impact of caregiving and the consequent risk of strain.

Disease Stage. Factors unique to each stage of Parkinson's directly impact the strain on the care partner. In early disease progression, worrying is a predominant feature of caregiver strain and can be significant. In the middle stages

264

to continue to emphasize the positive aspects of your relationship.

> " *I always say, 'It's your decision, not mine, but here's what I think.' My role is to give input. Once she makes the decision, I try to make sure we see it through and get the outcome she's looking for."*
>
> — MIKE

Hear more from Mike about how he helps Linda make decisions: 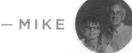 **dpf.org/mike**.

HEALTH RISKS

Care partners can experience more fatigue, depression, sadness and less satisfaction with life than people who don't have the same responsibilities.[5] Increased strain and decreased attention to self-care can negatively impact the physical and emotional health of the care partner.[6] Mood has been shown to be the most important factor influencing a care partner's perceived degree of strain and the decline in health related to that strain. The more severe the Parkinson's symptoms, the greater the negative impact on care partner mood.[7]

> " *As the non-motor symptoms progressed, the anxiety and stress of having to be the emotional support increased proportionately."*
>
> — SHERYL

8 Hooker, Karen, Manoogian-O'Dell, Margaret, et al. Does type of disease matter? Gender differences among Alzheimer's and Parkinson's disease spouse caregivers. (2000). *The Gerontologist*, Vol. 40(5): 568-573.

9 Carter, Julie H., et al. Does Age Make a Difference in Caregiver Strain? Comparison of Young versus Older Caregivers in Early-Stage Parkinson's Disease. (2010). *Movement Disorders*, 25(6): 724-730.

5 Aarsland, D., Larsen J.P., Karlsen K., Lim N.G., Tandberg E. Mental symptoms in Parkinson's disease are important contributors to caregiver distress. (1999). *International Journal of Geriatric Psychiatry*, 14:866–874.

6 Son, Juheui, et al. The caregiver stress process and health outcomes. (2007). *Journal of Aging and Health*, 19(6).

7 Martinez-Martín, P., Forjaz, M.J., Frades-Payo, B., et al. Caregiver burden in Parkinson's disease. (2007) *Movement Disorders*, 22(7): 924-931.

Overall, care partners are more likely than the general population to experience any of the following health complications associated with caregiver strain:

- Symptoms of depression or anxiety
- Chronic medical problems, such as heart disease, obesity, cancer, diabetes or arthritis
- Higher levels of strain hormones and/or a weaker immune response
- May be at higher risk for memory problems

RISKS TO THE RELATIONSHIP WITH YOUR LOVED ONE WITH PARKINSON'S

As Parkinson's changes, so too can your role as care partner. As time passes, you'll observe changes and become an expert in the disease and how it affects the person with Parkinson's. Your growing expertise and experience can help you understand, and perhaps even improve, how you deal with Parkinson's on a day-to-day basis. This acquired knowledge can also unintentionally increase the demands on you. You may take over control of the treatment and organization of care, find yourself in the role of advocate and become an equal or primary source of history for the doctors and wellness team. The information you can provide is valuable and can lead directly to important changes in treatment. Yet even if it's tempting to take over, be sure to balance your role in therapy with your loved one's need to remain in control of his or her own treatment and the need to attend to your own health and well-being.

> **"** *There's a fine line between caring for someone and stripping them of their independence. I have to make sure I give my husband enough space to make his own decisions."*
>
> — LILY

of Parkinson's, communication problems lead to frustrations and tensions, and the increased care requirements elevate the strain felt by the care partner. The later stages of Parkinson's lead to more financial concerns, feelings of being manipulated and incongruent expectations. It's important to remember that the strain is cumulative over the years.[10]

Care Partner Outlook. Finally, care partner outlook may affect the degree of caregiver strain and its negative impact on care partner health. One study found that a pessimistic outlook correlated with depression and poor physical health and led to a faster decline in care partner health.[11]

265

10 Carter, J. et al. Living with a person who has Parkinson's disease: The spouse's perspective by stage of disease. (1998). *Movement Disorders*, 13(1): 20-28.
11 Son, Juheui, et al. The caregiver stress process and health outcomes. (2007). *Journal of Aging and Health*, 19(6).

Certain symptoms associated with Parkinson's can increase the pressure on you to take greater control of care and treatment. These include increasing physical or mobility difficulties, change in cognition or speech, depression and apathy. Each of these symptoms is covered in this manual. If you observe any of these problems, be sure to talk about them with your Parkinson's doctor, since medication, counseling or rehabilitation can help.

As Parkinson's symptoms and care needs increase, so do the number of hours you spend providing care. This situation can lead to a buildup of strain or even to medical problems for you as the care partner. Some of the most difficult symptoms to manage at home are characteristic of advanced Parkinson's, including urinary incontinence, anxiety, confusion, hallucinations, paranoia, apathy and falls. Together, they create a complex combination of care needs that can increase beyond the skills of the care partner. If you don't have the time and energy to attend to your own well-being, managing these difficult symptoms can lead to depression and poor health. Hear how Mike cares for himself as a care partner: ■◀ **dpf.org/mike**.

Taking on a larger role and transitioning from care partner to caregiver can especially affect couples. It's challenging to juggle the demands of hands-on care while maintaining an intimate relationship.

- Be sure to set some time aside, even if it's just a few minutes, to connect as a couple. (If you are the care partner for a parent with Parkinson's, take time to nurture your parent-child relationship outside the context of Parkinson's.)

- Seek counseling before the strain on the relationship becomes too great.

- Eat a healthy diet, get enough sleep, exercise and make your own medical issues a top priority.

TOOLS TO PREVENT CAREGIVER BURNOUT

Research has identified factors that lead to burnout. A decline in social support, psychological well-being, marital satisfaction and the independence level of the person with Parkinson's will aggravate caregiver strain.[12]

Untreated caregiver strain can lead to a medical condition called caregiver burnout. Warning signs of caregiver burnout include feeling overwhelmed, feeling angry or irritable, sleeping poorly, fatigue, worsening medical problems and self-medicating with alcohol or prescription medications.

---

12   Edwards, NE and Scheetz, PS. Predictors of burden for caregivers of patients with Parkinson 's disease. (August 2002). *Journal of Neuroscience Nursing*, 34(4): 184-190.

Strategies to ease the strain of caregiving and prevent caregiver burnout include:

- Establishing a social network of support

- Feeling prepared as a care partner

- Feeling a sense of taking action to improve Parkinson's

- Maintaining a quality relationship with the person with Parkinson's

It's important to devise a plan to lessen the impact of stress and strain and to prevent caregiver burnout. As a first step, learn to understand the situations and symptoms that place you at risk and to recognize the impact of strain. The American Medical Association (⌕ ama-assn.org) provides an online overview of caregiver health as well as a caregiver self-assessment tool and recommendations. The self-assessment is intended to facilitate communication and problem solving during a medical appointment. Using this simple tool is another good first step toward opening a discussion about caregiver strain with your family and medical provider.

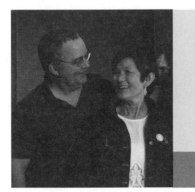

> " *It didn't work for me to be the taskmaster, so now I model the behaviors I want to see. For instance, if I want Brian to exercise or eat healthy, the best thing for me to do is to model those behaviors first. It helps both of us.*"
>
> — LILY

COPING STRATEGIES FOR PARKINSON'S CARE PARTNERS

By Jessica Shurer, LCSW

If you are reading this, you are probably a Parkinson's care partner. This means that you can recognize that, similar to people with Parkinson's, care partners face changing roles, relationships and lifestyles throughout the progression of Parkinson's. You may have noticed difficult and evolving emotions during these changes and transitions: guilt that you're "not doing a better job," regret about things that happened in the past, sadness related to your loved one's diagnosis, anger at the universe, family members or even your loved one with Parkinson's. These emotions are a normal and understandable part of the experience. Give yourself the space and energy to cope with them.

"But I'm Fine."

Perhaps you're thinking, "I'm fine, I don't need coping strategies." No matter how well you're doing, it can still be beneficial to find time for self-care and self-reflection. You might not want anyone to worry about you, or you may feel selfish for bringing attention to your own needs because you're not the one living with Parkinson's. There also can be stigma around on mental wellness and a tendency to believe that going it alone equates to strength. Care partners getting stuck in this perception is very common, often feeling, "No one can do it like I can," or "If I am not here, something will go wrong." This stalwart attitude and refusal to give necessary care and space to yourself can lead to feeling run down and frazzled, which isn't beneficial for anyone.

COPING STRATEGIES TO FOSTER BALANCE AND WELLNESS

There are a number of coping strategies that many Parkinson's care partners have found to be effective. These can provide some guidance as you seek ways to proactively balance your own well-being and needs with those of your partner living with Parkinson's.

- **Check in with yourself.** We tend to ask others how they're doing, but forget about ourselves. Doing regular self-check-ins fosters self-awareness. Ask yourself, "How am I doing with this? What has been my attitude towards Parkinson's? Am I missing out on things that are important to me and that I enjoy? What would be helpful for me at this point in time?" When you attend to your own feelings and needs as a *person*, you are better able to do the things you want to do as a *care partner*.

- **Look for signs of burnout.** Any role can feel overwhelming and leave you feeling down at times, but if this becomes the norm, it can lead to burnout. Try to notice if you've been more irritable or angry, socially withdrawn, have had difficulty concentrating, experienced anxiety or depression, missed your own medications or medical appointments or have had trouble sleeping at night. These are all red flags that the current care situation may not be sustainable. If you notice that your own health — physical, emotional or social — is compromised in any way, now is the time to make positive changes or reach out for additional help.

- **Be your own advocate.** You are the expert when it comes to your unique care partner experience. As you advocate for your loved one with Parkinson's, remember to stand up for yourself, as well. Assert your rights, share your knowledge, determine your goals, recognize your limitations and negotiate and communicate your needs. You may find that self-advocacy is quite empowering!

- **Embrace "me time."** People with Parkinson's and care partners often find themselves spending more and more time together. For some, this can increase intimacy and connection; for others, it can put stress on the relationship or erode the care partner's sense of self. Try to intentionally carve out periods of time in which you are the priority, even if they are brief. Some examples could be relaxing with a book for 30 minutes twice per week, going to the movies on a Friday night, even going on a cruise for a week – do whatever you need to do to recharge your batteries and return with more energy and a clearer head.

268

- **Ask for help.** What aspects of your support system could you continue to build? What if you need additional assistance down the road? You might worry about being a burden if you ask for help or accept help that is offered, but remind yourself you and your loved one with Parkinson's do not have to go it alone. Think of ways that others can help, whether it is taking your dog for a walk on a day when you have too many appointments or hanging out with your Parkinson's partner while you run an errand or take a period of respite. If you have not done so already, it might be a good time to try a Parkinson's support group. Care partners are often surprised by the relief they feel meeting other people with whom they can relate. Learn about other available resources, such as professional in-home care and mental health counseling, that may provide additional support now or down the road.

- **Have a laugh.** Life doesn't stop being funny with a Parkinson's diagnosis. Too many of us take ourselves too seriously! Enjoy the humor in the moments life presents, and laugh when something silly occurs. It's okay to laugh at the strange situations Parkinson's can sometimes cause, too. In fact, laughing can be cathartic, especially in those awkward moments.

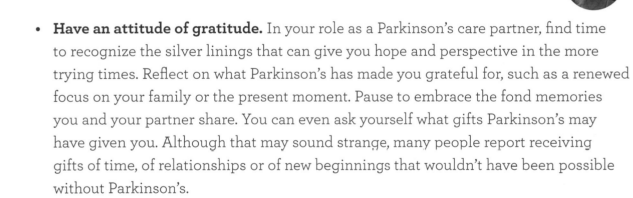

" *We tell a lot of Parkinson's jokes and try to laugh as much as we can. Nothing is really off limits.*"

— SHERYL

- **Have an attitude of gratitude.** In your role as a Parkinson's care partner, find time to recognize the silver linings that can give you hope and perspective in the more trying times. Reflect on what Parkinson's has made you grateful for, such as a renewed focus on your family or the present moment. Pause to embrace the fond memories you and your partner share. You can even ask yourself what gifts Parkinson's may have given you. Although that may sound strange, many people report receiving gifts of time, of relationships or of new beginnings that wouldn't have been possible without Parkinson's.

- **Practice communication, find connections.** Adapting to life with Parkinson's is a partnership between you and your loved one, so it's important to remain on the same page. Good communication fosters closeness and connection. Create times to connect and enjoy one another when the focus is not on Parkinson's. Practice open, honest communication about each of your care needs, big decisions and your future together.

- **Recognize your strengths.** Whether your loved one has been diagnosed with Parkinson's for one month or 25 years, recognize the fact that you survived, even thrived. What's given you strength through this period? In what ways have you surprised yourself? What skills have you gained? Take strength from them, and celebrate them!

- **Find meaning.** Every experience is a learning opportunity. You may not be conscious of it, but adapting to life with a complex and chronic condition can lead to personal growth. Think about your Parkinson's story and what this journey has meant to you. Many care partners can find a sense of purpose in supporting their loved one with Parkinson's. When you are faced with new challenges and transitions, try to see the big picture, and focus on what matters most to you.

- **Stay flexible.** A Parkinson's care partner once sent me this quote: "Blessed are the flexible, for they shall not be bent out of shape." Sometimes, when everything else is unpredictable, the only thing that is in your control is the choice to "go with the flow." Care partners who practice resiliency and can adapt to changes as they come have an easier time coping with Parkinson's and a more positive overall mindset.

- **Be kind to yourself.** It can't be said too often: you are doing the best you can, and that is more than good enough!

DEFINING YOUR ROLE AND SETTING EXPECTATIONS

Both the person with Parkinson's and you, the spouse or care partner, may feel very familiar with Parkinson's and also be affected significantly by the disease. Your observations and experience may lead you to identify and prioritize very different issues than those the person with Parkinson's may wish to raise with his or her doctor. Yet the typical medical appointment may focus solely on the person with Parkinson's. As a care partner, your concerns can suddenly feel minimized, even though you, too, are experiencing the consequences of Parkinson's. Being heard during a medical appointment can foster a sense of control over the disease and help you cope. Everyone, including your doctor or other healthcare professional, can benefit greatly from an open discussion about who is on the wellness team and the role each member will take (with the understanding that these roles will evolve over time). Let them know that you intend to be an active member of the team. Setting these expectations as soon as possible will help smooth out many of the inevitable bumps in the road during the long haul with Parkinson's.

These tips can help you as you shape your role as care partner:

- **Talk** about the extent to which you expect or wish to be involved in care. Be sure to discuss how you'll deal with any differences between these expectations and those of the person with Parkinson's. For example, if you tend to take control and find yourself pushing the person with Parkinson's to be more active than they're ready to be, take a moment to consider whether your actions could possibly add to the overall stress of caring for your loved one.

- **Make sure your loved one understands and accepts** your concerns and desire to help and support them. You might think about your role of care partner as one of "Parkinson's coach," someone who provides ongoing feedback about things like standing taller, speaking louder or taking larger steps.

- **Set up rules** or even agree on a "catch phrase" that the person with Parkinson's can use to let you know when they feel that your guidance and encouragement have become unwanted nagging.

- **Accompany your loved one to medical appointments and be heard.** Write down the three most important things that you would like the Parkinson's doctor to address in order to ensure that your concerns are heard, too.

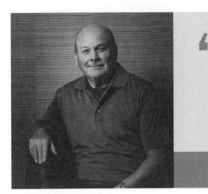

> *It's easy for me to forget my wife has Parkinson's because she's in such good shape, so I've been doing more reading to learn about all the different aspects of Parkinson's, especially the emotional effects."*
>
> **— SCOTT**

NOTES FROM THE TRENCHES: AN EXPERIENCED CARE PARTNER'S PERSPECTIVE

By Carolyn Allen Zeiger, PhD

When your loved one is diagnosed with Parkinson's disease, your whole world is suddenly turned upside down. Of course in reality, you probably knew that something was amiss and things have not been quite right for a while. Yet, living with a progressive disease that has an unpredictable course means that you can't go back to life as it was, and you will need to adapt your life accordingly. In the beginning, it's hard to even grasp what that might mean.

Having been in your shoes – and still walking in them today – I can emphatically tell you that yes, you will face many challenges ahead, but take heart: life does go on, and *your* life can still be rich and meaningful, perhaps even in new and different ways.

I am not saying that it is always going to be easy, but with perseverance and an open mind and open heart, it is doable and rewarding. I know. I have been and still am in that situation both personally and professionally. Every day I live and work with courageous and inspiring people with Parkinson's and their families, who share their challenges and wisdom with me. We link our arms and hearts together and keep on moving!

CARE PARTNER? CAREGIVER?

Our local support group calls itself Parkinson's Partners, and defines partners as "anyone walking beside someone with Parkinson's." This includes spouses, children, siblings, parents, friends and even professional caregivers. There are many kinds of support that partners offer their people with Parkinson's, and the form it takes depends on the particular situation, the stage of the Parkinson's and the relationship between the people involved.

We encourage both members of the partnership to maintain the give-and-take of partners as much as possible, for as long as possible. This is the most empowering relationship for both. Realistically, however, there might come a time when the *care partner* becomes a true *caregiver*, tending to even the most basic physical needs. It's important to stay alert to what the actual needs are as they change, and negotiate with each other — and other family members — about how they will be handled as time goes on. Like all important life decisions, it can be helpful to have these discussions early, when you are both healthy and can consider these questions without the added burden of emotions that emerge when times get tough.

CARE PARTNER AS ADVOCATE

The manifestation of Parkinson's, and therefore its treatment, varies so much from one person to another that there are no standard guides to living with Parkinson's as either patient or care partner. Consequently, it is imperative that you learn as much as possible about Parkinson's, available treatments and how it affects your person with Parkinson's. There is more and more information available in books, websites, conferences and workshops. Using these resources to become a well-informed advocate will improve the quality of life for everyone involved.

One of the key features of the disease is that the symptoms are sometimes not as apparent to the people with Parkinson's as they are to others, especially those closest to them. Even though my husband Paul is a yoga teacher, he was unaware of losing his arm swing and likewise oblivious to the fact that his walk was often more of a shuffle. People with Parkinson's often complain that everyone else is becoming deaf when actually, their friends notice that their voices are becoming a whisper. Consequently, to help your partner get the most effective treatment, you need to become a careful observer who goes along to neurology appointments to share your observations and concerns. As an advocate, you also can help by asking questions, clarifying treatment recommendations and taking notes.

My husband and I keep a list of symptoms (similar to the worksheets in this manual) that we go through together, before every appointment with the neurologist. For each symptom, we mark our independent judgments as to whether he is better, worse or the same. We also add any new symptoms we notice. Then we compare notes and talk about any differences in our perceptions. Our neurologist finds this very helpful — although he does smile at the Excel spreadsheet. But, hey, Paul is a computer scientist after all.

I do recommend finding a neurologist who specializes in movement disorders. These specialists have the particular expertise and wealth of experience needed to customize treatment for the individual.

MORE THAN A MOVEMENT DISORDER

Although Parkinson's is still called a "movement disorder," it also has non-motor and cognitive symptoms that can be as troublesome as the motor symptoms. Remember that Parkinson's manifests in many ways, so don't rely on your doctor to always ask the "right" questions; bring up everything you are concerned about, whether you think it has to do with Parkinson's or not.

Another important reason to understand these symptoms is that they can create big challenges for the care partner, as well as for the person with Parkinson's. Choking and constipation can become medical emergencies if measures are not taken to keep them in check; neurologically-based apathy, anxiety or depression affects both partners; someone whose handwriting has become tiny and illegible cannot continue writing checks, so maybe someone else needs to do it. Personally, I hate working with numbers, so Paul now prints checks out on the computer. We all find our own solutions, and you come to find solutions that make sense for your situation.

CARING FOR YOURSELF

Another reason you need to take on the observer-advocate role is to mitigate the impact on your own health and well-being. Every resource on caregiving you find will tell you to take care of your physical, mental and spiritual health. The trick is *doing* it! And *continuing* to do it. It is easy to get caught up in the day-to-day challenges of re-ordering your life, maintaining your household, and caring for your loved one — pushing yourself to the limit until you collapse literally or figuratively. One way to stay on track is to enlist the aid of someone you trust to give you regular feedback about how you are doing: Overtired? Irritable? Depressed? Find ways to make some changes.

DEALING WITH OTHERS' REACTIONS

There is no telling how others will react to the news that your loved one has Parkinson's. For starters, most people know very little about it. I was stunned by a friend who said angrily, "Why are you so upset? Parkinson's is nothing but a little tremor." I was also surprised (and delighted) to discover friends who reached out and showered us with love and compassion. Those you expect to be the most sensitive or well-informed may prove to be the least so and vice versa. Don't take it personally if you get a reaction based on their fears or lack of knowledge about Parkinson's. You can just let it go, or take it as a "teachable moment" and pass on some information about the disease, including referring them to your favorite website or blog.

GETTING SUPPORT

A woman recently told me she was reluctant to ask for support because, "things are not so bad." At every stage of Parkinson's, care partners need support! Things do not need to be "bad." Being heard and understood by others who know what we are dealing with is a great comfort in itself. And when you are stretched to the max, it is really critical. There was a time when my husband went through repeated hospitalizations and trips to the ER, due to medical problems associated with Parkinson's. I finally broke down and wept with exhaustion and frustration in a doctor's office. I will always be grateful to the physician who put his arm around me and said, "Call me any time you need help. Even if it is outside my medical specialty, I will help you get what you need." I wish I had *asked for help* sooner and more directly.

It has been helpful to me to go to support groups to understand Parkinson's better and to see how people go about living well. I think it is also valuable for Paul and me to go by ourselves sometimes, so we can speak freely without fear of upsetting or hurting the other person.

Look for a care partners' support group. In our group, we really let it "all hang out." To live well with Parkinson's, you need to be honest with yourself about how you are doing, and be open to others' ideas and suggestions. In addition, sometimes our group has speakers address topics that we think we need to understand better.

" *We tend to connect when we're really struggling. You realize that somebody is going through the exact same thing with kids at home, or a husband leaving his job, etc. Lots of similarities. The opportunity to connect with others in similar situations when you need it, whether in a regular support group or online, is really good.*"

— SHERYL

The first time you go to a support group, it can be a little daunting. It is important to find the right group for you. If your person with Parkinson's has young onset Parkinson's, for example, you will have more in common with others in this category who are likely to be working or raising children, as opposed to older retired people facing challenges more common to senior citizens. Go to different groups in your area to see where you feel most comfortable — or create your own group! Maybe it is just two families; do what works for you. Internet blogs and websites also can be tremendous resources for both information and heart-to-heart sharing with others in your situation.

The value of professional counseling should not be overlooked. One session with a skilled grief counselor got me through the worst of my distress when Paul was diagnosed. I came to terms with the fact that although previously I was the one who had serious health problems, my exceptionally healthy and fit husband and I had now switched roles. I had to face the loss of our imagined future life together and revise my scenarios. You, too, might discover that you are sad, depressed, or angry and resentful. You might also feel guilty about these reactions.

Psychotherapy can be expensive, so check your health insurance to see if it is covered. If not, look for reduced-fee services through your local Parkinson's association or mental health center. Some university graduate programs for psychologists or social workers have training clinics. I look forward to the day when these services are offered to both the person with Parkinson's and care partner as part of the standard treatment for Parkinson's.

Your person with Parkinson's can be one of your most valuable sources of support. Doing everything they can for themselves and expressing their appreciation for all you do can really keep you going. In addition to managing his own meds, Paul looks for opportunities to help me out. He hunts for TV programs he knows I would enjoy, encourages me to take time to myself and hangs in there doing all the household chores he can still manage.

EMBRACING CHANGE

Although Parkinson's is a progressive disorder, don't get in the mindset that it is all going to be downhill from here on out. Changes in medication, life circumstances, reduced stress, the addition of exercise and nutrition can maintain your partner on a plateau for a long time, or even make things better. Yes! Sometimes the change is for the better. Be prepared for it, and embrace it!

So much is unpredictable in this Parkinson's life. The more flexible you remain, the more you are able to go with the flow, the easier it will be for everyone. "Going with the flow" has ease built into it. Many new doors open; so keep your eyes open for new opportunities. Paul and I could never have guessed that his and my professional work would come together for a new career for both of us, late in life.

CONTINUING TO LIVE YOUR OWN LIFE

Your partner is not just someone with Parkinson's and you are not just a Parkinson's care partner. Continue with activities you enjoy; move on from activities and relationships that no longer nurture you. Find new interests and activities that give you energy. Avoid isolation; human beings are social creatures. Stay engaged with existing communities or find new ones, bearing in mind that you might need to change to less demanding roles. If you say you are too tired or too busy to lead any kind of independent life, then you need to reach out to others to help you change that.

BECOMING A SKILLED CARE PARTNER

With the progression of the disease, you may find yourself more in the role of a true care*giver*, as opposed to care *partner*. Be reassured that should you need them, there are valuable resources on how to assume this role, including books, websites and local workshops and resource centers. Parkinson's support groups and Parkinson's caregiver support groups can be invaluable resources here. In our groups, we constantly share our solutions with each other, and share laughter over our failures. In addition, at this point, you really need to reach out to all those people who have offered help, being willing to tell them exactly what you need and when. Without this guidance from you, well-meaning people will hold back because they don't know what to do and don't want to be intrusive.

LOOKING AT BOTH THE SHORT-TERM AND THE LONG-TERM

To get off on the right foot, it is good to know about some moves you'll want to make now, as well as to be aware of some you'll need to make in the future – perhaps, the near future. I have noticed that when people keep "waiting until later" to even think about, let alone plan for later stages of the disease, they almost always wait too long. At that point, they are usually in crisis and unable to make good decisions, or they find that the help or services they need right away are not available or affordable.

While it might be difficult territory to navigate, especially if you are currently young and healthy enough for these issues to seem remote, it will serve you well to do some thinking ahead about such matters as wills and trusts, financial planning, medical powers of attorney, long-term care insurance for the care partner, possible nursing care for the person with Parkinson's, moving into a simpler, easier living space, paying for additional helpers, etc. If you start planning early, a crisis won't catch you unprepared. Many people actually find that the prospect of delving into these topics can be more uncomfortable than the doing. Knowledge is power. There can be real peace of mind in knowing that a plan is in place, should future circumstances make implementing it become necessary.

EDUCATING YOURSELF

Learn about Parkinson's to help understand the sources of your stress and to avoid or limit the negative consequences of being a care partner. Reading the essays and comments from care partners in this manual is a good start and will help you gain some perspective. Other sources of information include your doctor, nurse or social worker. Most hospitals have a health help line and/or social work department to assist you in getting more information on support and connections in your community.

SEEKING PROFESSIONAL ASSISTANCE

For those living in the US, most metropolitan areas have an Area Agency on Aging (AAA) that provides information about services in your community. In addition, the National Eldercare Locator is a public service of the Administration on Aging and a valuable resource for finding state and local community assistance. It maintains a search engine for in-home services, a respite locator, fact sheets about caregiving and resources for programs that may provide some financial assistance (eldercare.gov). Some services may be covered by Medicare or Medicaid (medicare.gov). If you are living outside of the US, reach out to local resources to see what organizations might offer comparable assistance.

If financial resources don't allow you to hire professional caregivers, reach out to family members and investigate community resources that may provide assistance. Some common care partner programs include respite in-home care, adult day centers, short-term nursing and home health services. These services are more commonly needed during the more advanced stages of Parkinson's. As Parkinson's advances, more time and energy is required to manage it. In-home care can make a significant, positive impact on your level of strain as a care partner.

When you first consult with a social worker, home services agency or facilities manager, the initial goal will be determining your level of need. During the consultation, risk assessment, medical needs and personal assistance questionnaires will help you decide on the right level of assistance. Financial resources may dictate the level of service available to some people.

If you need to leave home during the day or for an extended period of time, ask specifically about assistance with transportation for you or the person with Parkinson's and about daytime companionship (if needed) for your loved one. If you have medical issues that impact your ability to do household tasks, ask about assistance with domestic chores, shopping and cleaning. Depending on the level of mobility challenges, you may want to ask for a home modification consultation to learn where to place grab bars, safe floor surfaces, extra lighting or how to ergonomically arrange your kitchen, bathroom or closets. Occupational therapists can also help you evaluate your home for safety modifications.

CONCLUSION

As a care partner, you can only feel as good as your general health allows. Taking the time to prioritize your physical and emotional health and wellness will benefit you and the person with Parkinson's. Seeking comfort in the support of others – and giving comfort, as well – is particularly helpful. Finding the right balance for your situation may take time and energy, but the payoff will be better health and deeper energy reserves when you need them the most.

Everyone chooses an approach that suits the individual and the person with Parkinson's in their life. The common thread is recognizing the importance of maintaining the identity, health and well-being of both the person with Parkinson's and their care partner. Doing so leads to better outcomes for both people.

CARE PARTNER SUPPORT: LEARNING TO FIND WHAT YOU NEED

By Angela Robb

SETTLING INTO LIFE WITH PARKINSON'S

My relationship with Parkinson's began with a mouse click.

I met my husband, Karl, in an America Online chat room 21 years ago. Our first discussions were mostly comprised of getting to know one another and playing 20 questions.

Our conversations were easy, and his dry sense of humor came shining through our instant message exchanges. Within the first week or so, he told me that he had had Parkinson's disease for more than four years. His disclosure did not alarm me, and I remember asking, "Don't older people usually get Parkinson's disease?"

I married Karl, never having known him without Parkinson's. I love him, but I do not love the disease. We acknowledge that it is part of our life, but we do not allow it to be all of our life. We decided early on in our lives together to start our own business and work from home. At the time, we were in our mid-30s, and we didn't want to postpone our desire to own our own business. Since the progression of Parkinson's is unpredictable, we decided to grab the bull by the horns and pursue our dreams.

We have adapted our goals and plans to account for the unpredictability of Parkinson's, which can change by the day or even by the moment. We do our best to plan, but we usually have a back-up strategy – not just for Karl, the Parkinson's or his medications – but for me, too. We ask ourselves questions: Do we have enough energy to tackle that task? Would we be more prepared to take on that task tomorrow, with more energy or stamina? Communication, honesty and self-awareness allow us to share how we are really feeling and come up with a mutually agreeable approach.

That's why I've always considered myself a care partner. Karl and I had a few discussions about our roles in this part of our life together, and we consider ourselves partners on the journey of living with Parkinson's. Others may think of themselves as caregivers, and indeed, it's up to individuals to determine which term (or any other) best fits their personal preference and specific responsibilities. For the purpose of simplicity here, I'll use the term care partner to describe any person who has primary responsibility for assisting with the care and decision-making for a person living with Parkinson's.

Care partner is not my primary identity (although I've become rather knowledgeable on the subject and do my best to pass on what I've learned to others). When I meet people, it's not the first thing I tell them, but I think I would be doing myself a disservice to not acknowledge the fact that it is one of the hats I wear. My husband says, "If you don't accept your diagnosis, fighting illness becomes even harder." I believe that the same idea holds true for care partners. Acceptance does not mean giving in to Parkinson's; it means being prepared for the road ahead and wherever it takes you.

There is some peace to be found in acknowledging this role, but it doesn't mean that I have to give up another part of myself to make room. Parkinson's is not going to define Karl, and it's not going to define me, either. I'd like to share some of the things I've learned with you so that you can find your own peace in caring for someone living with this disease.

CARE PARTNERS NEED NURTURING, TOO

Anyone who has cared for another knows the temptation to forego one's own needs when someone else's needs seem more pressing. For many years, as I visited with other care partners, I stressed my strong belief that we needed to take care of ourselves first so that we could care for our loved ones with Parkinson's.

It's so easy to put ourselves last on the care list. We put our children, spouses, family, home, work, pets and so on way ahead of "me." When a chronic disease like Parkinson's is part of the equation, there's an even greater tendency for us care partners to make our loved ones the number one priority. Yet, if we don't care for ourselves, who will?

> ***I don't compartmentalize wife and care partner, but I know it's important to take time for myself. I play tennis a couple times a week, I babysit and enjoy the grandkids.*"**
>
> — NANCY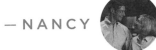

It is vitally important that care partners have a depth of self-knowledge and be willing to ask, "How am I doing today?" or "How am I doing in this moment?" My own realization of this fact came from my study of Reiki and mindfulness meditation. My self-knowledge evolved over time, and I'm so happy that it did. I only wish that I had come to it sooner! I find myself checking in on my mental, emotional and physical awareness. This really is something that you have to do by yourself, for yourself. As much as your loved one, family or friends may ask you how you are doing, they may not be prepared for your honest answer. Most care partners will not respond truthfully anyway. The real answer is found in being with yourself and reflecting honestly on the whole package.

I find that posing some personally meaningful questions to myself can be helpful. Once you begin an internal dialogue with yourself, you will find questions that are suited to you and your personal needs. Here are some examples of mine:

- How do I physically feel today? Are there areas that need some attention?
- How balanced do I feel mentally today?
- How much time can I make for myself to meditate and exercise today?
- How can I best care for myself today?

This personal reflection helps me acknowledge my own needs and gives me pause to make sure that I attend to them. It's a simple exercise, but it really works. I encourage care partners to try it.

IF YOU NEED HELP, GET IT

I encourage all care partners to have a contact list of family and/or friends who can help out in both emergency and non-emergency situations. So often, friends and neighbors say, "What can I do to help?" Please view these generous offers as sincere, and take people up on their willingness to help. Some care partners even have a prepared list of tasks that need to be done (mow the lawn, fix a broken door handle, come over and sit with the person with Parkinson's while you're away at a doctor's appointment). You may just find out that you have resources you were unaware of, and you will give your friends a meaningful way to give of themselves.

279

It is also important for the care partner to realize when he/she may need outside or professional assistance. Help may come in the form of a paid caregiver, household help, a driver, etc. We all want to be a superhero, but even Wonder Woman and Superman are part of the Justice League! Don't let yourself get overextended before you acknowledge that you need additional help. I learned the hard way when I tried to run a business, keep up on household chores and stay involved with Parkinson's activities for many years without help. I felt physically and emotionally drained trying to keep all these balls in the air. I finally arranged monthly housekeeping services to help me take better care of my home and to allow me more time for myself and for my husband.

Don't be afraid to also seek additional help or support from your wellness team. You may want to visit with your loved one's neurologist or movement disorder specialist in a separate meeting to discuss issues important to you, or you may want to visit with a nurse, social worker or case worker at the neurologist's office to seek more information and resources. Developing a support team within the medical community can be a great asset to living with Parkinson's effectively. At one point in my care partner journey, I saw a therapist to discuss some difficulties that I was experiencing. I found great benefit in talking with someone who was outside of my life sphere. The therapist gave me valuable tools and life skills that I used to overcome my personal hurdles. I would encourage anyone to seek out professional help if you find yourself needing additional support. Check with your health insurance provider to see if the cost of a therapist may be covered.

THE VALUE OF SUPPORT GROUPS ESPECIALLY FOR CARE PARTNERS

Five years into my marriage, I decided that I wanted to attend a support group after work hours. I inquired at the local Parkinson's organization and found that there were no evening care partner groups in my area. So, I started one myself. There are care partners-only groups and general Parkinson's disease support groups that welcome both the person with Parkinson's and their care partner. I decided to make the group a care partners-only support group because I wanted the kind of focused discussion that this format allows. Care partners-only groups lend themselves to:

- "You're Not Alone" – shared experiences, even though no two Parkinson's care partner journeys are the same.

- Carving out time for the care partner to nurture him or herself.

- Giving those participating an opportunity to share their true feelings with one another, without any concerns or fears about the person with Parkinson's disease hearing these comments.

- Vitally important confidentiality – what is discussed within the group stays within the group.

- Building trust among participants. It is important for the support group leader, professional (social worker, psychologist, psychotherapist) or volunteer, to set this expectation from the start of the first meeting and at every meeting.

- Developing camaraderie between care partners and allowing for an exchange of information that helps foster relationships that go beyond the support group meeting.

Some Parkinson's support groups may be more geared to information exchange, or they can be topic or speaker-oriented. Which type is best for you is a matter of personal preference. If you try one group and do not find the support you need, try another. As with any type of gathering, you may need to "shop around." Don't hesitate to look around for the group that fits your needs best.

" *Brian and I co-lead a support group in our area. I get to see Brian happy as he's teaching and doing something he loves. I'm learning how to step out of my own little boxes that I've put myself in as Brian encourages me to get more involved with the care partners as the co-director. I do feel inspired by our support group: there's a special camaraderie, hopefulness and energy."*

— LILY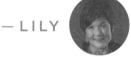

Hear more about Lily's experience leading a support group with Brian: 🎥 **dpf.org/lily**.

Check with your local Parkinson's organization or Parkinson's center to see if they provide a support group in your area. You may also check with the regional or national Parkinson's organizations, hospital, neurologist or movement disorder specialist's office, Parkinson's therapy providers (physical, occupational, speech, for example), retirement community or assisted living/nursing center to see if they provide a group that fits your needs. If no appropriate groups exist, you can do what I did – start your own!

STARTING A SUPPORT GROUP FROM SCRATCH

There are many ways and methods to develop a support group. Here are some questions you should consider before starting a group:

- Will the group be care partners only or a general Parkinson's support group that includes those who have Parkinson's and their care partners, family or friends?

- Will the group meet during the day, in the evenings or on weekends, and for how long and how often?

- Will there be speakers for each meeting, an open discussion group, or a simple gathering tied to a social activity? Perhaps it will be a combination of these.

- Will the group be small or large?

- Where will the group meet? Will the venue be a free space or rented, and is there a size restriction for the meeting space?

- Are there others who can help you shape the group and get started?

I was fortunate that our local Parkinson's organization was very supportive of my efforts to start a support group. They provided materials about how to start a group, access to their staff psychotherapist who acted as a coach and they publicized the details about the support group meeting. I found a local library that had a room available at no charge and was available for a once-monthly, two-hour evening meeting. I emailed care partners that I had I met at Parkinson's events and told them about the new group. I started this group without additional support but over time, attendees of the support group began volunteering to help find speakers, provide snacks and water, suggest discussion topics and publicize our meetings.

When you start a group, there are bound to be bumps along the way. There were some evenings that I sat by myself or when only one person would arrive for the meeting. This was the hardest lesson I had to learn. My support group leader coach warned me about this scenario. As the group leader, you need to let the care partners know that you will be there, but the care partners have to commit to making the time to attend a meeting. Attendance may fluctuate each month.

My group was small and mostly discussion-based, with occasional speakers. The group stayed together for two years. Care partner attendance started to decline for a variety of reasons: inability for some to drive at night, loved ones with Parkinson's that couldn't be left alone, job commitments, etc. I decided to discontinue the group and put my efforts into creating a new Parkinson's support group with my husband, closer to home.

For 13 years, Karl and I facilitated a support group that was a mix of people with Parkinson's, their care partners, loved ones, family and friends. More than 20 people consistently attended monthly meetings. The group moved from a general discussion format to a mix of speakers, discussion and social time. Every support group member was encouraged to suggest or arrange a speaker and bring a topic for discussion. Discussions include medication management, speech therapies, exercise, complementary and holistic therapies, physical therapy, assistive devices, local/state/national programs, clinical trials, doctors and more. Many members keep in touch with each other between meetings. In 2016, we closed our support group, but continue to find support through attending other groups in our area and by attending Parkinson's events.

FINDING YOUR NICHE

I cannot say enough to encourage every care partner to get involved with a support group. Find one that works for you or create one made up of like-minded people. Meeting and sharing with others who understand your journey will help you to realize that you are not alone in this journey.

Support need not always be formal. In addition to attending a monthly support group, I also receive support by meeting for coffee on an "as needed basis" with three to four care partners. We are all at different stages in our Parkinson's care partnering journey. We gather to discuss our lives and to nurture each other.

> **Having people say, 'If you ever need anything, we're here for you,' gives us comfort."**
>
> — NANCY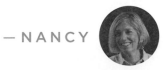

Everyone can benefit from some form of "talking support," whether it is a group of friends you gather for lunch, a sport in which you participate, walking at the mall, spending time with extended family members or possibly seeing a professional counselor. It is vital that you have some outlet for self-expression and discussion.

Remember – your best strategy for being the best care partner you can be is to be the healthiest, happiest, most supported person you can be first.

Hear Connie Carpenter Phinney's tips for care partners about setting appropriate boundaries and saying no: ◼ **dpf.org/boundaries** ◼ **dpf.org/saying-no**.

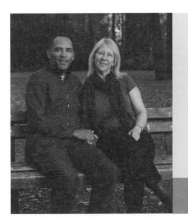

> **We try to have time where we go out and Parkinson's is not allowed to come. We just go and have fun, we won't talk about symptoms or how he is feeling. We've made it very deliberate, kind of to keep some romance in our relationship."**
>
> — SHERYL

283

■ PARKINSON'S AND CHILDREN

A parent's diagnosis of Parkinson's has a profound impact on children, no matter the age. For those diagnosed with young onset Parkinson's (before the age of 50), though, children are usually younger and living at home, creating an entirely different dynamic than those whose children are grown and living on their own.

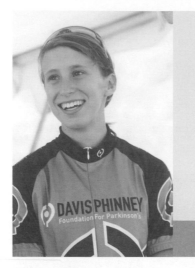

" *I used to go with my dad to the store when he was really shaky so I could help him with the shopping cart and to make change more easily. He needed extra hands, and I was happy to help him – even when I was little, like 9 or 10 years old.*"

— KELSEY PHINNEY

Kelsey in 2009

How children handle a diagnosis of Parkinson's will be unique and evolve as the disease progresses. However, often kids will take on a role as secondary or even primary care partners, supporting both the parent living with Parkinson's and the care partner. Maintaining an ongoing dialogue between parent(s) and children about Parkinson's and the continued impacts of the disease is essential to living well. In this chapter, you'll find links to videos and podcasts of stories from children of people living with Parkinson's as well as tips from others living with Parkinson's about how to intentionally keep an open conversation with kids about the effects of Parkinson's and the changes it brings.

KIDS AT HOME

Listen to Dave discuss managing his wife's Parkinson's with young kids at home: 📹 dpf.org/dave.

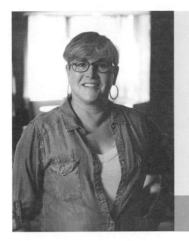

" *I remember my youngest son was in late elementary school when I came and did a presentation for his class. One of the kids in the class asked him why I was shaking so much and my son became really upset and embarrassed. He'd grown up seeing me tremor, so for him it wasn't anything abnormal.*"

— JILL

" *We wanted our kids to be just normal kids and not have to do anything different because of Parkinson's.*"

— SHERYL

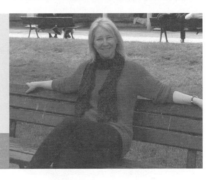

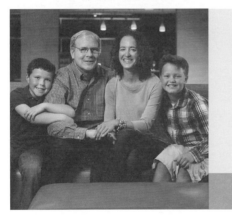

" *All I want is to give my kids as normal a childhood as possible. We take it one day at a time with our boys. I don't know how much they really are affected by it. There's never been anything I feel like I can't do with them, whether it's skiing, hiking, biking, etc.*"

— LIZ

" *As the kids got older, we basically just answered any questions they had. If they asked, we answered. Otherwise, we tried not to make Parkinson's a central focus of their lives. They were regular kids growing up and we wanted to protect that for them.*"

— JILL

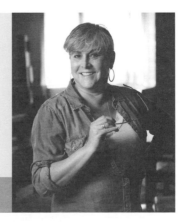

PARKINSON'S AND THE FAMILY

ADULT CHILDREN

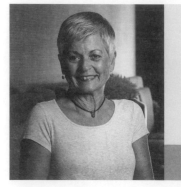

> *I don't burden my daughters with all the little details. I figure they'll look up what they need to know and if I'm having a problem, we'll talk about it. It's on a need-to-know basis right now."*
>
> — EDIE

> *Our girls are really supportive and interested, and I know they're going to be there for us in the future. It's mostly emotional support, caring and love."*
>
> — NANCY

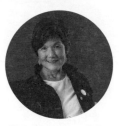

Listen to more stories about involving adult children in life with Parkinson's:

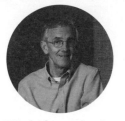
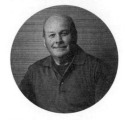

🎥 dpf.org/mike

🎥 dpf.org/scott

🎥 dpf.org/lily

Hear a variety of adult children who have or had a parent living with Parkinson's share their experience and what they've learned: 🔊 dpf.org/kids-and-pd.

Watch Connie Carpenter Phinney discuss tips for communicating with adult children about Parkinson's: 🎥 dpf.org/communicate-kids.

GRANDKIDS

> *With my grandchildren, I try not to overdo it and swamp them with information. I want grandpa to be grandpa. If something comes up, though, I will use it as a coachable moment. Keep it simple and straightforward, but share it."*
>
> — RYAN

Hear Nancy talk about how she and Steve discuss Parkinson's with their grandkids: 🎥 dpf.org/nancy.

MY PERSPECTIVE: KIDS AS CARE PARTNERS

By Robert Villa

I was 12 or 13 when my dad told us he had Parkinson's. It's pretty difficult explaining to a child that a parent is sick, and I don't really think I had an immediate reaction to the news. What I do remember is that, little by little, over time, my father's lifestyle changed.

Change is something that we all have to deal with, no matter where we are in our lives and if we learn to embrace change before it happens, we will not find it as unsettling. Having a family member with Parkinson's has taught me to appreciate the little moments in life, and it has taught me to value things that many of us take for granted. My father was diagnosed at the young age of 40. I don't think that even now I can wrap my head around how he must have felt that day, but I do know that he did not stop fighting and living. He has continued to live his life as normally as possible, and my family has helped him stay on course for living a healthy and worry-free life.

Although there are many aspects of our lives that are constantly changing, it's important to focus on the things that are within our control. Growing up with a parent with Parkinson's has taught me the importance of staying positive, staying healthy, staying knowledgeable and also staying aware. It has helped me to reach out to a community with similar experiences. My advice to others is to get out and find a group that shares a similar background and understands what you and your family are experiencing. I came to my group with my questions and concerns about my father's Parkinson's. Sometimes we forget that when we share our thoughts and ideas and also carefully listen to others, we can experience the incredible power of connecting with another person.

Today my family is closer than we have ever been. We communicate, we help each other and we face obstacles and barriers together. I would be lying if I said I never felt afraid about the future. But what I've found to be even more important is that it is this same fear that increases my ability to live in the moment with my family, staying strong and positive.

> " *As a child of someone living with Parkinson's, there will be times when you feel helpless and alone and even angry.*"

It helps me to remember that everything will be okay. During times of pain and distress, I try to remain calm and optimistic, not only for myself, but also for my other family members. They're counting on me! Don't ever be afraid to reach out for help or to communicate with your family members living with Parkinson's by encouraging them and helping them stay active. Supporting each other will bring you closer, help ease the road when it gets bumpy and keep the focus on living well for many years to come.

Hear from other kids like Robert who have a parent living with Parkinson's: ◆》**dpf.org/kids-and-pd**.

■ PARKINSON'S WHEN YOU LIVE ALONE

While Parkinson's does impact the entire family, many people living with Parkinson's may not reside with a spouse acting as a care partner or have children close by who are willing to help. When you live alone, staying informed, being engaged in your own health and remaining connected to your community of friends and support become even more critical.

> " *I don't have a spouse or children; I live alone. I have lots of friends, but I'm on my own to determine how to live and handle Parkinson's. Living alone has actually given me strength to handle this diagnosis.*"
>
> — BRENDA

Hear more from Brenda about living alone with Parkinson's: ◼ **dpf.org/brenda**.

Care partners and support come in many forms. Your wellness team, friends, other family members and adult children who are available to assist you in various ways are all part of your Parkinson's care network and should be considered valuable resources you can call upon to help. If you need extra assistance either inside or outside of the home (or both), research available options in your area for support. This could include paid professionals, such as home health nurses or house cleaners, or it may involve connecting with volunteer services like Meals on Wheels to meet needs you may have.

288

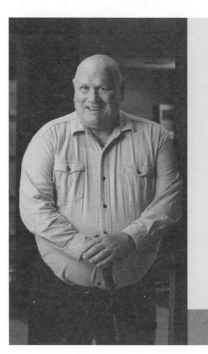

> " *I live alone, but I certainly have people that are close to me: my doctor, my social worker, my pharmacist, my dentist, my occupational therapist. I make the analogy that I may be up in the plane alone, but someone pre-checked the flight, someone put the gas in and there is ground control as I travel along, so I'm never really on my own.*"
>
> — RYAN

PRACTICAL PLANNING FOR THE FUTURE

Living well with Parkinson's is a long-term proposition that starts with a strong commitment to self-care. Quality of life, however, encompasses more than just physical, cognitive and emotional health. It also includes financial health, retirement planning and preparing for long-term care. (Detailed information about disability and other retirement planning can be found in the "Family, Relationships and Work" chapter of the **What You Need to Know About Parkinson's** section).

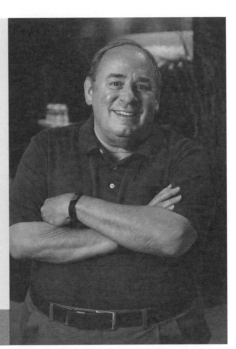

> *Anyone with Parkinson's has to face the reality that life could change – maybe not for a long time, but financial planning becomes much more important than before. The clock moves faster than you'd anticipated. I recently left my job of 15 years, though I didn't anticipate fully retiring quite yet, so I've had to look at other options."*

— JOHN

It's important to plan for the financial impact of living with Parkinson's and to consider now, before circumstances force a decision, how you would like to be cared for in the future and what options you have for meeting your needs.

> *Planning is very, very important. Anybody with Parkinson's thinking about retiring should sit down with a financial advisor and look at how to scale things so you're living at a level within your means. Social security is a lot further off for someone with young onset Parkinson's."*

— STEVE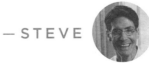

By Donald L. Haisman, CFP®

MY PERSONAL PARKINSON'S STORY

It was a bright, sunny Florida day on the outside, but not so on our insides. Our minds, our hearts and our full beings suddenly became overcast.

I traveled with my wife of 43 years on that sunny, 2.5 hour drive east. We arrived and strode through the lobby and rode the elevator to the third floor. The door opened onto the Neurology department of the Cleveland Clinic Florida. It all seemed like a routine visit to a physician's office until it happened.

"You know you have Parkinson's," she said, looking at my wife. "NO, we didn't know!" my inner voice quickly shouted. Those words from the neurologist's mouth seemed to echo in the room.

I hardly remember the drive back across the miles of Everglades sawgrass to the west side of the state. I am not sure if I even had my sunglasses on because between the discussions the two of us were having, my inner voice kept asking, "What now?"

I was supposed to be the expert planner. For three decades, I was a Certified Financial Planner (CFP). I flashed back to the many meetings with families over the years, where I had provided my list of "to do's" for them to accomplish so they would be prepared for various unforeseen events that only God could predict. Now, on that drive back, I was mentally checking off that "to do" list while looking not into the eyes of a client, but into a mirror in my mind. Was I the cobbler with no shoes, or had I followed my own financial planning advice in my own life? One of those unforeseen events of life had just happened to me, to my wife...to us.

WHAT TO DO: THE FINANCIAL PLANNING STEPS

Once you receive the diagnosis of Parkinson's, you need to prepare your own "to do" list. Since I am a US citizen, I am familiar with US legal protections and procedures. If you reside elsewhere, the basic planning concepts still apply, although you might need to look into the specifics in your country. Here are the items that I recommend you should consider:

Legal Preparations

This should be quite high on your list, probably even number one. Do not put it off; the sooner the better. Your legal preparation should consist of various documents that will lay out your plans now that Parkinson's is in your family health mix. An estate planning attorney friend of mine reminded me that in addition to a will and maybe a trust, it is very important to have a Durable Power of Attorney and a Designation of Healthcare Surrogate in place to avoid guardianship. If you live in the US or Canada, this collective group of legal documents is frequently called advanced directives. If you live elsewhere, familiarize yourself with the legal documents that allow you to designate a loved one to make healthcare decisions on your behalf, should you become unable to do so yourself. US residents might also want to review Medicaid benefits and determine how those fit into the plan.

Your advanced directives will lay out the foundation of your estate plan, which is an orderly plan for your family into the future. Do not rely on legal documents that you created years ago, since changes to the laws and statutes where you live are common. Your legal documents need to be updated to comply with those changes and the new health reality of your life. If you are considering relocating due to Parkinson's, consider having your legal documents drawn in your intended eventual place of residence, because much of your planning will be specific to that area, especially legal documents.

Many times, I have run across the situation that the person living with Parkinson's was previously named to be a legally responsible party, like a trustee or maybe custodian of a child's education fund. With the new diagnosis, this responsibility may better be transferred to another person.

Appraise Your Financial Situation

You do this by listing, in detail, all your things of value that you and your family own or in which you have any financial or legal interest. For example, this might be all investments, real estate, retirement accounts, business interests, hobbies of value or automobiles. Make note who is the legal owner of each. I will bet there are many items that you do not remember who the owner is. I have found that most families do not remember who even owns the house they live in. Locate the deed. Do not trust your memory.

Locate all insurance policies. This includes life, disability, long-term care, homeowners and auto (also known as property and casualty). Do not forget that general liability or "umbrella" liability policy, if you have one.

Now here is a difficult question: who or what OWNS the policies? Yes, most insurance policies have owners and this is critical to know. The owner has control of the policy. In that same vein, who or what is the beneficiary of those policies? This is probably one of the most overlooked financial planning issues. Are the beneficiaries (and the owners) appropriate now that you have the diagnosis? Also, know that most insurance policies have a person you can designate to be notified if premiums are not being paid. It is probably a good idea to implement this service.

Your retirement plans require special attention because they have distinct and unique rules and tax ramifications. Beneficiary designations are of special importance here and remember to name secondary beneficiaries. Listen as Dave describes their long-term financial planning as a result of Liz's young onset Parkinson's: ◼ **dpf.org/dave**.

Prepare, Prepare, Prepare

As a start, do the following:

- Gather all your individual and family original legal documents (or at least copies).

- Prepare that detailed list of all things you have of value along with the ownership information.

- If you and your wellness team have prepared a healthcare plan, have a copy available.

- Collect all your insurance policies together.

- Prepare that list of current beneficiaries of all retirement plans and insurance policies.

- Tell your executor or a trusted friend or family member how and where to access this information. Be sure to advise them of all passwords necessary to get inside any computers, Internet sites and cellphones.

FEEL OVERWHELMED? HELP IS AVAILABLE!

I know that all this seems like a monumental task to organize, coordinate and administer. Remember how we are educated that people living with Parkinson's need a devoted care partner or group of care partners and a team of medical professionals to have the best outcome? This same concept applies to your financial planning. You should consider a team of "financial" care partners to assist you. Who should you consider to be on your financial "team"? Your financial "team" should be made up of the following functions (Specific US-based designations in parentheses):

- Accountant (I prefer a Certified Public Accountant, CPA)

- Attorney that specializes in estate planning

- Financial planner (I prefer a Certified Financial Planner-Professional, CFP)

- Investment advisor (many times this is also the CFP)

- Insurance agent (I prefer a Certified Life Underwriter, CLU)

Share your honest concerns with those professionals on your team; they likely have years of experience assisting families in your situation. The next step is that someone on your team needs to be the coordinator of all these professionals. This is very important because these disciplines overlap and contribute to your personal estate plan. Of the professionals I have suggested, the CFP is most likely to have the overall training, experience and background to be your coordinator or quarterback. Often, if you start with a CFP, they can refer you to the others, if necessary.

YOU CAN DO THIS

Yes, I know this all sounds like a lot of work, and it is. However, once you get organized and develop a plan with your financial care partners, you will feel peace of mind, and it is well worth the effort. The goal is to get your entire financial house in order, simplify your financial life and make smart money decisions, so you can focus more on things you enjoy doing to live well today.

ONLINE RESOURCES

An excellent source for planning information is the National Institute on Aging, found at 🡕 **nia.nih.gov**.

CONSIDERING ASSISTED LIVING ARRANGEMENTS

The discussion about needing help at home or about assisted living should occur well before an event leaves you in crisis mode and compromises your ability to process options calmly. Have a thoughtful discussion with your loved one's doctor about his or her prognosis. Your doctor can warn you when Parkinson's is reaching a point that requires increased supervision. He or she can let you know when a higher level of medical help at home would be advisable. For instance, the onset of hallucinations and paranoia that cannot be addressed by medication may signal the need for constant supervision. If blood pressure becomes erratic and treatment options do not address the issues, a home nurse or nursing home placement may be advised. Many of the advanced symptoms of Parkinson's can be managed at home with the appropriate assistance; however, be aware that the strain of care on the care partner significantly increases with these increasing demands. Plan ahead together for the onset of some of the more demanding symptoms. This will reduce some of the strain of the difficult decision-making associated with advanced Parkinson's.

Your physician can help by discussing the natural progression of Parkinson's and letting you know where your loved one is in the process. Cognitive and mood-related symptoms typically require more hands-on care than some of the mobility challenges of Parkinson's. It's crucial for you as a care partner and for your family to anticipate and recognize worsening symptoms that are unlikely to improve with medication therapy. This knowledge will prepare you to take appropriate steps when care needs increase.

❝ *You could live for many years and not need this, and yet you don't know — you could have cognitive factors or depression that prevent you from making the decisions you would have when you were at your best. Getting this information early on is very important."*

— JOHN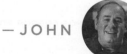

LONG-TERM CARE PLANNING FOR PEOPLE WITH PARKINSON'S

By Jessica Shurer, LCSW

While no one can predict the future, we do know Parkinson's is progressive and as Parkinson's progresses, aging is also happening. As a result, it is possible that people with Parkinson's and their care partners will require more daily help and support over time than they presently need. Although aging and living with Parkinson's are out of your control, taking steps now to maintain quality of life and plan for care in the future is an action that people with Parkinson's and their care partners can control.

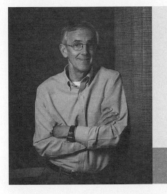

> " *It's the instability of what the future may bring, but we've still got to learn and keep digging for answers. We can't let uncertainty frighten us. We've got to be serious about it, but we've also got to keep our sense of humor.*"
>
> — MIKE

Often people prefer not to think about the future until they feel they have to. This means people can find themselves faced with big decisions that need to be made quickly and in an emotionally-charged situation. For example, someone falls suddenly, ends up in the hospital and a decision is made to move to a long-term care facility instead of returning home. Doing the research, understanding the options and making decisions before they are needed can leave you feeling better prepared. It is possible that the long-term plans you make will not be needed, but the research and conversations will have been completed while you were calm and in a position to take the time you need for these important decisions.

KNOW YOUR OPTIONS AND LONG-TERM PLANNING TERMS

What is the difference between assisted and skilled nursing? What defines a retirement community? Keep in mind that the definition of types of care can vary area to area and sometimes, from facility to facility. Furthermore, insurance coverage, private pay costs and eligibility criteria are subject to change. In general, however, there are six common types of long-term care communities:

- **Continuing care retirement communities (CCRCs).** CCRCs offer multiple levels of care, including independent, assisted and skilled nursing in the same community. For many CCRCs, you begin residence in the independent living area, moving into areas with greater assistance and supervision as your needs change and you require more care. The policies vary regarding eligibility, but it is common for CCRCs to require up front "buy-in" fees and a doctor's report stating that you will remain independent for at least five years.

- **Independent living.** These facilities can overlap with planned communities geared for those over 60. There may be certain services and activities offered, such as transportation, a restaurant and exercise equipment or classes, but for the most part, you are expected to live independently and safely, without monitoring. Many independent living facilities are free standing, some are part of golf or beach communities, and a few may be on the same campus as an assisted living or memory care facility.

- **Assisted living.** This level of care is ordinarily for people who need some assistance with everyday tasks for safety and to maintain engagement, but remain relatively independent in other ways. Residents of assisted living frequently require help with meal preparation, bathing, household tasks like laundry and overall safety monitoring, but may not need help with mobility or eating. Services vary widely, as do costs. Some facilities charge flat rate fees, while others bill a minimum rate with "add-ons" or "a la carte fees," depending on additional services needed, such as a bath more than twice per week or help with medication management. Some assisted living communities will allow someone to stay on, even if they progress to needing skilled nursing level care or hospice. Others may require residents to find other accommodations if they have progressed beyond what services are offered by the facility.

- **Family care homes.** These typically offer assisted living level of care, but in a smaller setting, often in a house with fewer residents. Assisted living facilities can have 30-80 residents, compared to a family care home, which may have only 3-15.

- **Skilling nursing.** This level of care is most appropriate for people who need help with three or more "activities of daily living," which include dressing, bathing, grooming, mobility, feeding and toileting. Additionally, someone may benefit from a skilling nursing facility if they follow a complex medication regimen, have multiple medical diagnoses (for example, Parkinson's AND rheumatoid arthritis or diabetes), a feeding tube, pressure wounds or catheters.

- **Memory care.** These "special care units," as they are often called, cater to people with more complex care needs related to cognitive impairment or dementia. This can include regular confusion, delusions or paranoia, disorientation, wandering, combativeness and difficulty with task follow-through (for example, understanding how to get dressed).

Now that you are familiar with the various long-term care options, here are some tips for finding the best long-term care for yourself or your loved one:

- **Think about what kind of care is appropriate.** Take a moment to think about what types of assistance you or your loved one needs at this time, as well as areas and levels of independence in daily functioning. When deciding what level of long-term care is necessary *now*, also consider what may be needed in the not-too-distant *future*, in order to avoid multiple residence moves in a relatively short period of time.

- **Understand the costs and financial options.** Depending on the level of care and where you live, the cost of long-term care can vary greatly. For some, it is financially within reach while for others, it is cost prohibitive. It is very surprising for many to learn that most health insurance, including Medicare, does not cover long-term care. In the US, most long-term care is paid for by Medicaid, long-term care insurance or veteran's benefits. If you have long-term care insurance, look into your policy to know what kinds of care it covers and for how long, and how to activate it when you are ready. If you are a veteran in the US, contact the local Veterans Administration's benefits services to see if you may qualify for long-term care benefits. If you are not sure whether you are eligible for Medicaid for long-term care or special assistance programs, contact your county's Department of Social Services. You may also want to work with a financial advisor and/or elder law attorney to better understand what you may be able to afford and explore asset protection options for yourself or your partner.

- **Reflect on your priorities for long-term care.** Choose three main aspects of a long-term care community that will meet your or your partner's needs, lifestyle and comfort level. Examples include location, cost, quality of food, activities they offer, staff turnover, options they offer for activities outside of the facility and other people with Parkinson's living there. Have your priorities in mind when you evaluate them to know what you are looking for and asking about.

- **Visit _at least_ two facilities.** Schedule a tour and inquire about the costs. Observe the staff in action. Do the residents look clean, happy and engaged? In addition to nurses and nursing assistants, find out if they have extra staff such as a social worker, music or art therapist, or exercise specialist and what activities are offered to residents. View the bedrooms, common rooms, outside spaces and surrounding neighborhood. Inquire about whether they have done any Parkinson's trainings for their staff. Getting a feel for the living environment and services offered will help you to know in which place you or your loved one will fit best.

- **Check out the reviews.** Because assisted living and skilled nursing are regulated by government entities, you can often find lists of facilities and ratings online. The Medicare website (medicare.gov) has a nursing home comparison tool and many state- or county-level agencies, such as the state Department of Health & Human Services or Agencies on Aging, will provide credible information about reported quality of care at assisted living facilities and family care homes. Be wary of social media-style review sites or sites that accept paid advertising or have few reviewers. These sites might not always project an accurate picture and therefore, the reviews published there should be considered with a grain of salt and investigated further. You can also ask your friends, religious community members and support group goers if any of them are personally familiar, either positively or negatively, with a long-term care community. Keep in mind that experiences and chemistry with facilities are very individual, and yours could be different from what you hear or read.

- **Talk with your family.** Have a frank discussion, speaking candidly about all the factors related to long-term care decisions. Reflect together on the physical and mental health of the primary care partner and whether he or she would "burn out" if responsible for the long-term care of the person with Parkinson's at home. Including other family members in the decision process can provide additional insight and add a team perspective that considers the well-being of both people impacted most. Consider the convenience of the location of the long-term care community for other family members. If you have not yet done so already, now is also a good time to complete a healthcare Power of Attorney and Living Will so that the person living with Parkinson's can designate someone to make medical decisions on his or her behalf and can document his or her beliefs around medical treatment and interventions. These documents will be kept on record at the long-term care community and inform the staff of the resident's wishes.

- **Consult your wellness team.** Depending on which level of care you chose, you may be required to have a physician complete some forms. This can be a family doctor or neurologist — whoever knows the symptoms, treatment plan and safety concerns the best. It is helpful to give your primary Parkinson's doctor a heads up when you are thinking about long-term care. Your doctor will benefit from having seen you recently so that he/she can better explain your situation when filling out the form. Plus, you might want to brainstorm with your doctor about the type or level of long-term care that meets your care needs best. Additionally, your physician or social worker may be able to lend insight into which facilities generally have good reputations among their patients and colleagues and/or which offer Parkinson's-specific services.

- **Understand the alternatives.** Your options might include moving to a long-term care community or "aging in place" at home. Find out what "aging in place" would mean for you and require of your care partner. A good place to start is to have an occupational therapist perform an in-home safety evaluation. It is possible that you would need to make home modifications, such as installing a ramp, widening doorways and installing grab bars, so try to understand whether such modifications are feasible and what those costs would look like. Also consider if there are adult day care centers or professional in-home care nearby and whether they are affordable for you, in case you need help in the home or a periodic respite that your current support system could not provide.

295

The biggest factor in deciding what type of long-term care accommodation is right for you is determining what is safe and sustainable for the person with Parkinson's AND for the care partner, both now and in the future. There can be a lot of guilt and a sense of lost independence associated with shifting to residence in a long-term care community, especially when the care partner remains at home and the person with progressing Parkinson's symptoms moves out. It's okay to express and process these emotions as a normal part of the transition, while at the same time being aware of your practical limitations and needs.

Additionally, try to acknowledge the peace of mind that can come from embracing long-term care. For example, many people with Parkinson's and their care partners are pleasantly surprised that the quality of their time together actually improves after the move to long-term care, because now that time can be spent enjoying one another's company or an activity instead of being focused on providing care. Overall, what is important is that you know the options that are available to you so that you can make informed decisions *beforehand* that will support your safety, encourage as much independence as possible and facilitate the best possible quality of life.

■ WORKSHEETS

One of the most important things you can do to live well with Parkinson's is take action. This section will help you identify what you need, determine which steps to take and track your progress. Additional copies of any of these worksheets can also be downloaded and printed out at ⌇ **dpf.org/worksheets**.

There are three different kinds of interactive tools to help you develop greater awareness of your needs, learn self-care approaches to address specific symptoms and organize your thoughts so you are better prepared to make the most of your appointments with the various specialists on your wellness team about your care:

1. 💗 **Wellness and lifestyle self-assessments.** Designed to help you evaluate your needs, set priorities and take positive steps toward living well with Parkinson's. There are also worksheets to help you track your progress so that you can see the effects over time of changes you've made and set new goals for the future.

   a. Parkinson's Care Questionnaire

   b. Goal Summary for Doctor Visits

   c. Daily Medication Log

   d. Overall Medication Log

   e. Wellness Self-Assessment

   f. Pre-Exercise Self-Assessment

   g. Exercise Journal

   h. Nutrition Self-Assessment

   i. Parkinson's Psychosis Self-Assessment

   j. Deep Brain Stimulation (DBS) Self-Assessment

   k. Our Relationship Self-Assessment

2. ☑ **Symptom checklists.** These worksheets encourage you to become more aware of how and when symptoms are problematic, offering recommendations for simple things you can do to minimize and manage symptoms. Completing these worksheets will also help you organize your needs and concerns so that you can clearly communicate them to your wellness team.

   a. My Symptoms Worksheet

   b. Bladder Worksheet

   c. Cognitive Wellness Worksheet

   d. Constipation Worksheet

   e. Dental Worksheet

WORKSHEETS AND RESOURCES

    f. Dyskinesia and "Off" Time Log

    g. Emotional Wellness: Anxiety

    h. Emotional Wellness: Depression

    i. Fatigue Worksheet

    j. Gait, Balance and Freezing Worksheet

    k. Insomnia and Sleep Worksheet

    l. Low Blood Pressure and Dizziness Worksheet

    m. Speech and Communication Worksheet

    n. Swallowing Worksheet

    o. Sexual Dysfunction Worksheet

3. 📷 **Medical information snapshots.** These documents are intended to organize important information about you for your wellness team, including specialists such as a DBS programmer, dentist or a hospital wellness team. The "Medical Summary for Your Doctor Appointment" worksheet is a one-page document that organizes the most important information about you for your doctor's appointment. The "Prepare for Your Hospital Stay" worksheet collects all your current and essential Parkinson's information into a single document for the doctors, nurses and aides that will be caring for you during your stay.

    a. Clinical Appointments Summary

    b. Current Symptoms Summary

    c. Wellness Team Contact Information

    d. Medical Providers

    e. DBS Medical History

    f. Prepare for Your Hospital Stay

    g. Medical Summary for Your Doctor Appointment

    h. Medical Summary for Dentists

For your convenience, all of these resources can be downloaded and printed out at ⌐ **dpf.org/worksheets**. Print additional copies for your wellness team as well as care partner to use, as he or she might have different observations that are important to bring up at appointments.

♥ PARKINSON'S CARE QUESTIONNAIRE

Name: _____ Age: _____

Date of Birth: _____

Healthcare Provider Name: _____

What are your goals for this appointment?

_____

_____

_____

_____

List your current or most bothersome problems or symptoms:

_____

_____

_____

_____

Did you make the changes recommended during your last visit?

_____

_____

_____

_____

Were your last treatment changes helpful? Explain: _____

_____

_____

_____

WORKSHEETS AND RESOURCES

List any new medical problems or allergies since your last visit: _____

_____

_____

_____

Do you experience dyskinesia? (circle one) Yes / No

Do your medications wear "off" or stop working? (circle one) Yes / No

If yes, on average how long does each dose last? _____ hours

Have you had any falls since your last visit? (circle one) Yes / No

List any changes in your living arrangements: _____

_____

_____

_____

List prescription refills you need: _____

_____

_____

_____

_____

Circle any problems that you had in the past month related to each specific area:

Movement

Tremor	Stiffness	Slowness
Imbalance	Walking Problems	Frequent Falling
Movement Freezing	Involuntary Movements	Muscle Spasm/Cramping

Other (Explain): _____

▶ Speech/Swallowing/Gastrointestinal

Speech Changes	Swallowing Problems	Drooling
Pneumonia	Weight Loss	Weight Gain
Aspiration	Nausea	Vomiting
Abdominal Pain	Facial Masking	

Other (Explain): _____

Bowel or Bladder/Autonomic/Other

Bladder Problems	Constipation	Diarrhea
Chills/Sweats	Fatigue	Leg Swelling
Dizziness/Lightheadedness	Fainting or Loss of Consciousness	
Sexual Dysfunction		

Other (Explain): _____

Cognitive/Behavioral

Anxiety	Depression	Apathy
Sleep Problems	Daytime Sleepiness	Fatigue
Memory Loss	Confusion	Hallucinations
Paranoia	Delusions	Mania

Impulsive Spending, Sex or Gambling

Executive Function Difficulties (planning, decision-making, etc.)

Sudden, Uncontrolled Sleep "Attacks"

Other (Explain): _____

Other

Fever	Chills	Hearing Loss
Headache	Joint Pain	Back Pain
Neck Pain	Palpitations	Chest Pain
Cough	Hearing Loss	Vision Change
Numbness/Tingling	Driving Challenges	

List any other concerns or problems that you have: _____

_____

_____

_____

WORKSHEETS AND RESOURCES

♥ GOAL SUMMARY FOR DOCTOR VISITS

The best way to improve your health is by being an active participant. Complete this form during and between each visit with your Parkinson's doctor or other healthcare professionals on your wellness team. Record your action steps and progress between visits. Review your results with your wellness team at each visit.

My goals for today's visit (date) ____ / ____ / ____ *are:*

1. _____
   _____
   _____
   _____

2. _____
   _____
   _____
   _____

3. _____
   _____
   _____
   _____

Action steps I will take to meet these goals are:

1. _____
   _____
   _____
   _____

▶

EVERY VICTORY COUNTS

2. _____

_____

_____

_____

3. _____

_____

_____

_____

Progress I have made toward these goals:

1. _____

_____

_____

_____

2. _____

_____

_____

_____

3. _____

_____

_____

_____

WORKSHEETS AND RESOURCES

Obstacles or areas for improvement needed to reach these goals are:

1. _____
_____
_____
_____

2. _____
_____
_____
_____

3. _____
_____
_____
_____

**MAKE A FILE FOR COPIES OF THIS AND OTHER FORMS TO
REFER BACK TO AS MARKERS OF YOUR TREATMENT OVER TIME.**

EVERY VICTORY COUNTS

♥ DAILY MEDICATION LOG

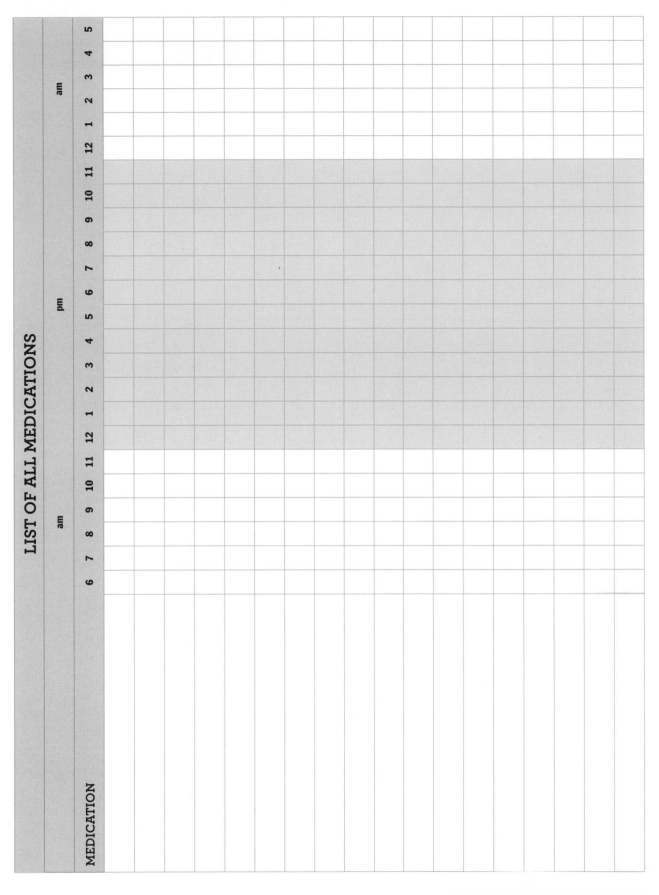

♥ OVERALL MEDICATION LOG

LIST OF ALL MEDICATIONS

MEDICATION	Started Medication	Ended Medication	Positive Effects	Negative Effects	Other Side Effects

EVERY VICTORY COUNTS

♥ WELLNESS SELF-ASSESSMENT

Complete this self-assessment after reading the **Living Well Now** section.

For each section below, record two areas you would like to improve and steps you will take for improvement. For instance, if you have not seen your primary care physician in the past year for a yearly physical, this can be listed with the action step to make an appointment within the next month.

Then, pick the top three items (from any category) you listed that you would like to achieve in the next month.

General Healthcare   *Check if Priority Item* ☐

This section focuses on general health items, such as preventative health screenings and blood pressure management.

1. Area of concern _____

   Actions to take _____

2. Area of concern _____

   Actions to take _____

Parkinson's Self-Care   *Check if Priority Item* ☐

This section focuses on preparing for your doctor's visits, emergency and hospital stays. It can also include taking the steps to take charge of your medications and learning about specialists who can be on your wellness team.

1. Area of concern _____

   Actions to take _____

2. Area of concern _____

   Actions to take _____

Physical Exercise

Check if Priority Item ☐

This section focuses on participation in exercise programs, improving symptoms such as pain, balance, decreased stamina and pursuing physical therapy.

1. Area of concern _____

   Actions to take _____

2. Area of concern _____

   Actions to take _____

Diet and Nutrition

Check if Priority Item ☐

This section focuses on changes you would like to make in your diet.

1. Area of concern _____

   Actions to take _____

2. Area of concern _____

   Actions to take _____

Emotional Health

Check if Priority Item ☐

This section focuses on treatment of depression, anxiety, apathy, stress reduction, relaxation, social engagement and spiritual growth.

1. Area of concern _____

   Actions to take _____

2. Area of concern _____

   Actions to take _____

♥ PRE-EXERCISE SELF-ASSESSMENT

Pre-exercise screening is a process allowing a doctor to review your medical and exercise history and assess risk factors that may impact your health and safety when engaging in an exercise program. If you are not exercising now and wish to begin, your primary care physician may call for pre-exercise testing, especially if you have heart or lung disease, high blood pressure or diabetes. With a neurological condition like Parkinson's, pre-exercise screening should be completed by a family doctor, clinical exercise specialist, clinical exercise physiologist or cardiologist.

Before starting a new exercise program, talk with your Parkinson's doctor about whether there are any safety concerns that specifically relate to your situation. This worksheet will allow you to assess both motor and non-motor symptoms that can impact your exercise. Although exercise is essential to living well with Parkinson's, it is important to consider and discuss with your doctor before you start or change your exercise routine.

Use the space below to check and describe symptoms or concerns you have related to exercise, as well as to record any recommendations from your wellness team about these concerns.

Motor Symptoms

☐ Dystonia (muscle spasms) worsens before, during or after exercise.

Concern: _____

Recommendation: _____

Ask your physical therapist to test your walking and balance and recommend exercises to include, as well as any to avoid.

☐ Exercise seems to worsen my dyskinesia.

Concern: _____

Recommendation: _____

Inform your doctor and discuss how to address your symptoms. You may be more prone to muscle tears during bouts of uncontrolled dyskinesia.

☐ I'm unsure whether I should exercise when I am in an "off" state.

Concern: _____

Recommendation: _____

If your medications wear "off," ask your doctor if you should avoid exercising when medications are not working well. Typically, stiffness, slowness and walking are worse when the medications are wearing "off," which can increase risk of injury.

WORKSHEETS AND RESOURCES

Non-Motor Symptoms

☐ I have difficultly falling or staying asleep.

Concern: _____

Recommendation: _____

Sleep problems can be improved with regular exercise, although avoid exercising close to bedtime. If you're taking sleep medications, ask your doctor if your medications can be reduced if exercise improves your sleep problems.

☐ Exercise-induced fatigue is a problem for me.

Concern: _____

Recommendation: _____

If fatigue is limiting your exercise plans, talk to your primary care doctor. Fatigue has many causes and may require an in-depth discussion to determine how to treat it.

☐ If my anxiety or depression symptoms improve with exercise, should I change my medications?

Concern: _____

Recommendation: _____

Exercise can have positive effects on emotional wellness. Ask your doctor whether mood control medications are still necessary if you are experiencing improvements as a result of exercise.

☐ I feel tired during the day, making it difficult to exercise.

Concern: _____

Recommendation: _____

Ask your doctor about ways to improve daytime sleepiness so that you can be more ready for exercise. You might need to plan exercise around times of day when you feel most alert and refreshed, as well as consider timing and nutrition of meals and snacks.

☐ Overactive bladder limits my ability to exercise.

Concern: _____

Recommendation: _____

Talk to your doctor if overactive bladder is limiting participation in exercise. Ask about minimum and maximum fluid intake per day for optimal hydration.

▶ ☐ Could my medications influence my blood pressure while exercising?

Concern: _____

Recommendation: _____

Talk to your doctor about whether the combination of your medications and exercise could alter your blood pressure. You might need to exercise at specific times of day to avoid either very low or high blood pressure.

☐ I have low or fluctuating blood pressure.

Concern: _____

Recommendation: _____

Low or fluctuating blood pressure can get worse if the intensity of your exercise is too much, so you may need to avoid certain exercises. Ask your doctor if your blood pressure is a concern to address when making your exercise plans.

☐ I have attention or concentration difficulties.

Concern: _____

Recommendation: _____

You might want to avoid complicated exercises and work individually with a trainer who can supervise you and keep you on task. Ask your doctor or physical therapist to determine whether your exercise program should be supervised.

☐ I experience cognition problems (sometimes or often).

Concern: _____

Recommendation: _____

Talk to your doctor about whether your cognitive health limits your exercise choices. For instance, you might not be able to swim alone or might need to use a treadmill only with supervision for safety.

Exercise Readiness

☐ I want to start a new exercise program.

Concern: _____

Recommendation: _____

Ask your doctor for a referral to see a physical therapist before starting a new exercise program.

Describe your current level of activity:

☐ I exercise regularly.

☐ I don't exercise regularly, but my lifestyle is somewhat active.

☐ I'm mostly sedentary.

What do you do to exercise or to stay active?

_____

_____

_____

How often do you engage in physical activity?

_____

What fitness concerns do you have?

☐ I want to increase my stamina and endurance.

Activities I'd like to improve through increased cardiovascular fitness:

_____

☐ I want to get stronger.

Activities I'd like to perform better through increased strength:

_____

☐ I want to be more flexible.

Activities or mobility I'd like to improve through increased flexibility and balance:

_____

Notes:

_____

_____

_____

_____

_____

EVERY VICTORY COUNTS

12

❤ EXERCISE JOURNAL

Use this journal to record your daily exercise activity. Download and print additional copies at ⌁ **dpf.org/worksheets** to help you keep track of your progress over time.

Week of: _____

DAY		CARDIOVASCULAR	STRETCHING	STRENGTHENING	OTHER
Sunday	Activity				
	Duration				
Monday	Activity				
	Duration				
Tuesday	Activity				
	Duration				
Wednesday	Activity				
	Duration				
Thursday	Activity				
	Duration				
Friday	Activity				
	Duration				
Saturday	Activity				
	Duration				

Example	Activity	*Walked outdoors*	*Seated stretches, standing stretches*	*10 lunges, 5 arm raises with 1 lb. weights*	*Took stairs to second floor office instead of using elevator*
	Duration	*20 minutes*	*10 minutes a.m., 10 minutes p.m.*	*15 minutes*	*—*

WORKSHEETS AND RESOURCES

♥ NUTRITION SELF-ASSESSMENT

Complete this self-assessment to determine what changes you can make in your diet to improve your wellness. Following these general guidelines can help you feel your best and address some common Parkinson's symptoms, such as constipation, fatigue, weight fluctuations and even various cognitive challenges. Refer to the "Diet and Nutrition" chapter in the **Living Well Now** section for detailed explanations of the nutrition information highlighted here. Be sure to discuss with your doctor and wellness team before making major changes to your diet.

See how your current diet stacks up with the recommendations below. If you can't check all the boxes in the first section, plan for what actions you will take to improve your basic nutrition. Which additional suggestions for optimal nutrition can you incorporate into your diet? Take a trip to your grocery store, local farmer's market or natural foods market to explore the possibilities. Make a list of new foods and supplements you'll incorporate into your diet. Exploring new flavors and cuisines can be fun!

GENERAL GUIDELINES
Daily Recommendations for Basic Nutrition

☐ Take a general multivitamin with calcium, phosphorous, vitamin B and D.

☐ Drink at least eight cups of fluid per day, including when you take your medication for general health and to avoid low blood pressure and constipation.

☐ Select healthy snacks such as fruits, nuts, yogurt, oats, milk or soy.

☐ Avoid processed foods high in sugar, "bad fats," unwanted chemicals and additives. These foods actually rob you of energy.

☐ Choose fresh, local and organic products if you can. This will increase the freshness, level of nutrients and limit pesticides or unnecessary additives.

☐ Be sure to consume adequate protein. Ask your doctor how much protein is right for you each day and when to best consume protein if you experience interactions with your medications.

☐ Avoid fad diets and supplements in high doses.

Additional Suggestions for Optimal Nutrition

☐ Consuming antioxidants is essential brain and heart health. See below for suggestions on antioxidants to include in your diet.

▶

EVERY VICTORY COUNTS

- [ ] Add omega-3s into your diet. Salmon, halibut, tuna, walnuts, almonds, ground flaxseed and fish oil tablets are good choices for omega-3s.

- [ ] Aim for 20–30 grams of fiber daily from fruits, vegetables and wheat products to help with digestion and constipation.

- [ ] Discuss with your doctor if you experience weight gain or weight loss. Some medical conditions can cause weight changes.

- [ ] Determine whether you are getting adequate levels of calcium and vitamin D, which are important supplements for bone strength.

- [ ] Consult the "Constipation Worksheet" and "Low Blood Pressure or Dizziness Worksheet" for more specific information tailored to these problems.

ANTIOXIDANTS

The following high-nutrient foods are also high in antioxidants thought to be helpful in maintaining brain and heart health:

Vitamin C: green vegetables, tomatoes, strawberries, broccoli, citrus fruits and juices, apple juice, potatoes, kiwi, green, red and yellow peppers

Vitamin E: whole grains including brown rice, green vegetables, nuts, seeds, vegetable oils, wheat germ, papayas, avocados, sweet potatoes and peanut butter

Vitamin A (Carotenoids): sweet potatoes, carrots, tomatoes, kale, collard greens, apricots, cantaloupe, peaches, pumpkin, broccoli and pink grapefruit

Selenium: eggs, garlic, chicken, fish, grains, wheat germ and bran, Brazil nuts, shellfish and beans

Lignans: flaxseed and oil (omega-3 fatty oils), rye, oatmeal and barley

Flavinoids: soy, dark chocolate (70% cacao), red grapes, cranberries, green or white tea and pomegranate

Lycopene: watermelon, pink grapefruit and tomatoes

Lutein: spinach, kale, broccoli, kiwi, Brussels sprouts and other dark green vegetables

Recommended foods that are rich in antioxidants and offer other health benefits:
- Ground flaxseed (provides fiber, omega-3 fatty acids and lignan)
- Salmon (provides omega-3 fatty acids and selenium)
- Soy products (provide protein and good source of all the essential amino acids, calcium, zinc, iron, magnesium, phosphorus, omega-3 fatty acids, fiber and B vitamins)

315

- Whole grains (provide B vitamins, vitamin E, iron and magnesium)
- Berries (provide vitamin C, folate, fiber and high antioxidant properties)
- Green vegetables (provide vitamin A and C, calcium and iron)

CoEnzyme Q10: A 2014 study did not show added benefit when used early in Parkinson's. However, CoQ10 has not been shown to be harmful. Discuss with your doctor before adding this supplement to your diet.

Antioxidant supplements are also available, but should not be used in place of a healthy diet. Speak with your doctor about appropriate choices and brands when taken into consideration with your current medications.

Make a list of items you will add to your regular diet:

1. _____   6. _____

2. _____   7. _____

3. _____   8. _____

4. _____   9. _____

5. _____   10. _____

♥ PARKINSON'S PSYCHOSIS SELF-ASSESSMENT

Sometimes Parkinson's itself or side effects of medications can change your perception of reality, resulting in Parkinson's psychosis. Parkinson's psychosis typically takes the form of hallucinations (experiencing things visually or otherwise that are not really there), delusions (a false belief or impression that you hold to firmly, even though it is irrational or illogical) or both. Some people are aware what they are experiencing is not actually real, while others are not.

Review the statements below together with your care partner and discuss with your doctor if you are experiencing any of the following:

For People Living with Parkinson's

☐ I've seen, heard or smelled things, such as people, animals or objects, that weren't actually there.

☐ I've had experiences, such as the vivid sensation of someone in the room with me or a brief vision of movement, when there was nothing actually there.

☐ I've looked at something and seen it appear briefly as something else. For example, words on a page appearing as insects.

☐ I've had beliefs or fears, such as my loved one abandoning me, being unfaithful or stealing from me.

For Care Partners and Family Members

☐ My loved one has seen things, heard things or felt things that weren't actually there.

☐ My loved one has experienced any false beliefs toward me or others, such as believing someone is stealing from them or that I'm being unfaithful.

☐ These false beliefs or visualizations have affected our daily lives.

Content used with permission from ACADIA® Pharmaceuticals

WORKSHEETS AND RESOURCES

♥ DEEP BRAIN STIMULATION (DBS) SELF-ASSESSMENT

DEFINING AND ASSESSING EXPECTATIONS

One of the most important discussions you can have with your doctor and your family before considering or undergoing DBS surgery is about defining realistic expectations. You should ask your doctor about how DBS will change **your** symptoms and motor function, not just about how DBS can help Parkinson's symptoms in general. Setting appropriate expectations before surgery can help pave the way for greater satisfaction with results in the many years that follow. Complete this self-assessment and use it to guide the discussion with your doctor and family.

What Parkinson's symptoms do you expect to be improved by DBS in order for you to be satisfied with the procedure outcome?

1. _____   4. _____

2. _____   5. _____

3. _____   6. _____

Considering all your Parkinson's symptoms, place them in the appropriate categories below:

Symptoms That Improve with Medication (most likely to respond to DBS)	Symptoms That <u>Do Not</u> Improve with Medication (not likely to respond to DBS)	Other Bothersome Symptoms Not Listed (discuss further with your doctor)
_____	_____	_____
_____	_____	_____
_____	_____	_____
_____	_____	_____
_____	_____	_____

▶

▶ The symptoms that respond favorably to Parkinson's medications typically respond well to deep brain stimulation, with tremor being the exception. Even if tremor does not respond well to medications, it will typically respond well to stimulation. Stiffness, slowness, posture, gait shuffling and tremor generally improve noticeably with stimulation. People who have DBS typically experience more "on" time and less dyskinesia and "off" time, once the stimulation settings have been optimized.

Completing this worksheet can help guide you through the important process of determining whether DBS may be appropriate for you. Although each individual experiences varying symptoms and severity, understanding how your symptoms may or may not be managed by DBS is a key factor in determining whether or not you are a candidate for the surgery and whether the benefits you can reasonably expect merit undergoing the procedure.

Other questions to think about and to discuss with your doctor:

1. Do my Parkinson's symptoms bother me enough to undergo brain surgery?
2. Do I understand the risks associated with the surgical implantation of the hardware?
3. Have I asked the surgeon about his/her specific rates of surgical complications?
4. Are my expectations reasonable enough to proceed with a DBS work-up?
5. Do I have any medical conditions that increase my risks of complications during DBS surgery?
6. Do I have adequate access to medical professionals that can adjust the stimulation settings once I have the implantation (helping with my maintenance over time)?
7. Are there any medical, environmental or exercise considerations after DBS?
8. How long will the implanted neurostimulator last?
9. How long will I need to take off work?
10. How long will I be restricted from driving?
11. What is the process leading up to surgery like?
12. What can I expect during the surgery?
13. What can I expect after surgery?

♥ OUR RELATIONSHIP SELF-ASSESSMENT

Parkinson's can affect many of your relationships, especially with your partner. Communication is crucial: make time to talk openly and honestly with your partner about your relationship. Questions to consider as you have a candid conversation with your partner include:

What has changed in our relationship that we are reluctant to discuss?

_____

_____

What could I do to make the relationship stronger?

_____

_____

What am I doing that is causing unnecessary stress on the relationship?

_____

_____

What is working well?

_____

_____

What needs more attention?

_____

_____

Could we meet with a specialist for guidance?

_____

_____

EVERY VICTORY COUNTS

☑ MY SYMPTOMS WORKSHEET

Use this body map to circle symptoms or problem areas that you would like to discuss with your doctor or other member of your wellness team. While most of these are symptoms of Parkinson's itself, some are side effects of Parkinson's medications. On the next page, indicate how bothersome each symptom is for you.

Bring the worksheet to discuss with your doctor at your next appointment.

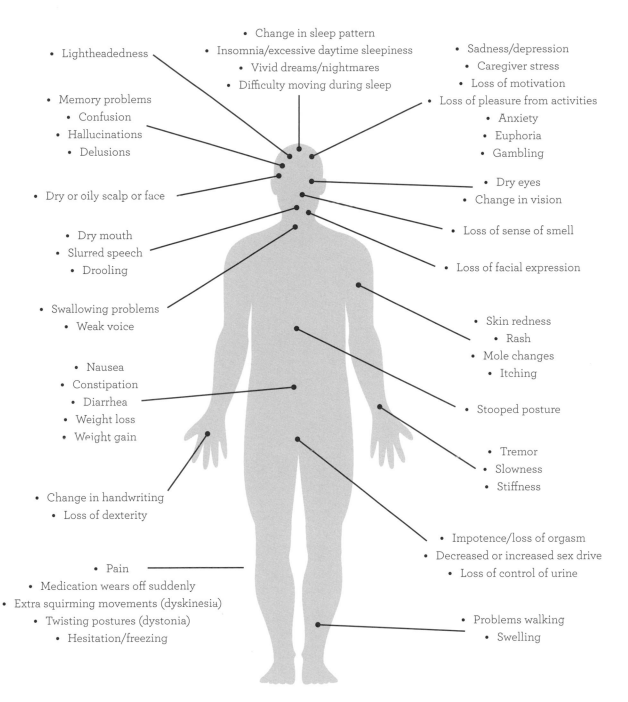

- Lightheadedness
- Change in sleep pattern
- Insomnia/excessive daytime sleepiness
- Vivid dreams/nightmares
- Difficulty moving during sleep
- Sadness/depression
- Caregiver stress
- Loss of motivation
- Loss of pleasure from activities
- Memory problems
- Confusion
- Hallucinations
- Delusions
- Anxiety
- Euphoria
- Gambling
- Dry or oily scalp or face
- Dry eyes
- Change in vision
- Dry mouth
- Slurred speech
- Drooling
- Loss of sense of smell
- Loss of facial expression
- Swallowing problems
- Weak voice
- Skin redness
- Rash
- Mole changes
- Itching
- Nausea
- Constipation
- Diarrhea
- Weight loss
- Weight gain
- Stooped posture
- Tremor
- Slowness
- Stiffness
- Change in handwriting
- Loss of dexterity
- Impotence/loss of orgasm
- Decreased or increased sex drive
- Loss of control of urine
- Pain
- Medication wears off suddenly
- Extra squirming movements (dyskinesia)
- Twisting postures (dystonia)
- Hesitation/freezing
- Problems walking
- Swelling

32

WORKSHEETS AND RESOURCES

Rate how each symptom or area of daily life bothers you by circling a number on a scale from 0 to 5.

0 = No Problem or No Concern   **5 = Severe Problem or Biggest Concern**

Anxiety	0	1	2	3	4	5
Bathing, Dressing	0	1	2	3	4	5
Bladder Problems	0	1	2	3	4	5
Chest Pain or Palpitations	0	1	2	3	4	5
Chills	0	1	2	3	4	5
Constipation	0	1	2	3	4	5
Cough or Sore Throat	0	1	2	3	4	5
Delusions	0	1	2	3	4	5
Depression	0	1	2	3	4	5
Double or Blurred Vision	0	1	2	3	4	5
Dyskinesia	0	1	2	3	4	5
Falls	0	1	2	3	4	5
Fatigue	0	1	2	3	4	5
Fine Motor Movement, like folding clothes or opening mail	0	1	2	3	4	5
Freezing	0	1	2	3	4	5
Hallucinations	0	1	2	3	4	5
Headache	0	1	2	3	4	5
Hearing Loss	0	1	2	3	4	5
Heartburn or Upset Stomach	0	1	2	3	4	5
Impulsivity	0	1	2	3	4	5
Joint Pain	0	1	2	3	4	5
Leg Swelling	0	1	2	3	4	5
Lightheadedness	0	1	2	3	4	5
Motivation	0	1	2	3	4	5

Muscle Spasm	0	1	2	3	4	5
Nausea/Vomiting	0	1	2	3	4	5
"Off" Time	0	1	2	3	4	5
Pain	0	1	2	3	4	5
Rash or Bruising	0	1	2	3	4	5
Rigidity	0	1	2	3	4	5
Seizures	0	1	2	3	4	5
Sexual Function	0	1	2	3	4	5
Sleep	0	1	2	3	4	5
Slowness of Movement	0	1	2	3	4	5
Speech	0	1	2	3	4	5
Swallowing	0	1	2	3	4	5
Sweating	0	1	2	3	4	5
Thinking	0	1	2	3	4	5
Tremor	0	1	2	3	4	5
Walking	0	1	2	3	4	5
Writing	0	1	2	3	4	5

WORKSHEETS AND RESOURCES

☑ BLADDER WORKSHEET

Bladder problems can occur as a result of how Parkinson's affects the nerves that control emptying the bladder. This can lead to an overactive bladder in people living with Parkinson's, and/or incontinence, the accidental or involuntary loss of control of urine or bowel movements. This can range from occasional minor leakage to complete loss of control of urine or bowel movements. Review this worksheet for ideas of changes you can make to improve bladder problems, checking those you can implement right now.

Dietary Changes

☐ Drink fluids for general health, but limit after 5:00 p.m. if you urinate frequently at night.

Lifestyle Changes

☐ Wear pads to reduce stress, anxiety and increase your freedom to go out.

☐ Be safe. Talk with an occupational therapist about safety measures to take at home, such as grab bars in the bathroom, night lights to illuminate your path at night, a bedside commode or urinals when appropriate.

Treatments

☐ See your doctor about abrupt changes in bladder control, since this could signal a bladder infection. Also, an abrupt decline in movement or thinking functions can be the first sign of a bladder infection.

☐ Physical therapy can help with pelvic floor exercises to improve incontinence.

☐ Occupational therapy can help with bladder therapy, bathroom and hygiene, as well as offer many safety techniques to reduce falls.

☐ Review bladder control with your doctor. Certain medical conditions affect bladder control. Some medications cause muscle weakness and can therefore weaken bladder control.

☐ A urologist can help if incontinence continues despite treatment.

☐ Be sure to tell your doctor if you have memory or thinking problems, as certain bladder control medications can worsen memory.

EVERY VICTORY COUNTS

☑ COGNITIVE WELLNESS WORKSHEET

Thinking and processing can be improved in many enjoyable ways. Brain games, physical activity and social engagement all boost your brain health, which leads to increased cognitive wellness. Visit your community center, senior center or local community college to see what programs are available to you and your family. Many libraries, universities, school districts and online outlets also offer adult learning programs covering a wide range of interests. You can also ask your healthcare provider for a referral to an occupational, recreational, art, music or physical therapist for more focused cognitive wellness programs.

Make the commitment to schedule activities that challenge your brain into your routine. Choose things and people you enjoy, pace yourself and remember to have fun.

Increase Physical Activity

☐ Consult with a physical therapist to develop the best, safest exercise program for you.

☐ Exercise three to five times a week. Personal trainers can motivate and help you stick to your routine.

☐ Don't exercise alone: involve your family or a buddy, walk in the park, go to a group exercise class. Getting to know others in exercise classes can provide a sense of connection and accountability to go.

☐ Yoga and tai chi give extra benefits of relaxation and improve balance.

☐ Dance and music add fun, joy and allow creative expression.

Flex Your "Thinking Muscles"

☐ Read or listen to documentaries, and/or books on tape.

☐ Do brain teasers, such as video games, word games, sudoku or puzzles.

☐ Play cards. Bridge, poker, euchre or solitaire are some examples.

Engage Socially and Creatively

☐ Attend support groups.

☐ Take an art, music, drama, crafting or dancing class.

☐ Attend a poetry or book group.

☐ Join or organize your own coffee hour, dinner group or movie night.

☑ CONSTIPATION WORKSHEET

Digestive health and specific problems, like constipation, can be improved through dietary and lifestyle changes. Check the items listed on this worksheet to indicate actions you can take to improve your constipation. Discuss any problems that may persist with your doctor.

Dietary Changes

☐ Drink at least eight cups of fluid per day.

☐ Be sure you are eating 20–30 grams of fiber per day. Good examples are prunes, pears, nuts, grains, ground flaxseed and bran.

☐ Eat a well-balanced diet with plenty of fruits, vegetables, multigrain breads and cereals. Eat smaller meals several times per day, rather than three large meals.

☐ Avoid high-sugar foods and snacks.

☐ Choose high-fiber bread (>5 grams fiber) instead of refined white or wheat bread.

☐ Try homeopathic herbal teas blended to help relieve constipation.

☐ Try drinking a caffeinated warm beverages with earlier meals, but avoid carbonated beverages if bloating is a problem.

Lifestyle Changes

☐ Exercise! At least take a walk daily, if possible. A physical therapist can help you get started with an exercise routine that's right for you.

☐ Try to maintain good posture while doing cardio or strengthening exercises.

Medication Recommendations
(Note: talk to your doctor before beginning)

☐ Stool softeners once or twice a day can help. You can also try a stool softener with a stimulant if you experience moderate to severe constipation.

☐ Glycolax powder (like Miralax) can be purchased over the counter and is very effective, has few side effects and can be used daily if needed.

☐ Consider taking once-a-day supplements, such as fish oil, flaxseed oil or magnesium.

☐ Avoid excessive use of fiber supplements such as Metamucil or Citrucel as they can sometimes worsen constipation and lead to obstruction.

EVERY VICTORY COUNTS

▶ Other Treatment

☐ Ask your doctor about medications you may be taking that can worsen constipation, such as amantadine, amitriptyline and sedatives.

☐ Consider seeing a gastroenterologist, a specialist who treats constipation.

☐ Occupational therapy can help establish a bowel routine or regimen.

☐ Ask your doctor for a nutrition consult if you need more help with dietary changes.

WORKSHEETS AND RESOURCES

☑ DENTAL WORKSHEET

Dental care is an integral part of living well with Parkinson's. Regular dental care can minimize your risk of experiencing pain and discomfort, but most importantly, it can reduce the risk of infection, which can be a significant stressor on the body when coupled with Parkinson's-related challenges.

Dietary Changes

☐ Choose a nutritious snack between meals like cheese, milk, plain yogurt, fruits, vegetables or nuts. Sugary snacks (like candy), soda and sticky food (like dried fruits) can put you at risk for cavities and other oral health problems.

☐ Citrus fruits and other acidic foods (like oranges, tomatoes and red meat) should be eaten as *part* of a meal instead of separately, since the acidity of these foods can have a negative effect on tooth enamel.

☐ Talk with your primary care physician about including cheese, milk, calcium-fortified tofu, leafy greens, almonds, meat, poultry, fish and eggs in meals. These have high calcium, nutrient and phosphorus levels and may assist in dental health but prevent medication absorption.

☐ Drink your daily intake of fluids to avoid dehydration and dry mouth.

Lifestyle Changes

☐ Schedule tooth brushing around medication "on" times.

☐ Replace your toothbrush or toothbrush bristles every 3–4 months, after you've been sick or when it starts to show signs of wear such as frayed bristles.

☐ Brush your teeth three times a day or after each meal for two minutes to remove sugars and food particles from your teeth.

☐ Floss daily. Instruments like a flossing proxy brush can help ease the process, or a care partner can assist.

☐ Use moisturizing mouth spray, non-alcohol based mouthwash, a fluoride rinse or oral swab brushes daily if you experience dry mouth or inflammation (common Parkinson's medication side effects).

☐ Use a wide handle toothbrush or add an adaptive device to facilitate easier grip on the toothbrush handle.

☐ Consider an electric, ultrasonic or specialty toothbrush to maximize brushing benefits.

▶

EVERY VICTORY COUNTS

- [ ] ▶ Ask your dentist about using a biteguard if you have bruxism (grinding of teeth).

- [ ] Ask your dentist about prescription strength, topical stannous fluoride gel treatments and toothpastes, as these can be good preventative strategies.

Treatments

- [ ] Visit your dentist every 6 months for regular, short (45 minutes or less) check-ups.

- [ ] Complete the "Daily Medication Log" in this section, and bring it to your dental visit to address important risks of medication interactions during your dental appointment. Anesthesia and novocaine can cause increased sedation, imbalance or confusion.

- [ ] Schedule your appointments during your medications "on" time and when your dyskinesia is not generally bothersome.

- [ ] Ask to keep the dentist chair 45° incline or higher to enable comfortable swallowing.

- [ ] Request frequent suctioning to assist with saliva production and muscle weakness.

- [ ] Have your dentist or care partner assist you in and out of the dental chair to reduce the risk of a fall.

- [ ] Include your dentist in your wellness team, making sure they have an understanding of how Parkinson's disease may affect your oral health.

- [ ] Collaborate with your dentist to determine a signal for discomfort; for example, put your hand up to signal you need a break or are having trouble swallowing.

☑ DYSKINESIA AND "OFF" TIME LOG

Name: _____

Date: _____

1. In the Medications row, place an **X** under the hour that you took your medicine; draw a line though the hours that you are asleep.

2. In the Dyskinesia row, indicate the severity by entering the correct number. Use the guide below to determine which number is appropriate.

   0 = No extra movement
   1 = Mild extra movement
   2 = Moderate movement
   3 = Severe disabling movement

3. In the "Off" row, indicate if you felt that your medicine is not working using the following guide.

   0 = Feeling no symptoms
   1 = Mild tremor, stiffness or slowness without disability
   2 = Moderate tremor, stiffness or slowness, possibly requiring assistance
   3 = Severe tremor, stiffness or slowness requiring total assistance

TIME	am						am						pm						pm						am					
	6	7	8	9	10	11	12	1	2	3	4	5	6	7	8	9	10	11	12	1	2	3	4	5						
1. Medications (Place an **X** at the time of your dose)																														
2. Dyskinesia (See scale above)																														
3. "Off" (See scale above)																														

Keep this diary 3 days before your appointment and bring it with you.

EVERY VICTORY COUNTS

☑ EMOTIONAL WELLNESS: ANXIETY

Identify Triggers

☐ Keep a diary to identify triggers that worsen anxiety.

Some triggers I've identified are: _____

_____

☐ Record times when anxiety is worse. For instance, anxiety can increase when medications wear "off."

I've noticed my anxiety is worse when: _____

_____

Address Your Anxiety

☐ Talk with your doctor about treatment that can include medicine, relaxation techniques, counseling, mindfulness and coping strategies.

☐ Learn to breathe. Simple exercises consisting of 10–20 slow, steady deep breaths can be calming.

Reduce Stimulants

Avoid nicotine, diet or energy pills and caffeine.

Substance	Current Use	Goal for Reducing
Nicotine	_____x week	_____x week
Energy pills/drinks	_____x week	_____x week
Diet pills	_____ x week	_____x week
Caffeine	_____x week	_____x week

Implement Relaxation Techniques

☐ Try breathing exercises, guided imagery, biofeedback, meditation or prayer. Many community, recreation and senior centers offer meditation or yoga classes. There are also many good books from which you can learn more about these techniques.

☐ Plan relaxation breaks during the day. Take a moment to take a breathe deeply, slowly inhaling and exhaling 10 times to prevent an anxiety attack (or to calm one in progress).

☐ Use soft or meditative music, or guided meditation or yoga videos to help you relax. Establish a quiet space at home for relaxation. Try using aromatherapy, soft lighting and soothing surroundings to help you relax.

Change Your Habits

☐ Avoid taking on too many tasks or always saying "yes." Maintain a routine, and prioritize chores and commitments by making lists. An occupational therapist can help with this.

☐ Exercise to help relieve tension. Gentle stretching helps relax the face, shoulders and back. Try yoga or tai chi.

☐ Talk about your feelings of stress or anxiety with loved ones. Consider sharing your observations about what triggers these feelings, and talk about how they can support your efforts to reduce stress and anxiety in your life.

☐ Take a moment for yourself. Try a soothing cup of tea; chamomile, lemon balm or valerian root may have anxiety-fighting benefits for some people.

EVERY VICTORY COUNTS

☑ EMOTIONAL WELLNESS: DEPRESSION

Identify Triggers

☐ Keep a diary to identify triggers or thoughts that worsen your mood. Record times when depression is worse. For instance, depression can worsen when medications wear "off."

Some triggers I've identified are: _____

_____

Address Depression

☐ Talk with your doctor about treatment. This can include medicine (such as antidepressants), counseling, cognitive behavioral therapy or relaxation techniques.

☐ Obtain a general medical examination. Some medications, thyroid disease, heart disease and illness can cause or worsen depression.

☐ Explore light therapy if you suffer from seasonal/winter depression.

☐ If you are currently taking antidepressants, closely monitor with your doctor. Some studies have found that antidepressants may exacerbate other Parkinson's symptoms.

Add Positive Energy

☐ Spend five minutes a day thinking about or visualizing life's pleasures or what you are grateful for, such as family, grandchildren, pets.

☐ Spend time to reflect on the beauty of the natural world around you.

☐ Volunteer. It can be uplifting and rewarding.

☐ Laugh with others. Watch comedies. Children and pets bring a smile.

☐ Dance, paint, sing, share memories with others around you.

Change Your Habits

☐ Eat a well-balanced diet. Consult the "Nutrition Self-Assessment" in this section for more ideas of how to improve your diet.

☐ Take medications as prescribed.

☐ Tend to sleep habits. Consult both the "Fatigue Worksheet" and the "Insomnia and Sleep Worksheet" in this section for tips to improve your sleep hygiene.

Be Connected

☐ Attend classes, support groups, call a friend, join a positive chat group or a buddy program.

☐ Attend to your spiritual needs.

EVERY VICTORY COUNTS

☑ FATIGUE WORKSHEET

Complete this worksheet to determine if certain times of day or activities trigger your fatigue. Record observations you have about when you feel fatigued and what other things are happening when you do, and check the actions you can take right now to improve your energy.

I feel fatigued most often:

☐ Early morning

☐ Late morning

☐ Early afternoon

☐ Late afternoon

☐ Evening

☐ My mood or emotional state seems to make me feel more fatigued.

How often does this occur? _____

_____

Other situations I've noticed make me feel fatigued: _____

_____

Lifestyle Changes

☐ Exercise to improve strength and endurance. This improves mood and reduces the energy required to do daily activities.

☐ Exercise when you feel good, such as when the effects of your medications are at their best. Pace yourself, though. Don't overdo it.

☐ Pay attention to your sleep habits. Use short naps (between 10 and 20 minutes) during the day, if needed. However, limit naps. Sleeping excessively during the day can actually increase your sleepiness and fatigue, as well as make it more difficult to sleep at night.

☐ Avoid post-lunch fatigue by keeping your mind active with games, puzzles or hobbies or taking a walk outside.

WORKSHEETS AND RESOURCES

Dietary Changes

☐ Eat small, frequent meals instead of big, heavy meals. Don't skip breakfast. Be sure to get plenty of fluids.

☐ Snack on high-energy foods such as apples, oranges, pears, yogurt, walnuts, almonds, oats and whole-grain products. Avoid processed, high-sugar foods which can rob you of your energy.

☐ Caffeine can be helpful for midday fatigue or sleepiness if permitted by your doctor. Avoid caffeine after 3:00 p.m.

☐ See general dietary guidelines in the "Nutrition Self-Assessment" and in the "Diet and Nutrition" chapter in the **Living Well Now** section.

Treatment

☐ Take Parkinson's medications on time to avoid wearing "off."

☐ Avoid energy pills!

☐ See you doctor for a checkup. Anemia, malnutrition, sleep apnea, depression, thyroid and vitamin deficiencies can cause fatigue. Review your medications (prescription and over-the-counter) as some can cause fatigue and worsen daytime sleepiness.

☐ See an occupational therapist for energy conservation techniques and physical therapist or personal trainer for exercise guidance.

☐ Refer to the **Living Well Now** section for helpful tips on sleep, anxiety and depression. These are all problems that can reduce your energy levels.

☑ GAIT, BALANCE AND FREEZING WORKSHEET

Many of the main motor symptoms of Parkinson's—tremor, rigidity, stiffness and postural instability—can cause difficulties with walking and balance. Freezing, problems initiating movements that often results in feeling like your feet are glued to the floor, is especially common in the later stages of Parkinson's. This worksheet provides ideas to help improve gait and balance and to manage freezing. Check the options you can begin to implement right now and be sure to discuss any continuing challenges with your doctor and wellness team.

Physical Exercise and Training

☐ Perform balance exercises every day, even before you think you need them. Consider it part of your routine, like brushing your teeth. Balance is critical for walking. You can always improve your balance, even if it seems perfect right now! For more specific balance exercises, see the "Balancing Life, Exercise and Function for Optimal Health" article in the "Complementary Therapies" chapter of the **Living Well Now** section.

☐ Exercise daily. Include stretching, strengthening and exercises to help you get out of a chair, stand straighter and walk farther.

☐ See a physical therapist who specializes in movement disorders to develop a home exercise program, even if you have one. Ask your PT when you should be re-evaluated. Do not wait for your doctor to initiate it – you can ask for it. See the "Why Exercise Matters" chapter in the **Living Well Now** section for more details about at-home exercises to improve gait, balance and freezing.

☐ Practice making wide U-turns rather than pivot turns to avoid falling.

☐ Use a walking aid if you need help walking. It will help you walk better, keep you safe and remain independent longer. Be sure you see your physical therapist to choose the correct cane or walker. Using the wrong one can actually cause falls!

Lifestyle and Good Habits

☐ Get in the habit of daily exercise. Five minutes of exercise daily is better than 20 minutes once a week.

☐ Establish a routine. Write your goals and expectations on a calendar.

☐ Try to time your exercise to the time of day you feel best, such as when your medications are working.

WORKSHEETS AND RESOURCES

- [ ] Exercise with a buddy. Everyone in your family can benefit. Consider a "balance night" devoted to balance games. You do not need fancy video games for this. Make up your own challenges. Keep safety first, though. It is a good idea to involve your physical therapist before beginning.

- [ ] Avoid multitasking. Do one thing at a time. Avoid carrying multiple objects in both hands if you have trouble walking. This helps you focus on the task of walking if you have trouble.

Dietary Changes

- [ ] Dizziness and low blood pressure can cause weakness, fatigue, loss of consciousness and falls. See the "Low Blood Pressure and Dizziness Worksheet" as well as the and "Nutrition Self-Assessment" for additional treatment recommendations.

- [ ] Eat the high-energy foods explained in the "Diet and Nutrition" chapter in the **Living Well Now** section, rather than processed, high-sugar foods that rob you of your energy.

Treatment

- [ ] There is a tendency to blame difficulties solely on Parkinson's, but there are many causes of walking and balance problems. Fatigue, heart and lung conditions, muscle weakness, stroke, inner-ear problems, peripheral neuropathy, joint pain and arthritis are all examples of conditions that occur more often as we age. Talk with your doctor to be sure that these potential other problems are treated.

Tips for Freezing

Freezing (feet stuck to the floor) occurs in crowded, small places. Often, the act of initiating movement, such as when you stand and begin walking, make a turn or with any stop and start of movement, prompts freezing.

- [ ] Learn to make wide "U-turns." Avoid pivoting. If you use a walker, be sure your walker is the right type for freezing.

- [ ] See your physical therapist to review cueing strategies. Cueing from lasers, guided imagery, marching or even walking to the beat of a musical rhythm can help get you over or through a freezing spell. For instance, sing the first few lines of a common song like "Happy Birthday" in your head to help get "unstuck."

- [ ] See your occupational therapist to review areas that cause you to freeze. Can crowded spaces be identified, such as bathrooms or closets? Can these areas be modified by removing clutter?

EVERY VICTORY COUNTS

▶ ☐ Experiment with flooring and shoes. Shoes with soft rubber soles are comfortable, but may "stick" to the floor. Different flooring textures, color changes and patterns can precipitate freezing, such as changing from tile to carpet.

☐ Experiment with putting tape on the floor, a step distance apart. This can serve as a visual cue to help you lift your legs to walk over and through a tight space or threshold.

☑ INSOMNIA AND SLEEP WORKSHEET

Trouble falling asleep and staying asleep are very common in people living with Parkinson's. This worksheet provides a range of strategies for preparing your body for rest and for giving yourself the best possible sleep environment. Take a good look at your sleep routine using the list below. Note habits you'd like to change, and decide which recommendations you will incorporate into your routine in the future. Talk to your doctor about sleep concerns you may have, as well as strategies you've tried to improve your sleep.

Sleep Hygiene

☐ Remove TV, computers, tablets, cellphones and other technology devices from your bedroom. Keep the room dark and use night lights that can easily be turned on, such as motion-activated lights that will turn on when you walk to the bathroom.

☐ Establish a routine: go to bed and get up the same time each evening and morning.

☐ Avoid intense TV shows, video games or anxiety-provoking activities before bed. This is not the time to pay your bills! Try relaxing music, gentle stretching, aromatherapy, meditation and massage before bed.

☐ Avoid bright lights and screens at night. Many computers, tablets, smartphones and other devices have "blue light reduction" options you can either activate or download to reduce the impact of the specific light of computer screens that can keep you awake.

Dietary Changes

☐ Avoid stimulants such as caffeinated drinks after 3:00 p.m. Avoid alcohol completely or limit to one glass.

☐ Avoid heavy, starchy meals or snacks before bed. Try foods with tryptophan, such as poultry and milk.

Lifestyle Changes

☐ Take a warm bath to relax before bedtime.

☐ Limit catnaps during day to 10 to 20 minutes before 3:00 p.m.

☐ Avoid exercise at night, but do exercise daily.

▶

EVERY VICTORY COUNTS

Bed Comfort

- ☐ Use silk or satin pajamas or sheets if you have trouble turning.

- ☐ Consider a sturdy, secure headboard that you can use to help turn over in bed.

- ☐ Examine your mattress. Has it seen better days?

- ☐ An occupational therapist can also help with bed comfort.

Treatment

- ☐ See your doctor to optimize motor control and Parkinson's medication.

- ☐ Depression, anxiety, pain, restless legs syndrome, vivid dreaming, incontinence and sleep apnea can be treated. Discuss with your doctor.

- ☐ A sleep study may be needed to diagnose sleep apnea if you snore.

- ☐ Sleep medications can cause daytime sleepiness, confusion and weakness. You may not need them if you develop good sleep habits.

341

WORKSHEETS AND RESOURCES

☑ LOW BLOOD PRESSURE AND DIZZINESS WORKSHEET

Dizziness or lightheadedness can occur as a direct symptom of Parkinson's or as a side effect of some Parkinson's medications. You can also experience lightheadedness if you do not drink enough fluids or restrict salt in your diet.

Parkinson's may lower your blood pressure, as can the medications used to treat the movement symptoms of Parkinson's. This worksheet provides helpful lifestyle changes you can make to address low blood pressure and dizziness. Check the changes you can make now, but be sure to discuss with your doctor to identify root causes and other potential solutions. For more information about how to address low blood pressure and dizziness, consult the "Neurogenic Orthostatic Hypotension (nOH) in Parkinson's" article in the **What You Need to Know About Parkinson's** section.

Dietary Changes

☐ Increase fluid intake to eight cups per day. Caffeine can help, but use in moderation. Sports drinks and salty drinks such as Gatorade or V8 are helpful, but may not be safe if you have diabetes, hypertension or heart disease. Check with your doctor before you make any changes.

☐ Get in the habit of drinking a full cup of water every time you take a dose of your medication.

☐ Avoid alcohol.

☐ Add salt to your diet if approved by your doctor.

☐ Eat small meals to avoid blood pressure drops that can occur after large meals.

☐ Reduce your consumption of high-glycemic carbohydrates, like white breads, rice and pastas, sugary juices, cereals and sweets.

☐ Increase your consumption of low-glycemic index carbohydrates, like whole-grain breads, rice and pasta, fruits and nuts.

Lifestyle Changes

☐ Elevate the head of your bed by 30° by placing blocks under the legs of your bed or getting a mattress that can be easily adjusted. Simply adding more pillows may not help.

☐ Stand slowly to give your blood pressure time to adjust to a change in position.

▶

EVERY VICTORY COUNTS

- ▶ ☐ Wear compression stockings to help keep fluid in your blood vessels and reduce leg swelling.

- ☐ Avoid holding your breath or contracting your stomach muscles excessively when standing.

Treatment

- ☐ Review your medications with your doctor. Many medications, including Parkinson's medications, can reduce your blood pressure.

- ☐ Physical therapy can show you exercises that can reduce drops in blood pressure when standing, such as contracting your leg muscles before you stand.

- ☐ Talk to your doctor about medications to increase blood pressure if other measures are not helpful.

- ☐ If you take medications for high blood pressure, speak to your doctor about whether you still need them.

- ☐ Treat constipation, since straining may cause dizziness.

WORKSHEETS AND RESOURCES

☑ SPEECH AND COMMUNICATION WORKSHEET

Many people living with Parkinson's experience difficulties speaking and communicating. These challenges may show up as a quiet voice, unclear speech, trouble finding words or reduced facial expression. Review the worksheet below for ideas you can use to improve your speech and communication. Check the tips you plan to put into practice.

Speaking Tips

☐ Pace your words if you talk too fast.

☐ Begin talking by sitting up straight, taking a deep breath and opening your mouth.

☐ Singing is fun and helps keep your voice flexible and increases your breath support. Try karaoke or simply sing along to your favorite songs.

☐ Practice facial exercises like the sounds "ooh" and "ahh" with exaggeration in your mouth to reduce muscle stiffness.

Breathing Tips

☐ Open your chest by sitting up straight to allow for big, deep breaths. Breathing deeply helps increase your volume of speech.

☐ Practice deep breathing daily. Yoga, tai chi and meditation classes can all help you learn breathing exercises.

Communication Tips

☐ Improve communication with your care partner. A speech therapist and counselor can help with ideas such as active listening and other recommendations focused on staying engaged in communication and relationships, even when common verbal or non-verbal cues may be different because of Parkinson's.

☐ Get your hearing checked to ensure it is not impaired.

☐ Don't let conversation bypass you. If you are in a group setting, ask the group to pause, reminding them that you or your partner would like to speak and be heard!

☐ Use body language and hand gestures during a conversation to help tell your story, especially if your facial muscles do not express emotion like they used to.

▶

EVERY VICTORY COUNTS

▶ Treatment

☐ Seek out a speech therapist early in the course of Parkinson's. A speech therapist with experience working with people living with Parkinson's can help keep your speech strong before there is a problem or work with you to improve speech with any change.

WORKSHEETS AND RESOURCES

☑ SWALLOWING WORKSHEET

Parkinson's can present a variety of problems related to swallowing, ranging from minor complaints when swallowing pills to severe difficulty chewing tough foods like steak and hard breads. Swallowing issues are important to address because of the potential risk of aspiration pneumonia, caused when saliva, liquids or food is breathed into the lungs instead of being swallowed into the esophagus and stomach. Many swallowing issues can be easily addressed with specific swallowing exercises and minor changes in diet. It is a good idea to consult with a licensed speech language pathologist to identify problem areas and improve swallowing ability through intentional exercises. The worksheet below provides changes to help with swallowing challenges; check those you can incorporate into your daily routine now.

Swallowing Tips

☐ Cut food into smaller pieces.

☐ Take smaller bites when eating.

☐ Avoid gulping, big sips when drinking.

☐ Avoid straws if you have a swallowing problem, as using a straw may promote choking.

☐ Alternate food with sips of fluid to help your swallowing tract remain clear. This is especially helpful if you have dry mouth.

Lifestyle Changes

☐ Don't eat when overly tired. Try to eat before you reach that point.

☐ Eat at the table. This helps avoid distractions, allowing you to focus on eating.

☐ Eat sitting straight. A chair at the table is better for posture than the couch or recliner.

☐ Don't stop going to restaurants if this is enjoyable to you. Call ahead to discuss your concerns. Typically a chef can prepare your meal to meet your needs. You can ask for a specific table if you are self-conscious. Early-bird specials are not only cheaper, they're often less crowded and less noisy!

▶

▶ Dietary Tips

- ☐ Avoid dry, flaky foods like cornbread, toast, rice or cake unless it is moist. Sauces and gravy help keep your food tasty and moist.

- ☐ Switch to thicker liquids. Thin liquids and water are often more difficult to swallow. Mix pills in applesauce or yogurt if you have trouble swallowing.

- ☐ Try eating papaya fruit or drinking papaya juice to thin your saliva if it feels too thick.

- ☐ Drink adequate fluids, but give yourself more time to do so.

- ☐ Whether you have too much saliva in your mouth or not enough, try sucking on small suckers, lemon candy or chewing gum. Although this creates more saliva, it will prompt you to swallow more frequently.

- ☐ Ask for a swallowing evaluation if you are coughing, drooling, feeling like you have trouble clearing your throat or swallowing pills, are changing your diet due to swallowing concerns or are losing weight.

- ☐ Always report changes in swallowing to your doctor.

WORKSHEETS AND RESOURCES

☑ SEXUAL DYSFUNCTION WORKSHEET

Many people with Parkinson's experience changes in their sexual activity, including low libido, increased sex drive and even hypersexuality, difficulty achieving orgasm or pain during intercourse. Sexual changes and dysfunction can be caused by Parkinson's or side effects of certain Parkinson's medications. This worksheet will provide questions you can ask different members of your wellness team to start a conversation about improving sexual dysfunction as well as adjustments that may help improve your intimacy.

Ask Your Primary Care Physician:

☐ Are there diagnostic tests appropriate for sexual dysfunction?

☐ Do I need a referral to a gynecologist or urologist?

☐ Are my other medications impacting my sexual life? If so, are there treatments for this?

Ask Your Parkinson's Doctor:

☐ Are any of my Parkinson's or Parkinson's-related medications contributing to sexual dysfunction or hypersexuality/impulsivity problems?

☐ Discuss anxiety, depression, insomnia, restless legs, bladder problems, constipation, fatigue, personality changes or movement-related problems that are impacting your relationship. Medications and physical therapy may be helpful to treat symptoms and maximize strength and flexibility.

☐ Ask for a referral to a trained counselor or neuropsychologist.

☐ Ask for a referral to a speech therapist if challenges communicating verbally are affecting your relationship.

Other Tips:

☐ Take your medications on time to feel your best.

☐ Exercise to build up stamina, reduce fatigue and stress.

☐ Eat a balanced diet to maximize your health — body, mind and brain.

☐ Drink appropriate amounts of fluids to reduce fatigue and maintain your blood pressure.

☐ Reserve together time for you and your partner to focus on emotional and physical closeness.

☐ Be as independent as possible. Set guidelines when you want help.

▶

EVERY VICTORY COUNTS

▶ ☐ Show gratitude to your care partner, even the smallest of actions can make a huge impact.

☐ Set aside time each week to focus on your relationship.

📷 CLINICAL APPOINTMENTS SUMMARY

TAKE ACTION AT YOUR HEALTHCARE APPOINTMENTS

This section is focused on helping you get the most out of your healthcare appointments. You will get more out of these appointments if you are ready for them. ***Preparing and organizing information for your wellness team is often overlooked, but is time well spent.***

A key element to taking action is having the information available that you and your wellness team will need to discuss. The worksheets that follow will help you organize your information and will need to be updated occasionally, sometimes before each visit.

Healthcare appointments are intended to encompass visits with all of the following healthcare providers on your wellness team:

- Doctor (primary care physician, neurologist, movement disorder specialist)
- Specialist (gynecologist, urologist, sleep specialist, physical therapist, speech and language pathologist, occupational therapist, recreational therapist, art therapist, music therapist)
- Alternative therapist (acupuncturist, chiropractor)
- Dentist
- Optometrist
- Social worker
- Emotional health specialist (counselor, psychologist, psychiatrist)
- Dietitian

As you update your information, file older worksheets in a specific location so that you and your wellness team can refer to them later as a measure of your progress over time.

GET THE MOST FROM YOUR APPOINTMENT

As you learn to communicate your needs and current status with the various members of your wellness team, you will help each specialist better understand what you are experiencing. When you provide detailed information, you help your team be in the best position to improve both your quality of care and your quality of life.

Many things can cause your healthcare appointments to be less than satisfying. In some instances, you might not remember important details about a visit, especially if you are anxious, are learning things for the first time or have hearing problems, multiple medical problems or memory difficulties. In addition, you may have difficulty expressing yourself, forget what you were going to say or be hesitant to ask questions. ***These are all common***

▶

experiences, even for people who do not have Parkinson's. Utilizing the worksheets in this section will help you avoid these familiar pitfalls.

The following steps are provided to help optimize your time and enhance communication with your wellness team.

Step 1: Before Your Appointment

Write down your overarching goals for the appointment. It is very helpful to take some time and think about what is important to you. This will help you focus the appointment on your most pressing concerns.

- Complete the "Goal Summary for Doctor Visits" worksheet before your visit and bring a copy to share with your doctor.

Note specific questions and concerns before your visit. Sometimes you may forget to ask important questions during your healthcare appointment, so writing them down will remind you to ask.

- Prioritize your questions with the most important one first as you may not have the time to address everything in one visit.

- Allow space to write answers next to the question so you can refer to them later. It may also help to have your care partner or bring a friend or family member to the appointment with you to write the answers for you.

- If you are a care partner, your questions and concerns are important, too. Remember to add these to the list and be prepared to address them during the appointment.

Keep a record of any changes your doctor makes to your treatment for quick reference. Some ways to keep good records include:

- Keeping a dedicated notebook for your healthcare visits.

- Completing the "Daily Medication Log" and showing this to all members of your wellness team before starting treatment. This will lower risk of medication interactions.

- In the "Overall Medication Log," note how each medication you are currently taking or have taken affects you, being sure to mention any side effects you have experienced.

- Keeping copies of previous brain MRIs, CT scans and any other medical test or procedure you have had.

- Updating medical notes and contact information for current and previous healthcare providers (start by filling out the "Wellness Team Contact Information" sheet).

Step 2: Appointment Day

Maximize your time with your healthcare provider. Plan ahead, arrive early and complete forms accurately. These steps will save time for both you and your healthcare provider. Begin by asking your healthcare provider what information is needed from you. Ask questions that are important early during your appointment; don't wait until the end.

Complete the patient questionnaire forms provided by your healthcare provider. These forms can help improve communication, provide information for your record, allow your healthcare provider to spend more time on you and reduce errors and mistakes, especially when tracking your medications. Medications are a primary means of managing Parkinson's and accuracy can greatly affect how well your healthcare provider can control your symptoms.

If writing is difficult for you, ask your care partner or a family member or friend to assist you in completing the forms. In some cases, you might even be able to call and request the forms ahead of time, giving you more time to complete them at home before your appointment.

Remember these tips on the day of your appointment:

- Arrive at least 30 minutes early to complete any forms.

- Always bring a complete list of your medications (such as the "Daily Medication Log") to reduce errors that can occur from one visit to the next. Do not use statements like, "no changes," "same as last visit" or "the doctor knows what I am on." This is how errors occur!

- Visit the restroom before the start of your appointment to ensure comfort throughout the visit.

- Ask for extra copies of forms for future visits. Store them with your records and complete them at home before your next appointment.

- Schedule your appointments during your medication "on" times. This will reduce symptoms during the appointment. In some cases, it may be beneficial to schedule appointments during your "off" periods. For example, your neurologist might benefit from seeing you when your medication is "off." Talk with your doctor if you are unsure.

- Ask your doctor for permission to audio record your appointment for future reference.

- If applicable, bring your care partner with you to your appointment.

Ask questions and learn about your condition. To ensure a productive dialogue with your doctor, come prepared with questions you want to ask and note the answers. Important questions to ask include:

- What are the symptoms or problems that are related to my Parkinson's and what symptoms should I look for?

- Do I need medication? If so, what should I expect medication to change or improve?

EVERY VICTORY COUNTS

- What are the most common side effects of the medication you are considering for me?

- Are there any known drug interactions with over-the-counter medications?

- What symptoms or side effects should be reported immediately?

- How often should I make appointments? (Ask yourself how often you would like to see your doctor, then share this with them.)

- Where can I find accurate and comprehensive information about my symptoms?

- When should I see a physical therapist, occupational therapist, speech therapist, counselor or other specialist?

Step 3: After the Appointment

How often do you leave your healthcare appointment trying to remember what just happened? Do you have trouble following through with your treatment plan?

The following suggestions will help you stay on track between appointments:

- Bring a care partner, family member or friend to write down instructions and help you keep track of your next steps.

- Complete the remaining sections of the form "Goal Summary for Clinic Visits." You are more likely to follow through with changes if you review your goals and write down the action steps needed to get you there.

- Review the information in your "Goal Summary for Clinic Visits" with the other members of your wellness team to involve them in your treatment.

- Keep a journal or a calendar of your goals for the week and steps you have taken to reach them.

Between Appointments

- Keep a list of any changes that result from calls to your doctor about new symptoms experienced between appointments.

- Keep track of medication refill needs before you run out. Provide your pharmacy with your phone number, fax number and/or address for quicker refills.

- Keep a list of prior medicines that were tried and not effective or caused side effects so that they are not used again. You can do this in the "Overall Medication Log."

- Review your goals written in the "Goal Summary for Doctor Visits" worksheet and update on your progress.

- Ask each healthcare professional on your wellness team what information is important for you to bring to each visit so that you can work together as a team.

WORKSHEETS AND RESOURCES

Appointment Checklist

The following information will be helpful to you and your wellness team over time. The worksheets referenced in this section are intended for you to use to help organize your information and maximize the usefulness of your healthcare appointments.

- ☐ Complete your doctor's patient questionnaire, or use the "Parkinson's Care Questionnaire."

- ☐ Keep a list of medications to include name, strength, timing, generic or trade name. Consider using the "Daily Medication Log."

- ☐ Keep a list of all the medications you've tried over the course of living with Parkinson's, being sure to note side effects or reasons specific medications were discontinued. Consider using the "Overall Medication Log."

- ☐ Keep a list of all your treating healthcare professionals, including name, address and fax number. Consider using the "Wellness Team Contact Information."

- ☐ Keep a list of troublesome side effects to discuss with your doctor. Consider using the "My Symptoms Worksheet."

Remember to bring the following on appointment day:

- ☐ Updated "Daily Medication Log."

- ☐ Updated "My Symptoms Worksheet."

- ☐ Updated "Goal Summary for Doctor Visits" assessment.

- ☐ Updated "Current Symptoms Summary."

- ☐ Updated "Parkinson's Care Questionnaire."

- ☐ Updated "Dental Worksheet" and "Medical Summary for Dentists" if visiting a dental provider.

- ☐ List of questions to ask before your visit.

These steps require some effort on your part. They will, however, save time in the long run and most importantly, help you obtain the greatest possible benefit from your healthcare appointments.

◎ CURRENT SYMPTOMS SUMMARY

Name: _____ Date: _____

This document will summarize your problems or concerns, improving your team's understanding of you and your Parkinson's and helping them to effectively tailor your treatment.

I have trouble in the following areas that may be affected by my treatment, hospital stay or procedure:

Motor Problems

☐ Balance problems

☐ Communication and speech difficulties

☐ Dyskinesia – uncontrollable movements usually caused by medication

☐ Dystonia – involuntary muscle spasm, contraction leading to pain, flexion or twisting movements

☐ Freezing of gait or motor initiation problems (feet stuck to floor)

☐ "On/off" fluctuations – periods of time when my medications are "on" that I can move better and when my medications are "off" and I have difficulty moving. "Off" periods usually happen as my medication is wearing "off." To reduce this problem, **I must have my Parkinson's medications on time.**

☐ Swallowing problems

Non-Motor Problems

☐ Anxiety

☐ Apathy or trouble self-initiating tasks

☐ Bladder problems

☐ Constipation

☐ Depression

WORKSHEETS AND RESOURCES

- [ ] Cognitive problems
  - [ ] Memory problems or mild thinking difficulties
  - [ ] Dementia
  - [ ] Hallucinations or sensitivity to hallucinations with certain medications
- [ ] Drooling
- [ ] Excessive sweating or chills
- [ ] Fatigue
- [ ] Impulsivity problems
- [ ] Loss of smell or loss of appetite
- [ ] Pain in these areas: _____
- [ ] Sleep problems
  - [ ] Trouble staying asleep
  - [ ] Restless legs syndrome
  - [ ] Periodic limb movement disorder: repetitive movements, typically of the legs and feet
  - [ ] Sleep apnea
  - [ ] REM sleep behavior disorder: vivid, active, physical dreaming
  - [ ] Daytime sleepiness
- [ ] Sensations such as tingling, aches, pain, cold hands/feet
- [ ] Sexual dysfunction
- [ ] Vision problems

📷 WELLNESS TEAM CONTACT INFORMATION

Primary Care Physician

Name: _____

Address: _____

Phone: _____ Fax: _____

Neurologist

Name: _____

Address: _____

Phone: _____ Fax: _____

Other Provider _____ **Specialty:** _____

Name: _____

Address: _____

Phone: _____ Fax: _____

Other Provider _____ **Specialty:** _____

Name: _____

Address: _____

Phone: _____ Fax: _____

Other Provider _____ **Specialty:** _____

Name: _____

Address: _____

Phone: _____ Fax: _____

📷 MEDICAL PROVIDERS

Primary Care Physician

_____

_____

_____

_____

Primary Urgent Care

_____

_____

_____

_____

Alternate Urgent Care

_____

_____

_____

_____

Emergency

_____

_____

_____

_____

DBS Programmer

_____

_____

_____

_____

Neurologist

_____

_____

_____

_____

Optometrist/Opthamologist

_____

_____

_____

_____

Dentist/Oral Surgeon

_____

_____

_____

_____

EVERY VICTORY COUNTS

📷 DBS MEDICAL HISTORY

NO: Diathermy, Lithotripsy MRI or Ultrasound. Medical Consent Required.

PATIENT HISTORY

Name: _____ DOB: _____

Address: _____

Type of Residence: _____ Phone: _____

Marital Status: _____ Work Status: _____

Occupation (if employed): _____

Activity Level: ☐ Sedentary ☐ Moderately Active ☐ Very Active

Smoker: ☐ No ☐ Yes, Current ☐ Previous

Allergies *(check for YES)*:
☐ Aspirin ☐ Codeine ☐ Penicillin ☐ Local Anesthetics ☐ Acrylic ☐ Latex ☐ Metal

PATIENT PROGRAMMER

Device: _____ Manufacturer Contact: _____

Neurologist Contact: _____ Programmer Contact: _____

MEDICATIONS

NAME	DOSAGE	FREQUENCY	STRENGTH

PHYSICIANS

TYPE	DOCTOR NAME	HOSPITAL / CLINIC	ADDRESS CITY, STATE, ZIP	PHONE
Primary Care Physician				
Neurologist				
DBS Programmer				
DBS Surgeon				
Optometrist/Opthamologist				
Dentist				
Oral Surgeon				
OTHER				

EVERY VICTORY COUNTS

MEDICAL INSURANCE

PRE-AUTHORIZATION

Claim #:_____

Entitled to:_____

_____

Insurance Company:_____

Employee ID #: _____

Group Name:_____

Group Policy #: _____

Claim Inquiries: _____

_____

_____

_____

EMERGENCY CONTACTS

Name: _____

Relationship: _____

Home Phone: _____

Cell Phone: _____

Name: _____

Relationship: _____

Home Phone: _____

Cell Phone: _____

Name: _____

Relationship: _____

Home Phone: _____

Cell Phone: _____

IMMUNIZATIONS AND PREVENTATIVE SCREENINGS

TYPE	DATE
Flu	
Pneumonia	
Tetanus	
Hepatitis B	
Shingles	
Gardasil	

TYPE	DATE
Colonoscopy	
EKG	
Echocardiogram	
Eye Exam	
Physical Exam	
Neurology Exam	

SURGICAL HISTORY

SURGICAL PROCEDURE	REASON FOR SURGERY	DATE	SURGEON NAME	HOSPITAL	CITY, STATE

EVERY VICTORY COUNTS

📷 PREPARE FOR YOUR HOSPITAL STAY

BRING THE FOLLOWING INFORMATION WITH YOU:

Make copies of your completed "Daily Medication Log" to give to your nurses and doctors. Remember to update this each time your medications are changed.

List of Medications You Should Not Have

Common anti-hallucination and anti-nausea medications can worsen movement. Both nausea and hallucinations can occur with certain medications and during illness.

Note: This is not a complete list of medications to avoid. If you have questions about other medications, ask your pharmacist or doctor.

Anti-Hallucination Medications to Avoid

Note: The anti-hallucination medications Pimavanserin (Nuplazid), Quetiapine (Seroquel) or Clozapine (Clozaril) can be used for hallucinations and psychosis. The following should be avoided:

- Aripiprazole (Abilify)
- Chlorpromazine (Thorazine)
- Flufenazine (Prolixin)
- Haloperidol (Haldol)
- Molindone (Moban)
- Perphenazine (Trilafon)
- Perphenazine and amitriptyline (Triavil)
- Risperidone (Risperdol)
- Thioridazine (Mellaril)
- Thiothixene (Navane)

Anti-Nausea Medications to Avoid

- Metoclopramide (Reglan)
- Phenothiazine (Compazine)
- Promethazine (Phenergan)

WORKSHEETS AND RESOURCES

Medications to Avoid if You Are on Rasagiline (Azilect) or Selegiline (Eldepryl)

- Pain medications meperidine (Demerol), tramadol (Ultram) and methadone

- Antispasmodic medication (Flexeril)

- Dextromethorphan (cold medication) and ciprofloxacin (antibiotic)

Note: This is not a complete list of medications to avoid. If you have questions about other medications, ask your pharmacist or doctor.

If you have DBS: Bring the name and contact number for your neurologist, DBS programmer and device manufacturer, along with a document of tests, medications and procedures that require medical consent from your neurologist. Consider using the "DBS Medical History" form to collect and share this information.

Bring copies of the "Current Symptoms Summary," as certain symptoms such as swallowing, dizziness, constipation and confusion could worsen in the hospital and these symptoms could influence your treatment decisions.

Inform Hospital Staff

- Highlight your need for medications on time.

- Discuss what you can do when the medications are "on" and when they are "off," so that they are aware of any potential changes in your movement. This is an opportunity to reinforce the need to get your medications on time.

- Describe your dyskinesia and freezing episodes and when they occur, as these symptoms may be unfamiliar to your hospital treatment team.

What to Ask for During Your Hospitalization

- Physical therapy, occupational therapy, speech/swallowing therapy, especially if you have trouble with balance, swallowing and general mobility.

- Chaplain services or social work consult for support of you or loved ones.

What to Know or Ask Before Discharge

- Have your neurologist and primary care physician been notified of your condition while in the hospital?

- When should you see your primary care physician?

- Should you get additional rehabilitation such as physical therapy?

- What important tests, procedures or new diagnosis have you had?

- What medications have been changed and why?

- How do you get a copy of the hospital records sent to your doctor?

▶ Advanced Directives

The following advanced directives ensure that your rights and personal wishes are respected in the event of a medical emergency or change in your health status in which you are unable to make decisions for yourself. Many options are available to help you determine these, and each document should be reviewed by your attorney to ensure your wishes are accurately recorded. Check with the department of health in your state or country for additional guidance.

Medical Power of Attorney: This document gives a designated person the power to make medical decisions for you in the event that you are incapacitated and unable to do so.

Durable Power of Attorney: This document gives a designated person the power to make certain legal, financial and disability decisions for you in the event that you are incapacitated and unable to do so.

Living Will or Healthcare Directive: This is a written document that specifies what type of medical treatment you desire if you become incapacitated.

It is a good idea to also bring a signed statement identifying a friend or family member who your doctors can talk to about your treatment.

Summary of Hospital Document Checklist
- Bring "Daily Medication Log"
- List of medications to avoid
- Bring "Current Symptoms Summary"
- Advanced directives
- Bring "DBS Medical History" (if applicable)

📷 MEDICAL SUMMARY FOR YOUR DOCTOR APPOINTMENT

List your top three goals or concerns for your next doctor's appointment:

Note: You may wish to review the "Current Symptoms Summary" and "My Symptoms" worksheets to identify and help set these priority goals.

1. _____

2. _____

3. _____

Describe any treatment changes you have made since your last visit and how they have affected your symptoms:

_____

_____

_____

_____

List any new medical problems, allergies or hospitalizations since your last visit:

1. _____

2. _____

3. _____

Review the "Daily Medication Log" and "Overall Medication Log" to discuss any side effects of your medications.

_____

_____

_____

_____

📷 MEDICAL SUMMARY FOR DENTISTS

Bring the following information to your dentist to inform them of Parkinson's-specific dental issues and modification tips.[1]

About Parkinson's

☐ Parkinson's is a progressive, neurodegenerative movement disorder.

☐ Primary motor symptoms include rigidity, tremor, slow movement, postural instability, difficulty speaking, decreased facial expression and weakness of face and throat muscles.

☐ Primary non-motor symptoms include loss of smell, sleep disturbances, depression, excessive saliva, anxiety and cognitive issues.

☐ Parkinson's medication side effects commonly include dry mouth, low blood pressure, dizziness, confusion, nausea and an "on/off" cycle, when medication ebbs and flows in its effectiveness.

Communication

☐ Allow additional time for responses, as difficulty speaking and mild cognitive impairments can lead to a longer lead time in responding. Include the care partner (if present) in the discussion to ensure all information being understood is accurate.

☐ Collaborate with your patient to determine a signal for discomfort – for example, the patient may put his or her hand up to signal they need a break or are having trouble swallowing. Decreased facial expression can make it difficult to express discomfort in the chair.

❗ **Ask your patient what medications they are currently taking to reduce the likelihood of interactions with numbing medications or anesthesia.**

Treatments

☐ Use more frequent suction during cleaning, as the cough reflex may not be as strong.

☐ Offer an intraoral rubber bite block, as Parkinson's patients may have difficulty keeping their mouth open, managing saliva or restricting head and tongue movements.

☐ Use an aspirator tip placed under a rubber dam and stabilized by an assistant. This will assist the patient in managing saliva and protecting airways from the higher risk of aspiration.

---

1   Friedlander, A. H., Mahler, M., Norman, K. M., Ettinger, R. L. (2009). Parkinson Disease: Systemic and orofacial manifestations, medical and dental management. *The Journal of the American Dental Association*, 140(6), 658-669.

WORKSHEETS AND RESOURCES

- [ ] Look for excessive loss of tooth structure; Parkinson's tremors of the orofacial musculature and the use of levodopa medication may cause bruxism.

- [ ] Utilize glass ionomers and resin-modified glass ionomers.

- [ ] Keep the dental chair at an incline of 45° or higher to enable comfortable swallowing.

- [ ] The dental chair should be raised and lowered slowly to allow the patient to adapt to the position and prevent syncope episodes.

- [ ] Help your patient in and out of the dental chair slowly to reduce the likelihood of falls. Encourage them to sit up in the chair, plant their feet on the ground, stand up slowly and walk out of the room – pausing for around 20 seconds between each transition.

❶ **Ask your patient if they have had Deep Brain Stimulation surgery.**

Medications and Interactions

- [ ] If a patient is taking MAO-B inhibitors (selegiline, rasagiline), avoid meperidine (Demerol), tramadol (Rybix, Ryzolt, Ultram), droperidol (Inapsine), methadone (Dolophine, Methadose), propoxyphene (Darvon, PP-Cap), cyclobenzaprine (Amrix, Fexmid, Flexeril) and halothane (Fluothane).

- [ ] Administer no more than 0.05mg of epinephrine per 30-minute period, with careful aspiration to avoid intravascular administration.

- [ ] Be careful when using local anesthetic agents containing epinephrine in patients being treated with levodopa and entacapone, because these patients may experience an exaggerated effect on blood pressure and heart rate.

Deep Brain Stimulation (DBS) Therapy

- [ ] Patients should have a complete dental checkup and treatment prior to DBS surgery.

❶ **Ask your patient if they have had Deep Brain Stimulation surgery. If the answer is yes:**

  - [ ] Do not use diathermy (therapeutic ultrasound), as it is contraindicated and may lead to coma or death.

  - [ ] Ultrasonic cleaning that uses air and water will not interact with the device.

  - [ ] X-ray use is not contraindicated.

  - [ ] Laser technology use should be reviewed with the DBS device manufacturer.

  - [ ] Any electrical or magnetic device near the head, neck or chest should be approved for use by the device manufacturer.

  - [ ] Device labeling does not require pre-medication with antibiotics for dental treatment

EVERY VICTORY COUNTS

GLOSSARY

Acetylcholine: A brain chemical that acts as both a neurotransmitter and a neuromodulator and plays a role in muscle function, attention, arousal, memory and motivation. Acetylcholine is reduced in Parkinson's-related dementia.

Acetylcholinesterase inhibitors: Medications that block the breakdown of the neurotransmitter acetylcholine to help treat Parkinson's-related dementia.

Action tremor: Type of tremor that gets worse when trying to perform an action, such as picking up a coffee cup or eating with a spoon.

Activities of daily living (ADLs): Basic self-care skills, including eating, dressing, grooming, bathing and using the toilet. Occupational therapists often focus on improving ADLs.

Adaptive equipment: Devices used to assist with activities of daily living, such as bathing, dressing and using the toilet. Examples include tremor-management eating utensils, non-skid mats, adaptive writing utensils, button hooks, etc.

Advance healthcare directive: A legal document in which someone explains the actions that should be taken for their health if they are no longer in a capacity to make their own decisions. In the US, an advance healthcare directive has its own legal status.

Akinesia: Lack of movement caused by Parkinson's, such as loss of arm swing, that primarily affects walking or the hands and trunk area. A hallmark motor symptom of Parkinson's.

Alpha-synuclein: A protein found in the brain. While the role of alpha-synuclein in a healthy brain is unknown, alpha-synuclein clumps together in the brains of people with Parkinson's to form Lewy bodies, one of the hallmark features of Parkinson's. This has led to ongoing investigation into the role this protein plays in the development of Parkinson's.

Alternative brain pathways: Recruiting stronger brain circuits to execute similar functions that enables people to perform and gain strength in a difficult task. For example, people with speech problems may be able to sing or someone who struggles walking may be able to ride a bicycle.

Amantadine: A medication originally used to treat the common flu and later found to improve the symptoms of Parkinson's. Amantadine can be used alone or in combination with other Parkinson's medications. It is sometimes added specifically for the treatment of dyskinesia and can also improve freezing of gait. Also has a stimulant effect, which can help with fatigue.

Amino acid: The building blocks of protein.

Anticholinergics: A type of medication that interferes with the action of the neurotransmitter acetylcholine to try and restore the balance between dopamine and acetylcholine.

Anxiety: Excessive feelings of worry, nervousness, apprehension and unease. Can be associated with compulsive behavior or panic attacks.

Apomorphine: A dopamine agonist that helps improve motor function by stimulating dopamine receptors. It is a Parkinson's medication used to help with "off" episodes and to treat muscle stiffness, slow movements or movement difficulties associated with Parkinson's.

Art therapist: A type of therapist who uses art and creative expression as a healing tool to convey the inner self and emotions, strengthen concentration and executive function and reinforce mind-body connections.

Aspiration: When food or fluid enters the lungs.

Ataxia: A loss of muscle control or the ability to coordinate one's voluntary movements, such as walking. Ataxia signals the presence of an underlying condition and can affect various movements, leading to challenges with swallowing, speech and eye movement.

Basal ganglia: Clusters of neurons located deep in the brain that play an important role in movement. The basal ganglia includes the substantia nigra, and cell death in the substantia nigra contributes to signs of Parkinson's.

Benzodiazepines: A category of psychoactive medications used to treat anxiety and insomnia by slowing the central nervous system.

Biomarker: An early indicator that a person may have a disease, such as Parkinson's, that can be recognized before symptoms appear. Identifying biomarkers may lead to earlier interventions and treatment. Biomarkers could be a chemical, clinical or physiological change or found via imaging.

Blood brain barrier: The membrane separating the blood and the brain; a tight physical barrier that normally keeps immune cells, chemicals and drugs out of the brain.

Botulinum toxin: A neurotoxic protein that prevents the release of acetylcholine. Injections may help with dystonia. Commonly referred to as Botox.

Bradykinesia: The slowness of movement that can be caused by Parkinson's. One of the hallmark motor symptoms of Parkinson's.

Bradyphrenia: Slowed thinking that can be caused by Parkinson's.

Carbidopa: A drug given with levodopa. Carbidopa blocks the enzyme dopa decarboxylase, thereby preventing levodopa from being metabolized to dopamine. Since carbidopa does not penetrate the blood brain barrier, it only blocks levodopa metabolism in the peripheral tissues and not in the brain, thereby reducing side effects such as nausea, while increasing the effectiveness of levodopa.

Care partner: Anyone who provides help or support to a relative or friend living with Parkinson's.

Caregiver burnout: A medical syndrome resulting from untreated caregiver strain that includes feeling overwhelmed, angry, irritable, sleeping poorly, fatigue, worsening medical problems and/or self-medicating.

Caregiver strain: A medical syndrome resulting from the burdens and demands of caregiving.

Chronic: A condition of long duration. Chronic diseases typically appear gradually and progress slowly over time. The term does not imply anything about the severity of a disease. The opposite of a chronic condition is an acute condition.

Clinical trials: Experiments or observations done in clinical research on human participants. Clinical trials are designed to test the safety and efficacy of biomedical or behavioral interventions, including new medications, medical devices and supplements.

Cognition: Mental processes including attention, remembering, producing and understanding language, solving problems and making decisions.

Cognitive behavioral therapy (CBT): A type of treatment for anxiety and depression addressing behaviors and thought patterns. CBT is time-limited and skills-based, and may be used alone or in combination with medication.

Complementary therapies: Non-medical treatments used in addition to conventional medical and surgical treatments, such as physical therapy, occupational therapy, speech and language therapy, music and art therapies, etc.

Complex carbohydrates: Long chains of sugar molecules that require more complex digestion and are more slowly absorbed; includes starch and fiber.

COMT inhibitors: A type of medication that prevents the COMT enzyme from converting levodopa into a form unable to be used by the brain. When levodopa is taken, a portion of the COMT enzyme converts into a useless compound. COMT inhibitors prevent this, thus making more levodopa available for the brain to use to counteract symptoms of Parkinson's.

Compulsive behaviors: The overwhelming and often repetitive drive to act in a certain way to ease an urge or reduce worry or tension. Often, this behavior can be out of character for the person experiencing it and can be a side effect of certain Parkinson's medications.

Constipation: Infrequent or hard to pass bowel movements. A common problem for people living with Parkinson's that can be helped by increasing fiber in the diet.

Continuous subcutaneous infusion of apomorphine (CAI): An ongoing stream of apomorphine delivered into the bloodstream through a needle into the skin, similar to an insulin pump. This treatment is designed to limit the amount of "off" time experienced. It is currently not available in the US, but is in advanced clinical trials.

Controlled release drugs: Special preparations of drugs that release the drug into the body slowly and steadily, rather than all at once. This helps to keep the amount of the drug in the blood stream at a steadier level than the "ordinary" version of the same drug.

DaTSCAN: A nuclear medicine scan that measures levels of dopamine nerve cells in the basal ganglia. While this scan cannot determine if someone has Parkinson's or not, it was approved by the FDA in 2011 to help differentiate Parkinson's tremor from Familial or Essential Tremor (ET). It is also not able to distinguish Parkinson's from other forms of parkinsonism, nor is it used to track symptoms or progression.

Deep Brain Stimulation (DBS): A surgical procedure involving the implantation of electrodes in specific areas of the brain that produce electrical impulses to help regulate abnormal impulses or affect certain chemicals or cells in the brain. DBS is used to help a variety of neurological conditions, most commonly the motor symptoms of Parkinson's, including tremor, rigidity, stiffness, slowed movement and walking problems.

Dementia: A decline in cognitive function due to damage or disease in the brain beyond what might be expected from normal aging. Areas particularly affected include memory, attention, judgment, language, planning and problem solving.

Depression: A mood disorder that causes a persistent feeling of sadness and loss of interest. Depression can affect feelings, behavior and thinking, leading to various physical and emotional problems.

Designation of healthcare surrogate: A document naming another person as a representative to make medical decisions on one's behalf should one be unable to make them oneself. As in a living will, people can include instructions about treatments they do and do not want.

Dopa decarboxylase inhibitors (DDI): Parkinson's medications that block the actions of the enzyme dopa decarboxylase (DDC) to inhibit the metabolism of levodopa to dopamine in the bloodstream, allowing more levodopa to reach the brain and be converted into dopamine there. Includes carbidopa and benserazide.

Dopamine: A small chemical molecule that is one of the brain's neurotransmitters. It is found especially in cells within the substantia nigra and conveys messages in the brain to coordinate muscle movements. The motor symptoms of Parkinson's appear when 60-80% of the dopamine-producing neurons in the brain are damaged and unable to produce sufficient dopamine.

Dopamine agonist: A type of medication that acts like dopamine, but is not actually dopamine. These compounds activate dopamine receptors and can be used in both the early and later stages of Parkinson's. Dopamine agonists can cause side effects such as confusion, sleepiness, sleep attacks, ankle swelling, hallucinations and impulse control problems, like uncontrollable gambling, eating, obsessive behaviors and sexual urges.

Durable power of attorney: A document appointing an agent (usually a trusted relative or friend) to carry out specific health, legal and financial responsibilities on behalf of another. There are two types of power of attorney: POA for healthcare and POA for finances. The POA for healthcare gives the appointed agent authority to make healthcare decision on behalf of someone. The POA for finances gives the appointed agent authority to make legal/financial decisions on behalf of someone. At the time the documents for POA are signed, the person establishing a durable power of attorney must be physically and mentally capable of making the decision to seek assistance.

Dysarthria: A motor speech disorder characterized by slow or slurred speech. Dysarthria results from impaired movement of the muscles used for speech production, including the tongue, vocal folds, lips and/or diaphragm. The type and severity of dysarthria depends on which area of the nervous system is affected.

Dyskinesia: Uncontrollable, jerky and involuntary movements, often the result of levodopa medication wearing off.

Dysphagia: Difficulty swallowing.

Dystonia: Involuntary tightening or spasms of the muscles, often in the feet or lower legs, caused by a lack of dopamine.

Electrocardiogram (ECG): A test that measures the electrical activity of the heartbeat.

Employee assistance program (EAP): A voluntary, confidential program that helps employees navigate various life challenges that may affect their health, job performance and personal well-being.

End-of-dose wearing off: The phenomenon of medicine's effectiveness wearing "off" before the next dose, causing Parkinson's symptoms to re-appear or get worse before it is time to take the next dose of levodopa.

Erectile dysfunction (ED): The inability to achieve a sustained erection throughout intercourse. Can be a symptom of Parkinson's.

Executive function: Cognitive processes that allow one to plan, focus attention, remember and multitask.

373

Facial masking: A condition resulting in reduced facial expression that may additionally cause softer, more monotone speech. The technical term for this is "hypomimia" and often this is referred to as "mask-like" or "masked" face.

Family Medical Leave Act (FMLA): A federal act in the US entitling employees to an unpaid, extended leave of absence for specified family and medical reasons. It also ensures that employer-provided health insurance continues during leave. There are specific criteria that must be met to qualify for FMLA.

Festination: The tendency toward smaller, faster steps that pitch one forward.

Freezing of gait: Problems with initiating movements that often result in feeling like one's feet are glued to the floor. A motor symptom that is more common in later stages of Parkinson's.

Functional mobility: Ability to move around one's home and environment to perform daily activities, such as getting in and out of bed, bathing, sitting on and getting up from the couch or table, etc. Occupational therapists often focus on improving functional mobility.

Glutamate: An amino acid and the main excitatory neurotransmitter in the human brain. Glutamate plays a critical role in the development of the brain and helps with learning and memory. Excess glutamate in the brain is associated with neurological diseases like Parkinson's, Alzheimer's, multiple sclerosis (MS) and amyotrophic lateral sclerosis (ALS).

Glycemic index: A number measuring a food's effect on blood glucose after consumption. The GI represents the rise in a blood sugar level two hours after consumption and depends on many factors. GI is useful for understanding how the body breaks down carbohydrates.

Glycemic load: A measure related to the glycemic index that multiplies the glycemic index of a food by the carbohydrate content in the actual serving to put the glycemic index into appropriate context. For instance, watermelon has a high glycemic index, but a low glycemic load per the typical quantity consumed.

Gut microbiome: The complex community of microorganisms that live in the digestive tracts of humans and other animals.

Growth factors: Naturally occurring substances (usually proteins) that help maintain the health of neurons and encourage cell growth, proliferation and differentiation. Some growth factors are being looked at to try to promote the survival of the neural cells that are degenerating in Parkinson's.

Hallucinations: The experience of perceiving something that is not actually there. Hallucinations may be a symptom of Parkinson's or a side effect of certain Parkinson's medications.

Hypertension: Abnormally high blood pressure.

Hypersexuality: A clinical diagnosis describing extremely frequent or suddenly increased sexual urges or activity. Can be a side effect of certain Parkinson's medications.

Hypokinesia: Small movements that can come as a result of Parkinson's. One of the hallmark motor symptoms of Parkinson's.

Hypomimia: The decrease in facial expressions resulting in a masked-like face that can come as a result of Parkinson's.

Hypophonia: Soft speech caused by Parkinson's.

Idiopathic: A type of condition arising from an unknown cause. The majority of people living with Parkinson's are considered to have "idiopathic" Parkinson's, meaning there is no clear and definitive genetic or environmental cause for developing the disease.

Impulsive behaviors: The inability to resist the temptation to engage in a certain activity. Often, these activities give an immediate sense of pleasure, such as eating, gambling, increase in sexual thoughts or feelings, etc. Can be a side effect of certain Parkinson's medications.

Impulse control disorder (ICD): A set of psychiatric disorders characterized by an inability to control one's actions, particularly activities that could bring harm to oneself or others. This can be a side effect of certain Parkinson's medications. People taking dopamine agonists may experience ICDs, including compulsive gambling, eating, shopping and hypersexuality.

Instrumental activities of daily living (IDLs): Activities that include caring for others and pets, financial management, driving, one's ability to be active in the community, health and medication management, meal preparation, leisure activities, shopping, safety, etc. Occupational therapists often focus on improving IDLs.

Insoluble fiber: A type of fiber found in vegetables, whole grains, raisins and prunes that does not absorb water and passes through the gastrointestinal tract to reduce constipation.

Interdisciplinary care: Multiple healthcare professionals collaborating to provide care with a common perspective, often involving joint consultations. Sometimes referred to as "integrative care."

Leucine rich repeat kinase 2 (LRRK2): A large and complex gene that influences the production of proteins. Mutations in this gene are the most common cause of Parkinson's in the small percentage (~10%) of people with Parkinson's whose disease is linked to a genetic component. Mutations in the LRRK2 gene that can increase one's risk of developing Parkinson's are much higher in certain ethnic groups, such as Ashkenazi Jews, Basque and North African Berbers.

Levodopa (L-DOPA): A chemical that is the precursor to dopamine and one of the oldest and most effective medications for Parkinson's. It can pass through the blood-brain barrier where it is absorbed by dopamine nerve cells and converted to dopamine to replace lost dopamine in the brain.

Levodopa sparing strategy: Limiting the use of levodopa in an attempt to minimize wearing "off" problems and dyskinesia as Parkinson's progresses.

Lewy bodies: A pathologic hallmark of Parkinson's and dementia with Lewy bodies. Named for Frederic Lewy who first described them, Lewy bodies are seen microscopically as inclusions in neurons in several brain regions, including the substantia nigra.

Macronutrients: The three major food categories: carbohydrates, fats and proteins.

MAO (monoamine oxidase): A family of enzymes with two subtypes: MAO-A and MAO-B. These catalyze the oxidation of amine molecules, replacing the amine group with an oxygen molecule. MAO-B inhibitors are a type of drugs (such as selegiline, rasagiline) that inhibit the breakdown of dopamine via MAO-B enzyme and do not cause abnormally high blood pressure (hypertension).

Mediterranean diet: A type of diet consisting of traditional foods consumed in Mediterranean countries, emphasizing plant-based foods like fruits and vegetables, whole grains, legumes and nuts as well as moderate consumption of poultry and dairy. The diet replaces butter with fats such as olive oil and canola oil and uses herbs and spices instead of salt to flavor food.

Micrographia: Small, cramped handwriting that can be a symptom of Parkinson's.

Micronutrients: Vitamins and substances found in food that are needed in smaller amounts to promote cell health and catalyze biochemical reactions.

Mind-body medicine: An approach to medicine based on the belief that thoughts and emotions can influence physical healing and well-being.

Modified barium swallow (MBS): A radiology procedure that can show the passage of food or fluids from the mouth to the stomach.

Monounsaturated fats: Type of fat that is liquid at room temperature, but gets cloudy when refrigerated. Examples include olives and olive oil, canola oil, nuts and nut oils and avocado. These oils are a better substitute for saturated fats, and can reduce cholesterol levels and improve insulin activity.

Motor fluctuations: A complication of levodopa therapy characterized by periodic reemergence of Parkinson's symptoms that are normally controlled when the medication is working.

Motor skills: The degree of coordination provided by the brain's control of the skeletal muscles.

Motor symptoms: Symptoms that involve movement, coordination, physical tasks or mobility. These include resting tremor, bradykinesia, rigidity, postural instability, freezing, micrographia, facial masking, unwanted accelerations, stooped posture, dystonia, impaired motor dexterity and coordination, speech problems, difficulty swallowing, muscle cramping and drooling.

Movement disorder specialist (MDS): A neurologist with additional training in movement disorders like Parkinson's, essential tremor and ataxia.

Multidisciplinary care: Care given by multiple healthcare professionals, each approaching the patient from their professional perspective. This often involves separate, individual consultations.

Music therapist: Specialists who use music to help with movement.

Neurogenic bladder: Problems with nerve control of the bladder, including urinary frequency and sense of urgency.

Neurogenic orthostatic hypotension (nOH): A type of orthostatic hypotension caused by a neurological disorder like Parkinson's or multiple system atrophy (MSA) that triggers a sustained drop in blood pressure upon standing. An estimated 30-50% of people with Parkinson's experience nOH. The prevalence increases with both age and number of years living with Parkinson's. nOH can appear with or without symptoms, and common symptoms include dizziness, lightheadedness, blurry vision and occasional fainting.

Neurological conditions: A collection of disorders caused by damage or malfunctioning of the brain or nervous system.

Neurologist: A doctor who specializes in the diagnosis, care and treatment of disorders of the brain or nervous system.

Neuromodulation: The act of altering nerve activity through delivering a targeted stimulus in the brain, such as electrical stimulation. Neuromodulation devices use electrical signals, pharmaceutical agents or other avenues to stimulate nerves and modulate the abnormal neural pathway behavior caused by a neurological disease. Approaches to neuromodulation range from non-invasive techniques, such as transcranial magnetic stimulation, to implanted devices, such as a deep brain stimulation system for Parkinson's.

Neuro-ophthalmologist: A neurologist or ophthalmologist with fellowship training in the field of neuro-ophthalmology. These specialists have a particular appreciation for the intersection of the eyes and the brain, and perform comprehensive testing to determine the cause of visual or eye movement problems.

Neuroplasticity: Activity and experiences that cause the development of new nerve connections or the strengthening of old connections, resulting in improved brain function.

Neuroprotection: Mechanisms within the nervous system that protect neurons from dying as a result of a degenerative disease like Parkinson's or from other types of injury.

Neuropsychologist: A psychologist specializing in understanding the relationship between the physical brain and behavior.

Neurostimulator: A device that delivers electrical impulses through tiny wires placed in regions of the brain affected by Parkinson's.

Neurotransmitter: A chemical messenger in the nervous system that facilitates communication between two neuronal cells, normally across a synapse. The neurotransmitter is released from the nerve terminals on the axons. Examples of neurotransmitters include dopamine, acetylcholine, adrenaline, noradrenaline, serotonin, glutamate and GABA.

Non-motor symptoms: Symptoms of Parkinson's that do not involve movement, coordination, physical tasks or mobility. Common non-motor symptoms include loss of sense of smell, constipation, sleep disorders or disturbances, mood disorders, orthostatic hypotension, bladder problems, sexual problems, excessive saliva, weight loss or gain, vision and dental problems, fatigue, depression, fear and anxiety, skin problems and cognitive issues.

Occupational therapist: Specialists concerned with assessing a person's home or work situation to determine ways to make life more manageable. Occupational therapists can also advise on aids and adaptive equipment that may make everyday life easier.

Omega-3 fats: A type of fat necessary for brain cell function found in walnuts, flaxseeds, pumpkin seeds, purslane and cold water fish.

Omega-6 fats: A type of fat that includes sunflower oil, safflower oil, corn oil, most seeds and oil from grains.

"On/off" fluctuations: The clinical states of Parkinson's while being treated with levodopa, which can often fluctuate after a few years of treatment. The "on" state is when levodopa reduces Parkinson's symptoms. The "off" state is when the benefit has been reduced or lost. The most common type of "off" is referred to as "wearing off," and happens because of levodopa not lasting more than four hours after a dose. Sudden and unpredictable "off" states can also occur, but are less common. "Off" states usually will respond to another dose of levodopa.

378

Orthostatic hypotension (OH): A sustained drop in blood pressure that occurs after standing. OH can happen for a variety of reasons. When OH is caused by a nervous system disorder, like Parkinson's or multiple system atrophy (MSA), it is called neurogenic orthostatic hypotension (nOH). Symptoms can include lightheadedness, dizziness or feeling as though one is about to black out.

Overactive bladder (OAB): A sense of urgency and needing to urinate quickly and/or frequently, even if the bladder is not full.

Palliative care: An approach to care of chronic illness that is holistic and team-based, shifting the focus from an individual patient to the patient together with their family. Palliative care places a strong emphasis on enhancing quality of life and integrating psychological and spiritual aspects. Hospice is a subset of palliative care, administered in the US in the last six months of life.

Parkinsonism: A general term for group of neurological conditions displaying movement changes often seen in Parkinson's disease, such as slowness of movement, rest tremors, muscle stiffness and impaired speech. Not everyone who has parkinsonism has Parkinson's disease.

Parkinsonian gait: A slow, short-paced way of walking common in people living with Parkinson's. Often there is a tendency to shuffle and a decreased arm swing.

Parkinson-plus syndromes: A group of neurodegenerative diseases displaying the classic motor symptoms of Parkinson's disease (such as slowness of movement, rest tremors and muscle stiffness), but with additional features that distinguish them from typical Parkinson's disease. Parkinson-plus syndromes include multiple system atrophy (MSA), progressive supranuclear palsy (PSP), dementia with Lewy bodies (DLB) and corticobasal degeneration (CBD).

Partially hydrogenated oils: Primary source of artificial trans fat in processed foods. In 2013, the US Food and Drug Administration (FDA) made a preliminary determination that partially hydrogenated oils are no longer Generally Recognized as Safe (GRAS) in human food.

Periodic limb movement disorder (PLMD): A sleep disorder involving repetitive movements, typically in the legs and feet, that occur about every 20-40 seconds and cluster into episodes lasting anywhere from a few minutes to several hours. These movements can be brief muscle twitches, jerking movements or an upward flexing of the feet. PLMD often occurs in tandem with restless legs syndrome, with nearly three-quarters of people with RLS also experiencing PLMD.

Peripheral neuropathy: A condition caused by damage to peripheral nerves. This often results in weakness, numbness and pain, usually in the hands and feet, but can also affect other areas of the body.

379

Physical therapist: Specialists who use physical means such as exercise and manipulation to help prevent or reduce stiffness in joints and restore muscle strength. Physical therapists can also advise on aids and equipment to help with movement problems.

Placebo: A simulated or inert form of treatment without known proven benefit on a symptom or a disease. A pill serving as a placebo is often called a "sugar pill." When placebos provide benefit, this phenomenon is called a "placebo effect." Placebos are employed in controlled clinical trials along with the active drug being tested. The difference in responses between the two drugs is considered the true effect of the active drug.

Polyunsaturated fats: Type of fat that is liquid at both room temperature and when refrigerated. Can be divided into two types: omega-6 fats and omega-3 fats.

Postural instability: General balance issues that result from how Parkinson's delays reflexes related to posture. Although this typically shows up as problems with balance, there can be many different causes for balance challenges in Parkinson's.

Prudent diet: A modification of the Mediterranean diet that is rich in fruits, vegetables, nuts, whole grains, legumes, low-fat dairy products, fish and lean meats. A prudent diet is associated with reduced rates of many major diseases, including cancer, stroke, diabetes, heart attack and high blood pressure.

Receptor: A protein structure typically embedded in the cell membrane with which neurotransmitters and drugs interact.

Recreational therapist: Specialists who help people stay active in hobbies and play.

Rapid eye movement sleep behavior disorder (RBD): A sleep disorder that involves movement and abnormal behavior during the sleep phase with rapid eye movements, the stage of sleep in which dreaming occurs. In normal sleep, muscles are paralyzed during dreaming, except for eye movements. In individuals with RBD, the muscles are not paralyzed, so the dreamer is free to physically act out his or her dreams. RBD is common in people with Parkinson's and may precede the onset of motor symptoms.

Restless legs syndrome (RLS): A neurological disorder characterized by unpleasant sensations in the legs, like the feeling of ants crawling underneath the skin. These sensations usually occur in the late evening and during sleep. Walking around relieves the sensation, hence the term "restless legs." RLS interferes with sleep and is common in people with Parkinson's.

Rest tremor: A type of tremor that worsens when relaxing or resting.

Retropulsion: The tendency to fall backward, caused by postural instability.

Rigidity: A special type of muscle stiffness, which is one of the hallmark motor symptoms of Parkinson's. The muscles tend to pull against each other instead of working smoothly together.

Saturated fats: Type of fat that is solid at room temperature and found primarily in red meat, tropical oils (like coconut) and dairy. A diet high in saturated fats can increase cholesterol levels, one's risk of accumulating plaque in the arteries (called "atherosclerosis"), stroke and heart disease.

Seborrhea: Flaky, white or yellowish skin forming on oily areas of the scalp, forehead or ear. Can be an early, non-motor symptom of Parkinson's.

Selective serotonin reuptake inhibitors (SSRIs): A class of antidepressant medications that increases serotonin levels in the brain and can be used to treat depression and anxiety.

Serotonin: A neurotransmitter that contributes to feelings of happiness and well-being.

Serotonin-norepinephrine reuptake inhibitors (SNRIs): A class of antidepressant medications that increase the neurotransmitters serotonin and norepinephrine and are used to treat depression and other mood disorders.

Shuffling gait: Short, slow steps, with feet close to the ground or dragging along the ground. Often seen in people with advanced Parkinson's disease.

Simple sugars: Sugars that are only made up of one or two sugar units and can be used to fuel cells and provide energy to the brain. Simple sugars are absorbed quickly as they require little to no digestion. For instance, table sugar is a simple sugar comprised of the sugar units glucose and fructose.

Sleep apnea: A sleep disorder in which one's breathing stops and starts during the night. While sleep apnea is not more prevalent in people living with Parkinson's, it does occur more frequently as adults age.

Soluble fiber: A fiber type found in fruits, flaxseeds, oatmeal and psyllium in water that can slow digestion and cause feelings of fullness.

Speech language pathologist (SLP): Specialists trained to treat problems associated with speech and swallowing. Speech language pathologists can also advise on communication aids.

Starch: A long chain of carbohydrates that is digestible by the body and must be metabolized before absorbed. Starch does not cause glucose to rise as quickly as simple sugars do, resulting in steadier energy.

Stem cells: Special cells with the potential to develop into several different cell types in the body. When a stem cell divides, each new cell has the potential to remain either a stem cell or become another, more specialized type of cell, such as a brain cell or red blood cell. Stem cells are currently being researched as a potential disease-modifying treatment for Parkinson's.

Substantia nigra: An area located in the midbrain that looks like a dark streak in brain tissue, hence the Latin name meaning "black substance." The substantia nigra influences movement and coordination, and is additionally thought to also play a role in other functions and behaviors, such as learning, drug addiction and emotions. A large amount of the dopamine cells that die in the brain because of Parkinson's are located in the substantia nigra.

Subthalamic nucleus (STN): A small lens-shaped area of the brain (specifically located in the basal ganglia) involved in movement control. The STN is "overactive" in people living with Parkinson's and is a common target in deep brain stimulation for Parkinson's.

Supine hypotension: High blood pressure that occurs when lying down. Common in people with neurogenic orthostatic hypotension (nOH).

Trans fats: Type of fat found in two forms: naturally occurring in animals (such as meat and milk products) or made artificially by adding hydrogen to liquid vegetable oils. The primary dietary source for trans fats in processed food is partially hydrogenated oils. Trans fats raise LDL cholesterol levels and lower HDL cholesterol levels, increasing one's risk of developing heart disease, stroke and Type 2 diabetes.

T.R.A.P.: Acronym for four primary Parkinson's motor symptoms: tremor, rigidity, akinesia/bradykinesia and postural instability.

Tremor: Involuntary shaking, trembling or quivering movements of the muscles. In Parkinson's, tremor is usually a resting tremor, which lessens with movement and is aggravated by stress. It can occur in any part of the body, although it often begins in one hand or arm. Although tremor is one of the hallmark motor symptoms of Parkinson's, not everyone with Parkinson's will experience tremor.

Visuoperceptual: Understanding the location of objects around oneself.

Xerostomia: Lack of saliva or dry mouth.

Young onset Parkinson's disease (YOPD): A diagnosis of Parkinson's under the age of 50.